Register No[w]
Access to

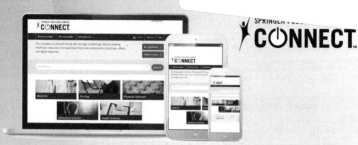

Your print purchase of *SITC's Guide to Managing Immunotherapy Toxicity* **includes online access to the contents of your book—** increasing accessibility, portability, and searchability!

Access today at:
http://connect.springerpub.com/content/book/978-0-8261-7215-0
or scan the QR code at the right with your smartphone
and enter the access code below.

CUK9S4SC

Scan here for quick access.

SITC's Guide to Managing Immunotherapy Toxicity

Editors

Marc S. Ernstoff, MD
Professor
Department of Medicine
Katherine Anne Gioia Chair
Senior Vice President for Clinical
    Investigation
Roswell Park Comprehensive Cancer
    Center
Professor of Medicine
Chief, Hematology and Oncology
Department of Medicine
Jacobs School of Medicine and
    Biomedical Sciences
State University at Buffalo
Buffalo, New York

Igor Puzanov, MD, MSCI, FACP
Professor of Medicine
Director, Early Phase Clinical Trials
    Program
Chief, Melanoma Section
Roswell Park Comprehensive Cancer
    Center
Buffalo, New York

Caroline Robert, MD, PhD
Professor of Dermatology
Chief of Dermatology Service
Co-Director of Melanoma Research Team
Institut Gustave Roussy, Villejuif
and
Paris Sud University, Le Kremlin-Bicêtre
France

Adi Diab, MD
Assistant Professor
Department of Melanoma Medical
    Oncology
Division of Cancer Medicine
The University of Texas MD Anderson
    Cancer Center
Houston, Texas

Peter Hersey, MD, PhD
Honorary Professor in Immuno-
    Oncology
Centenary Institute
University of Sydney
Sydney, Australia

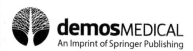

demosMEDICAL
An Imprint of Springer Publishing

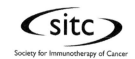

Society for Immunotherapy of Cancer

Visit www.springerpub.com and http://connect.springerpub.com

ISBN: 9780826172143
ebook ISBN: 9780826172150
DOI: 10.1891/9780826172150

Acquisitions Editor: David D'Addona
Compositor: Exeter Premedia Services Private Ltd.

Library of Congress Cataloging-in-Publication Data

Names: Ernstoff, Marc S., editor. | Puzanov, Igor, editor. | Robert,
   Caroline, editor. | Diab, Adi, editor. | Hersey, Peter, editor. | Society
   for Immunotherapy of Cancer, issuing body.
Title: SITC's guide to managing immunotherapy toxicity / editors, Marc S.
   Ernstoff, Igor Puzanov, Caroline Robert, Adi Diab, Peter Hersey.
Other titles: Guide to managing immunotherapy toxicity
Description: New York : Demos Medical Publishing, [2019] | Includes
   bibliographical references and index.
Identifiers: LCCN 2018049100| ISBN 9780826172143 | ISBN 9780826172150 (ebook)
Subjects: | MESH: Antineoplastic Agents, Immunological—toxicity
Classification: LCC RM370 | NLM QV 269 | DDC 615.3/7—dc23
LC record available at https://lccn.loc.gov/2018049100

Marc S. Ernstoff: https://orcid.org/0000-0002-8132-7069
Igor Puzanov: https://orcid.org/0000-0002-9803-3497
Caroline Robert: https://orcid.org/0000-0002-9493-0238
Peter Hersey: https://orcid.org/0000-0002-3064-737X

Printed in the United States of America.
19 20 21 22 23 / 5 4 3 2 1

This book is dedicated to our patients who provide us the opportunity to learn from their experiences and improve the health of future patients.

CONTENTS

CONTRIBUTORS

Maen Abdelrahim, MD, PhD, Assistant Professor, Institute for Academic Medicine and Weill Cornell Medical College, Houston Methodist Cancer Center, Houston, Texas

Noha Abdel-Wahab, MD, PhD, Instructor, Division of Internal Medicine, Section of Rheumatology and Clinical Immunology, The University of Texas MD Anderson Cancer Center, Houston, Texas; Lecturer, Department of Rheumatology and Rehabilitation, Faculty of Medicine, Assiut University Hospitals, Assiut, Egypt

Ala Abudayyeh, MD, Associate Professor, Division of Internal Medicine, Section of Nephrology, The University of Texas MD Anderson Cancer Center, Houston, Texas

Hamzah Abu-Sbeih, MD, Research Assistant, Gastroenterology Department, The University of Texas MD Anderson Cancer Center, Houston, Texas

Haroon Ahmad, MD, Fellow, Division of Neuro-Oncology, University of Virginia, Charlottesville, Virginia

Laurence Albiges, MD, Professor, Department of Cancer Medicine, Gustave Roussy, Villejuif, France

Nikolaos Andreatos, MD, Resident, Medicine Institute, Cleveland Clinic Foundation, Cleveland, Ohio

Paolo A. Ascierto, MD, Director, Unit of Melanoma, Cancer Immunotherapy and Development Therapeutics Unit, Istituto Nazionale Tumori IRCCS Fondazione "G. Pascale," Napoli, Italy

Shailender Bhatia, MD, Associate Professor, Department of Medicine, Division of Oncology, University of Washington, Seattle, Washington

Clifton O. Bingham III, MD, Professor, Division of Rheumatology and Allergy and Clinical Immunology, Johns Hopkins University, Baltimore, Maryland

Amy A. Case, MD, FAAHPM, Associate Professor; Chair, Department of Supportive Care, Roswell Park Comprehensive Cancer Center, University of Buffalo Jacobs School of Medicine, Buffalo, New York

George L. Chen, MD, Associate Professor, Department of Medicine, Roswell Park Comprehensive Cancer Center, Buffalo, New York

Ramona Dadu, MD, Assistant Professor, Department of Endocrine Neoplasia and Hormonal Disorders, The University of Texas MD Anderson Cancer Center, Houston, Texas

Camilo Fadul, MD, Professor, Division of Neuro-Oncology, University of Virginia, Charlottesville, Virginia

Jianjun Gao, MD, PhD, Assistant Professor, Department of Genitourinary Medical Oncology, The University of Texas MD Anderson Cancer Center, Houston, Texas

Elizabeth Gaughan, MD, Assistant Professor, Department of Medicine, Division of Hematology/Oncology, University of Virginia, Charlottesville, Virginia

Liliya Golas, MD, Shui-Chin Lee Vitreoretinal Surgery Fellow, Department of Ophthalmology and Visual Science, University of Chicago, Chicago, Illinois

Petros Grivas, MD, PhD, Associate Professor, Department of Medicine, Division of Oncology, University of Washington, Seattle, Washington

Eric D. Hansen, MD, Assistant Professor, Department of Supportive Care, Roswell Park Comprehensive Cancer Center, University of Buffalo Jacobs School of Medicine, Buffalo, New York

Jasmin Jo, MD, Resident, Division of Neurology, University of Virginia, Charlottesville, Virginia

Daniel H. Johnson, MD, Medical Oncology Fellow, Division of Cancer Medicine, The University of Texas MD Anderson Cancer Center, Houston, Texas

Douglas B. Johnson, MD, MSCI, Assistant Professor of Medicine, Vanderbilt University Medical Center, Nashville, Tennessee

Christine Kohn, PharmD, Senior Scientist, Hartford Hospital Evidence-Based Practice Center, Hartford; University of Connecticut, School of Medicine, Farmington, Connecticut

Mario E. Lacouture, MD, Professor, Director, Oncodermatology Program, Dermatology Service, Department of Medicine, Memorial Sloan Kettering Cancer Center, New York, New York

James Larkin, FRCP, PhD, Medical Oncologist, Skin and Renal Unit, Royal Marsden NHS Foundation Trust, London, United Kingdom

Alexander M. Lesokhin, MD, Assistant Member, Department of Medicine, Memorial Sloan Kettering Cancer Center, Weill Cornell Medical Center, New York, New York

Alberto J. Montero, MD, MBA, Staff Physician and Quality Officer, Taussig Cancer Institute, Cleveland Clinic Foundation, Cleveland, Ohio

Javid J. Moslehi, MD, Director, Cardio-Oncology Program; Assistant Professor of Medicine, Vanderbilt University Medical Center, Nashville, Tennessee

Ha Nguyen, MD, Fellow, Department of Endocrine Neoplasia and Hormonal Disorders, The University of Texas MD Anderson Cancer Center, Houston, Texas

Patrick A. Ott, MD, PhD, Clinical Director, Center for Immuno-Oncology and Melanoma Center, Dana Farber Cancer Institute, Brigham and Women's Hospital, Harvard Medical School, Boston, Massachusetts

Michael A. Postow, MD, Medical Oncologist, Memorial Sloan Kettering Cancer Center, Weill Cornell Medical College, New York, New York

Igor Puzanov, MD, MSCI, FACP, Professor of Medicine, Director, Early Phase Clinical Trials Program; Chief, Melanoma Section, Roswell Park Comprehensive Cancer Center, Buffalo, New York

Osama E. Rahma, MD, Assistant Professor, Center for Immuno-Oncology, Dana Farber Cancer Institute, Brigham and Women's Hospital, Harvard Medical School, Boston, Massachusetts

Caroline Robert, MD, PhD, Professor of Dermatology, Chief of Dermatology Service, Co-Director of Melanoma Research Team, Institut Gustave Roussy, Villejuif; Paris Sud University, Le Kremlin-Bicêtre, France

Vickie R. Shannon, MD, Professor, Department of Pulmonary Medicine; Director, Pulmonary Rehabilitation Program, The University of Texas MD Anderson Cancer Center, Houston, Texas

Rajeev Sharma, MD, FACE, Assistant Professor of Oncology, Roswell Park Comprehensive Cancer Center, Buffalo, New York

Natalia Shcherbakova, PhD, Associate Professor of Pharmacoeconomics, Department of Pharmaceutical and Administrative Sciences, Western New England University College of Pharmacy and Health Sciences, Springfield, Massachusetts

Dimitra Skondra, MD, PhD, Assistant Professor of Ophthalmology and Visual Science; Director, J. Terry Ernest Ocular Imaging Center; Department of Ophthalmology and Visual Science, University of Chicago, Chicago, Illinois

Lavinia Spain, MBBS, Research Fellow, Skin and Renal Unit, Royal Marsden NHS Foundation Trust, London, United Kingdom

Maria E. Suarez-Almazor, MD, PhD, Professor, Division of Internal Medicine, Section of Rheumatology and Clinical Immunology, The University of Texas MD Anderson Cancer Center, Houston, Texas

Ryan Sullivan, MD, Assistant Professor of Medicine, Harvard Medical School, Massachusetts General Hospital Cancer Center, Boston, Massachusetts

Pankit Vachhani, MD, Hematology/Oncology Fellow, Department of Medicine, Roswell Park Comprehensive Cancer Center, Buffalo, New York

Michelle Walter, DO, Associate Program Director, University of Buffalo Palliative Medicine Fellowship; Assistant Professor, Department of Supportive Care, Roswell Park Comprehensive Cancer Center, University of Buffalo Jacobs School of Medicine, Buffalo, New York

Yinghong Wang, MD, PhD, Assistant Professor/Director of Medicine-Induced Colitis and Enteritis, Gastroenterology Department, The University of Texas MD Anderson Cancer Center, Houston, Texas

Jeffrey Weber, MD, PhD, Deputy Director of the Laura and Isaac Perlmutter Cancer Center, Co-Director of Melanoma Program and Head of Experimental Therapeutics, Laura and Isaac Perlmutter Cancer Center, New York, New York

Jennifer Wu, MD, Lecturer/Attending Physician, Department of Dermatology, Chang Gung Memorial Hospital, Linkou, Keelung, and Taipei, Taiwan/Chang Gung University, College of Medicine, Taoyuan, Taiwan

FOREWORD

A BRIEF HISTORY OF TUMOR IMMUNOLOGY AND THE SOCIETY FOR IMMUNOTHERAPY OF CANCER

Tumor immunotherapy is now an established therapeutic option for an increasing number of patients with cancer. Immunotherapy differs from standard cytotoxic treatment options by eradicating cancer cells indirectly by recognizing the host immune system (1). When fully engaged, immunotherapy can induce long-term memory responses, which can in turn mediate durable protection and long-term survival against even widespread, metastatic cancers (2). The clinical implications of immunotherapy in the adjuvant and neoadjuvant setting are only now being explored with early evidence of therapeutic activity in melanoma. The real excitement, however, is evident that immunotherapy has now demonstrated antitumor activity across a growing number of solid and hematologic malignancies, suggesting the broad applicability of immunotherapy for many cancer patients. Despite the significant advances made over the last decade, not all patients respond to treatment, and there is now evidence that treatment resistance can occur (3). Furthermore, immuno-oncology treatment may be associated with side effects, including immune-mediated adverse events that require rapid identification and intervention. While the toxicities may be severe, early management can be associated with limited impact on organ function and quality of life. As patients are living longer with immunotherapy, the management of such side effects is also becoming more important. Thus, clinicians and all other healthcare providers must be familiar with the emerging indications for treatment, understand clinical treatment guidelines, and know how to recognize and manage the side effects of therapy to ensure optimal benefits for cancer patients being treated with immunotherapy.

The goal of this book is to provide the practicing physician and other allied healthcare providers with timely and authoritative access to the latest information and recommendations regarding adverse event management for patients treated with immunotherapy coupled with clinical pearls from an expert consensus panel, including leading authorities in the field from academia, industry, government, and patient advocacy groups. This was possible through a multi-disciplinary workshop convened in early 2018 by the Society for Immunotherapy of Cancer (SITC) and included representation from the American Society of Clinical Oncology (ASCO), National Comprehensive Cancer Network (NCCN), U.S. Food and Drug Administration (FDA), National Cancer Institute (NCI), and other stakeholder organizations and individuals. The workshop also invited subspecialty physicians in a variety of disciplines to add expert opinion on immune-mediated toxicity and patient management, thus providing the best consensus thinking in the field. In the Introduction, we will provide a brief description of the SITC and highlight how the Society has been a focus for bringing people together to advance the promise of immunotherapy and serve as a major resource for guiding the field forward over the last four decades. In many respects, the activities of the Society have mirrored the challenges and successes associated with the scientific and clinical development of the field of cancer immunotherapy.

The Early Years

The potential of using the immune system to treat human disease has been recognized for centuries. Early observations that previous exposure to a given infectious disease (or its close relative) could result in protection against the same disease later (the concept of immunologic memory) was well established at the end of the 18th century. The ability to move this critical observation into clinical practice established the field of immunology and is credited to British physician and epidemiologist, Edward Jenner (4). At the end of the 18th century, Jenner had developed vaccinia virus immunization as an effective way to prevent smallpox. The true potential of immunologic treatment would be later confirmed by the eradication of smallpox from the planet, which was eventually accomplished in 1984. Jenner's work also firmly established the role of the immune system in the pathogenesis and treatment of infectious diseases. Indeed, much of the 19th century, with the advent of the microscope, was spent classifying both infectious pathogens as well as cells found in the peripheral blood, which would be identified as part of the immune system. While the success in vaccination for prevention of infectious diseases was heralded as a major success for immunology, the molecular and cellular basis of immunology was largely unknown at the beginning of the 20th century.

William Coley, a New York physician and surgeon, is generally credited as the first to document the potential of using the immune system to treat cancer, through a series of scientific publications around the turn of the 20th century (4). Coley observed spontaneous tumor regression in several of his patients awaiting surgical treatment and noted that regression was often preceded by local infection and cellulitis around the tumor. He developed the concept that tumor rejection was driven by bacterial infection and devoted much of his remaining career trying to extract bacterial toxins, the so-called "Coley's toxins," believing that these were the molecular factors responsible for antitumor immunity. This was a strong line of research at that time since other microbiologists were beginning to unravel the association between bacterial toxins and clinical pathogenesis. Other observations of occasional spontaneous regression of established cancers in patients with influenza and other preceding viral illnesses were reported in the early 20th century, suggesting a link between antiviral immunity and cancer growth (5). Despite these important insights, much of the immunology community began to focus on how to inhibit immunologic rejection of organ allografts, which was emerging as the major barrier to successful organ transplantation.

In 1960, Burnet and Medawar were awarded the Nobel Prize for their discovery of how immune tolerance prevents recognition of the cells in the body by distinguishing between "self" proteins and "non-self" proteins (5). This breakthrough provided an explanation for why microbial pathogens could be recognized by mammalian immune systems, because they were derived largely from "non-self" proteins or antigens. However, it did not explain allograft rejection or spontaneous regression of established tumors. Further insight was obtained by a better understanding of how cell surface receptors interact between somatic cells and immune cells to regulate immune responses. The identification of the major histocompatibility complex elements, which serve to communicate the status of somatic cell proteins, presented a molecular mechanism for immunologic communication with cells in the body and hinted at how transplant rejection was occurring when major histocompatibility complex (MHC) mismatch was present (6). An improved understanding of how cell surface receptor interactions mediated immune homeostasis resulted in a Nobel Prize to Benacerraf, Dausset, and Snell in 1980. At that time, tumor rejection remained a conundrum. Many early attempts testing immunotherapy were unsuccessful, and therapy of metastatic cancer had largely been replaced by cytotoxic chemotherapy and radiation therapy. Nonetheless, murine models did support the potential for immunotherapy and careful studies in mouse tumor models focused attention on the role of T-cells in mediating tumor rejection (7). Rapid advances in cancer genomics were also occurring at this time and leaders in the tumor immunology arena began to discuss how to maintain interest in immunotherapy and promote ongoing basic and clinical research in the field.

The solution conceived in the early 1980s was the reason behind the creation of the Society for Biological Therapy (SBT), which was formally incorporated as a not-for-profit professional medical society in 1985 with six founding board members (Table 1). Following the initial founding of the organization, an illustrious group of leading physicians and scientists joined as charter members (Table 2), bringing strong scientific rigor and credibility to the Society. The name was later changed in 2002 to the International Society for Biological Therapy of Cancer (iSBTc) to reflect the international membership of the organization and cancer focus; and again in 2010, the name was changed to Society for Immunotherapy of Cancer (SITC) to better reflect the focus on the mission of improving patient outcomes through cancer immunotherapy.

TABLE 1 SITC Founding Board Members

- Richard V. Smalley, MD
- John Whisnant, MD
- Ernest C. Borden, MD
- Robert Bast, MD
- John Laszlo, MD
- Isaiah Fidler, DVM, PhD

TABLE 2 SITC Founding Charter Members

• Paul Abrams, MD	• Andrew Lister, MD
• Robert Bast, MD	• Michael Mastrangelo, MD
• David Berd, MD	• Enrico Mihich, MD
• Ernest Borden, MD	• Richard Miller, MD
• Robert Dillman, MD	• Malcolm Mitchell, MD
• Mehmet Fer, MD	• Herbert Oettgen, MD
• Isaiah "Josh" Fidler, PhD, DVM	• Robert Oldham, MD
• Kenneth Foon, MD	• Carl Pinsky, MD
• Allan Goldstein, PhD	• Ralph Reisfeld, PhD
• David Gordon, MD	• Jerome Ritz, MD
• Thomas Griffin, MD	• Ivor Royston, MD
• Jordan Gutterman, MD	• Seth Rudnick, MD
• Michael Hanna, PhD	• Gregory Sarna, MD
• Ronald Herberman, MD*	• Stephen Sherwin, MD
• Evan Hersh, MD	• Richard Smalley, MD*
• Hilary Koprowski, MD*	• Henry Stevenson, MD
• Mathilde Krim, PhD	• Gerald Vosika, MD
• Susan Krown, MD	• John Whisnant, MD
• John Laszlo, MD	• Jacob Zighelbolm, MD
• Hilton Levy, MD*	

*Deceased.

Since the beginning of the organization, the leadership recognized the importance of broad inclusion with representation from academia, industry, and government as a necessity to drive scientific and clinical development in the field. The core values of the Society include promoting interaction and integration within the field, fostering innovation, focusing in translation, and providing leadership in the area of tumor immunotherapy. The Society began with small annual meetings in 1986, bringing basic, clinical, and translational investigators together to learn the science and foster collaboration and vision for how to move the field forward.

The Cytokine Era

In the late 1980s, much of the focus was on understanding the basic science of tumor immunology with considerable attention on murine and other preclinical models. While murine studies supported the role of T-cells in mediating antitumor activity, the translation of this model to the clinic was significantly hampered by an inability to maintain human T-cells in culture ex vivo for longer than a few days. A serum factor called "T-cell growth factor" was essential for long-term survival of T-cells in vitro. In the late 1970s, T-cell growth factor was identified as interleukin-2 (IL-2), the gene was cloned, and recombinant IL-2 became available and was used to expand T-cell populations in vitro. In addition, other cytokines were being identified, and considerable investigation was focused on understanding the functional role of various cytokines in normal immune homeostasis and in disease pathogenesis. Around this time, the NCI Surgery Branch, led by Steven Rosenberg, was trying to develop T-cells in vivo for cancer treatment, mirroring the data from the mouse models. The

NCI group initially used adoptive transfer of leukocyte-activated killer cells, and later tumor-infiltrating lymphocyte cells, with the hypothesis that some patients may have preexisting tumor-specific T-cells, but these were present at insufficient numbers to mediate therapeutic responses (8). Since there were limited treatment options available for metastatic melanoma patients and given the reports of spontaneous regression in this disease, the Rosenberg group focused their studies on melanoma. An important conceptual advance made by this group was the increased T-cell yield with IL-2 exposure and later integration of IL-2 into the adoptive T-cell clinical regimen as a strategy to enhance T-cell survival in vivo. Following initial clinical trials, IL-2 alone was shown to have significant clinical activity in melanoma and renal cell carcinoma, findings that were confirmed by the extramural Cytokine Working Group, which led to FDA approval of IL-2 for the treatment of metastatic renal cell carcinoma and melanoma in 1992 and 1998, respectively (9). In addition, the pioneering work of John Kirkwood and Marc Ernstoff established a role for interferon-alfa in the adjuvant therapy of melanoma through a series of large, cooperative group clinical trials (10,31).

Interest in immunotherapy was maintained through advances in cytokine therapy but responses appeared to be limited to a small subset of high-performance status patients. Furthermore, high-dose cytokine treatment was associated with significant toxicity, limiting patient treatment to specialized centers of excellence. In the meantime, basic research was accelerating with the discovery of the T-cell receptor (TCR) by Reinherz, Marrack, Kappler, and Allison in 1983 (11,12). Deciphering the mechanism of how immune cells recognize viral infections in which the TCR is able to recognize viral peptides in the context of MHC expression on somatic cells, a finding by Doherty and Zinkernagel led to a Nobel Prize in 1996 (13). Another important advance was made by Ralph Steinman who identified a role for dendritic cells as "professional" antigen-presenting cells for stimulating adaptive immunity (14). His work also resulted in a Nobel Prize in 2011. During this era, SITC continued to bring basic scientists, clinicians, regulators, and industry members together to discuss the data and provide a structure for networking. The Society established the Smalley Award lectureship as the Society's highest honor, dedicated to the memory of founding member Richard V. Smalley. Notable recipients included Steven Rosenberg, James Allison, and Ralph Steinman (Table 3). However, the molecular mechanisms of tumor rejection, and why the immune system was not functioning sufficiently in most cancer patients, remained elusive.

Tumor Vaccines and Immune Monitoring

The identification that viral antigens that could be detected by MHC class I complexes on the surface of infected somatic cells led to the hypothesis that a similar mechanism could be underlying tumor immunity. This hypothesis was confirmed in preclinical models, and evidence of detectable immunity against mutated and overexpressed tumor-associated antigens began to appear in the early 1990s. In addition, the specific role

TABLE 3 Past Richard V. Smalley, MD Award Winners

- 2005 Recipient—Steven A. Rosenberg, MD, PhD, National Cancer Institute
- 2006 Recipient—Ronald Levy, MD, Stanford University School of Medicine
- 2007 Recipient—Ernest Borden, MD, Cleveland Clinic Foundation
- 2008 Recipient—Giorgio Parmiani, MD, Fondazione C.S. Raffaele
- 2009 Recipient—Isaiah J. Fidler, DVM, PhD, MD Anderson Cancer Center
- 2010 Recipient—James P. Allison, PhD, MD Anderson Cancer Center
- 2011 Recipient—Ralph M. Steinman, MD, The Rockefeller University (Deceased)
- 2012 Recipient—Theresa Whiteside, PhD, University of Pittsburgh Cancer Institute
- 2013 Recipient—Carl June, MD, University of Pennsylvania
- 2014 Recipient—Giorgio Trinchieri, MD, National Cancer Institute
- 2015 Recipient—Tasuku Honjo, MD, PhD, Kyoto University Graduate School of Medicine
- 2016 Recipient—Suzanne Topalian, MD, Johns Hopkins University
- 2017 Recipient—Paul Sondel, MD, PhD, University of Wisconsin–Madison
- 2018 Recipient—Philip D. Greenberg, MD, University of Washington

of CD8+ T-cells in recognizing MHC class I-restricted tumor peptides provided both a molecular explanation of how tumor immunity worked as well as a roadmap for vaccination against defined antigenic epitopes. Thus, major efforts were expended to identify the optimal tumor antigens with the hope that vaccination against such antigens would unleash the full potential of the immune system for treating cancer. During this era, innumerable strategies for vaccination were proposed and evaluated, including peptides and proteins, plasmid DNA, recombinant viral vectors, antigen-loaded dendritic and other immune cells, as well as both autologous and allogeneic whole tumor cell vaccines. Despite the initial enthusiasm, the only therapeutic vaccine to be approved by the FDA was an autologous antigen presenting cell vaccine loaded with prostatic acid phosphatase, a commonly overexpressed prostate cancer antigen, plus granulocyte-macrophage colony-stimulating factor (GM-CSF), a cytokine known to promote dendritic cell activation (Sipuleucel-T) (15). Although other therapeutic vaccines failed in randomized clinical trials, it is notable that a preventive cervical cancer vaccine utilizing human papilloma virus viral-like particles achieved approval based on the extensive work of Lowy and Schiller (16).

Although most vaccine studies were negative, several additional insights emerged from this intensive time in the field. A groundswell of interest in immune monitoring was established in which several ex vivo assays utilizing peripheral blood and tumor biopsy specimens were developed and standardized. This focus on immune correlatives became critical to the clinical development paradigm in immunotherapy (17). It provided a more biologic rationale for pursuing specific approaches that may have failed clinically in treating very advanced cancer patients which showed data supporting immunologic activity and expansion of antigen-specific immune responses. In addition, the more standardized approach to biomarker analysis resulted in several important findings. First, vaccination approaches were capable of inducing tumor-specific CD8+ cytotoxic T-cells; second, protein and longer peptides could activate CD4+ helper

T-cells which also had a therapeutic role; third, MHC and antigen loss could occur, suggesting immune editing and/or mutational evolution of tumors; fourth, costimulatory molecules such as B7-1, B7-2 (CD80 and CD86), and CD40 and cytokines like GM-CSF were important for antigen presenting cells and T-cell cross-talk (18). In addition, the general role of immune suppression in established cancer began to receive more attention. In 1995, Sakaguchi reported the existence of regulatory CD4+ T-cells defined by FoxP3 expression and demonstrated that such cells could limit antitumor immunity (19). Around this same time, James Allison also reported the functional role of the cytotoxic T-lymphocyte antigen 4 (CTLA-4) in blocking antitumor effector T-cells, showing that premature engagement of this "checkpoint inhibitor" could result in a loss of tumor-specific T-cells (20).

During this period, SITC began to attract interest from an increasing number of cell biologists, basic immunologists, clinicians, and most notably, translational investigators. The Society contributed to the field by forming task forces and working groups to address harmonization in immune monitoring and providing sessions at the annual meeting to dissect negative vaccine clinical trials. SITC members addressed how to optimize preclinical models and evaluate new technology designed to enhance antitumor immunity.

Breakthrough Treatment and Immune Checkpoints

In 2011, the first phase III randomized clinical trial of an anti-CTLA-4 monoclonal antibody alone or in combination with a gp100 peptide vaccine demonstrated a significant survival improvement in patients with advanced melanoma compared to vaccine alone (21). This pivotal study was significant for several reasons, including validation of immune checkpoint inhibition as a general therapeutic strategy in immuno-oncology and being the first phase III study to show a significant improvement in survival for patients with melanoma. The success of this study quickly led to additional evaluation of ipilimumab, the anti-CTLA4 antibody, in other cancers as well as testing new checkpoint inhibitor agents. As CTLA-4 was a T-cell surface receptor that blocked T-cell proliferation and activation, other cell surface receptors with similar functions were a priority for drug development. One such receptor known as programmed cell death 1 (PD-1) had been previously described by Gordon Freeman and Tasuko Honjo in 2000 (22). Studies of anti-PD-1 monoclonal antibodies resulted in unprecedented therapeutic activity in early phase I clinical trials and eventually would go on and demonstrate activity in a wide range of human cancers, including melanoma, renal cell carcinoma, head and neck cancer, bladder cancer, Hodgkin and non-Hodgkin B-cell lymphomas, non-small cell lung cancer, and microsatellite unstable solid tumors resulting in multiple regulatory approvals. Furthermore, pembrolizumab, one of the anti-PD-1 monoclonal antibodies, received the first FDA approval based on a molecular marker, microsatellite instability high (MSI-H) or mismatch repair deficient (dMMR) features in patients with disease progression after prior treatment, rather than based on a distinct histology (23). These unexpected results were quickly followed by approvals of several monoclonal antibodies targeting the programmed cell death ligand 1 (PD-L1) with evidence of activity in lung cancer, bladder cancer, and Merkel cell carcinoma (24). In many, patient responses were quite durable and the progress observed with checkpoint inhibition established immunotherapy as a bona fide treatment modality for cancer.

The success with single-agent checkpoint blockade in melanoma was rapidly followed by combination studies. In a pivotal randomized phase III study, Wolchok et al. (25) reported a 61% response rate with combination ipilimumab and nivolumab in metastatic melanoma patients who had not received prior treatment. This study, however, also reported a 54% incidence of grade 3 or greater drug-related adverse events including severe immune-related toxicity. While early detection of immune-related adverse events can often be managed by corticosteroids and brief treatment interruption, long-term follow-up has now concluded that some side effects may occur late and can be associated with chronic morbidity and, in rare cases, mortality (most notably from colonic perforation following autoimmune colitis and immune-related myocarditis) (26). Thus, while the clinical advances have proved dramatic, physicians and other healthcare providers caring for patients treated with immune checkpoint inhibition must now be aware of how to identify and rapidly manage emerging toxicities while patients are on treatment and during follow-up because toxicity may manifest late in some patients. Although research is needed to better understand the mechanisms of both antitumor activity and side effects associated with checkpoint blockade, SITC has provided expert consensus opinion in patient selection through a clinical immunotherapy guideline program that brings disease-specific expertise together in a tumor-specific manner to allow for integration of immunotherapy into the standard clinical treatment pathways for patients with cancer. SITC has also established a combination immunotherapy working group who have provided new perspectives into how to proceed with combination immunotherapy drug development (27). In addition, this handbook provides specific insights into toxicity identification and management incorporating both evidence-based data, where available, with the best consensus thinking by oncology and subspecialty experts. Finally, the FDA and other regulatory agencies should be applauded for recognizing the unique kinetics of immunotherapy and providing accelerated pathways for drug development and approval.

The Next Wave in Tumor Immunotherapy

While well-deserved enthusiasm surrounded progress with immune checkpoint blockade, several other recent advances continue to support an expanded role of other agents in the immunotherapy of human cancer. The first oncolytic virus, talimogene laherparepvec (T-VEC), an attenuated recombinant herpes simplex virus type 1 (HSV-1) encoding GM-CSF, demonstrated therapeutic activity in patients with surgically unresectable stage III and IV melanoma leading to approval in the United States, Europe, and Australia in 2015 (28). Additional studies are planned with several oncolytic viruses in melanoma and other cancers, and early data suggest a highly favorable interaction between oncolytic viruses and checkpoint blockade.

Another major advance has been the development of chimeric antigen receptor T-cells. Using a lentiviral vector to express a chimeric antigen receptor specific for CD19, a B-cell antigen, and an expression cassette from 4-1BB, a T-cell co-stimulatory molecule, Carl June et al. demonstrated an 81% remission rate within 3 months in children and young adults with CD19+ relapsed or refractory B-cell lymphoblastic leukemia (ALL). This led to FDA approval of tisagenlecleucel for ALL in patients up to 25 years of age and later also for refractory large B-cell lymphoma patients who failed previous treatments (29). Another CAR T-cell agent, axicabtagene ciloleucel was also approved for the treatment of certain types of large B-cell non-Hodgkin lymphomas (30). While these approvals represent important new options for patients with often refractory hematologic tumors, treatment is associated with unique toxicities and the therapy is expensive. To date, few, if any, cost-effectiveness or value analyses have been performed.

As the field has expanded, SITC continues to forge new territory, providing education to the experts in the field, to practicing physicians and nurses, and to patients who need information about immunotherapy treatments. The Society has now established strong programs in policy and patient advocacy and has become a leading voice in promoting the role of immunotherapy in clinical management. The provision of this handbook should provide healthcare providers with up-to-date guidelines for identifying adverse events associated with immune checkpoint blockade and provide expert rationale for effective patient management. As the oldest continuously operating professional membership organization dedicated to tumor immunotherapy, the Society has guided the field forward through a series of visionary and action-oriented leaders (Table 4)

TABLE 4 Past SITC Presidents

- 1984–1986: Robert K. Oldham, MD
- 1986–1988: Ernest C. Borden, MD
- 1988–1990: Richard V. Smalley, MD
- 1990–1992: Michael Mastrangelo, MD
- 1992–1994: Michael J. Hawkins, MD
- 1994–1996: Ronald B. Herberman, MD
- 1996–1998: David R. Parkinson, MD
- 1998–2000: Michael T. Lotze, MD
- 2000–2002: Robert O. Dillman, MD
- 2002–2004: Michael B. Atkins, MD
- 2004–2006: Ulrich Keilholz, MD
- 2006–2008: Jon M. Wigginton, MD
- 2008–2010: Bernard A. Fox, PhD
- 2010–2012: Thomas F. Gajewski, MD, PhD
- 2012–2014: Francesco M. Marincola, MD
- 2014–2016: Howard L. Kaufman, MD, FACS
- 2016–Present: Lisa H. Butterfield, PhD

and the unwavering support of the most dedicated and compassionate executive management team, led by Tara Withington. We hope you find this handbook useful and please monitor the SITC website at www.sitcancer.org for updates and new developments for helping your management of patients with cancer electing therapy with immuno-oncology.

Lisa H. Butterfield, PhD
President, Society for Immunotherapy of Cancer
University of Pittsburgh, Pittsburgh, Pennsylvania

Howard L. Kaufman, MD
Immediate-Past President, Society for Immunotherapy of Cancer
Massachusetts General Hospital, Boston, Massachusetts

ACKNOWLEDGMENTS

The authors wish to thank Tara Withington, the executive director and driving force behind the SITC, and her outstanding and highly dedicated staff. Her vision and insights allowed the Society to become the major influence in the field and has brought hope to cancer patients throughout the world. We also thank the patients and families that agreed to participate in clinical immunotherapy trials that made the advances in the field possible.

CONFLICTS OF INTEREST STATEMENT

H. Kaufman is an employee of Replimune, Inc. L. Butterfield has no relevant conflicts to declare.

REFERENCES

1. Pardoll D. Cancer and the immune system: basic concepts and targets for intervention. *Semin Oncol.* 2015;42(4):523–538. doi:10.1053/j.seminoncol.2015.05.003

2. Robert C, Ribas A, Hamid O, et al. Durable complete response after discontinuation of pembrolizumab in patients with metastatic melanoma. *J Clin Oncol.* 2018;36(17):1668–1674. doi:10.1200/JCO.2017.75.6270

3. Kim TK, Herbst RS, Chen L. Defining and understanding adaptive resistance in cancer immunotherapy. *Trends Immunol.* 2018;39:624–631. doi:10.1016/j.it.2018.05.001

4. Strassburg MA. The global eradication of smallpox. *Am J Infect Control.* 1982;10(2):53–59. doi:10.1016/0196-6553(82)90003-7

5. Brent L. The discovery of immunologic tolerance. *Hum Immunol.* 1997;52(2):75–81. doi:10.1016/S0198-8859(96)00289-3

6. Garcia MAA, Yebra BG, Flores ALL, et al. The major histocompatibility complex in transplantation. *J Transplant.* 2012;2012:1–7. doi:10.1155/2012/842141

7. Evans R, Duffy T. The immunological basis of tumor rejection: the absolute dependence of the effector arm on sensitized T cells after chemoimmunotherapy of a murine sarcoma. *J Immunol.* 1985;134(6):4255–4260.

8. Grimm EA, Mazumder A, Zhang HZ, et al. Lymphokine-activated killer cell phenomenon. Lysis of natural killer-resistant fresh solid tumor cells by interleukin-2-activated autologous human peripheral blood lymphocytes. *J Exp Med.* 1982;155(6):1823–1841. doi:10.1084/jem.155.6.1823

9. Rosenberg SA. IL-2: the first effective immunotherapy for human cancer. *J Immunol.* 2014;192(12):5451–5458. doi:10.4049/jimmunol.1490019

10. Tarhini A, Gogas H, Kirkwood JM. IFN-α in the treatment of melanoma. *J Immunol.* 2012;189(8):3789–3793. doi:10.4049/jimmunol.1290060

11. Reinherz EL, Meuer S, Fitzgerald KA, et al. Antigen recognition by human T lymphocytes is linked to surface expression of the T3 molecular complex. *Cell*. 1982;30(3):735–743. doi:10.1016/0092-8674(82)90278-1

12. Kappler J, Kubo R, Haskins K, et al. The major histocompatibility complex-restricted antigen receptor on T cells I. Mouse and man: Identification of constant and variable peptides. *Cell*. 1983;35(1):295–302. doi:10.1016/0092-8674(83)90232-5

13. Doherty PC, Zinkernagel RM. A biological role for the major histocompatibility antigens. *Lancet*. 1975;1(7922):1406–1409. doi:10.1016/S0140-6736(75)92610-0

14. Steinman RM, Nussenzweig MC. Dendritic cells: features and functions. *Immunol Rev*. 1980;53:127–147. doi:10.1111/j.1600-065X.1980.tb01042.x

15. Kantoff PW, Higano CS, Shore ND, et al. Sipuleucel-T immunotherapy for castration-resistant prostate cancer. *N Engl J Med*. 2010;363(5):411–422. doi:10.1056/NEJMoa1001294

16. Hildesheim A, Herrero R, Wacholder S, et al. Effect of human papillomavirus 16/18 L1 viruslike particle vaccine among young women with preexisting infection: a randomized trial. *JAMA*. 2007;298(7):743–753. doi:10.1001/jama.298.7.743

17. Butterfield LH, Palucka AK, Britten CM, et al. Recommendations from the iSBTc/FDA/ NCI workshop on immunotherapy biomarkers. *Clin Cancer Res*. 2011;17(10):3064–3076. doi:10.1158/1078-0432.CCR-10-2234

18. Slingluff CL, Petroni GR, Olson W, et al. Helper T-cell responses and clinical activity of a melanoma vaccine with multiple peptides from MAGE and melanocytic differentiation antigens. *J Clin Oncol*. 2008;26(30):4973–4980. doi:10.1200/JCO.2008.17.3161

19. Sakaguchi S, Sakaguchi N, Asano M, et al. Immunologic self-tolerance maintained by activated T cells expressing IL-2 receptor alpha-chains (CD25). Breakdown of a single mechanism of self-tolerance causes various autoimmune diseases. *J Immunol*. 1995;155(3):1151–1164.

20. Krummel MF, Allison JP. VD28 and CTLA-4 have opposing effects on the response of T cells to stimulation. *J Exp Med*. 1995;182(2):459–465. doi:10.1084/jem.182.2.459

21. Hodi FS, O'Day SJ, McDermott DF, et al. Improved survival with ipilimumab in patients with metastatic melanoma. *N Engl J Med*. 2010;363(8):711–723. doi:10.1056 /NEJMoa1003466

22. Freeman GJ, Long AJ, Iwai Y, et al. Engagement of the PD-1 immunoinhibitory receptor by a novel B7 family member leads to negative regulation of lymphocyte activation. *J Exp Med*. 2000;192(7):1027–1034. doi:10.1084/jem.192.7.1027

23. Topalian SL, Drake CG, Pardoll DM. Immune checkpoint blockade: a common denominator approach to cancer therapy. *Cancer Cell*. 2015;27(4):450–461. doi:10.1016/j.ccell.2015.03.001

24. Lee HT, Lee JY, Lim H, et al. Molecular mechanism of PD-1/PD-L1 blockade via anti-PD-L1 antibodies atezolizumab and durvalumab. *Sci Rep*. 2017;7(1):5532. doi:10.1038/ s41598-017-06002-8

25. Postow MA, Chesney J, Pavlick AC, et al. Nivolumab and ipilimumab versus ipilimumab in untreated melanoma. *N Engl J Med*. 2015;372(21):2006–2017. doi:10.1056/NEJMoa1414428

26. Johnson DB, Balko JM, Compton ML, et al. Fulminant myocarditis with combination immune checkpoint blockade. *N Engl J Med*. 2016;375(18):1749–1755. doi:10.1056/NEJMoa1609214

27. Ott PA, Hodi FS, Kaufman HL, et al. Combination immunotherapy: a road map. *J Immunother Cancer*. 2017;5:16. doi:10.1186/s40425-017-0218-5

28. Andtbacka RHI, Kaufman HL, Collichio F, et al. Talimogene laherparepvec improved durable response rates in patients with advanced melanoma. *J Clin Oncol*. 2015;33(25):2780–2788. doi:10.1200/JCO.2014.58.3377

29. Maude SL, Laetsch TW, Buechner J, et al. Tisagenlecleucel in children and young adults with B-cell lymphoblastic leukemia. *N Engl J Med*. 2018;378(5):439–448. doi:10.1056/NEJMoa1709866

30. Neelapu SS, Locke FL, Bartlett NL, et al. Axicabtagene ciloleucel CAR T-cell therapy in refractory large B-cell lymphoma. *N Engl J Med*. 2017;377(26):2531–2544. doi:10.1056/ NEJMoa1707447

31. Kirkwood JM, Strawderman MH, Ernstoff MS, et al. Interferon alfa-2b adjuvant therapy of high-risk resected cutaneous melanoma: the Eastern Cooperative Oncology Group Trial EST 1684. *J Clin Oncol*. 1996;14(1):7–17.

INTRODUCTION

It is now over 20 years since basic immunologists began the further interrogation of the immune synapse identifying additional receptors and ligands that regulate the activity of T-cells beyond the T-cell receptor and second signal CD28-CD80/86 necessary for T-cell activation (1). Blocking of the first of these molecules, cytotoxic T-lymphocyte antigen 4 (CTLA-4), identified in 1996 by Jim Allison's group, demonstrated enhanced tumor responses in mice (2). Ensuing work by many led to the approval of the anti-CTLA-4 antibody ipilimumab as the first immune checkpoint inhibitor (ICI) to treat cancer. At the time of writing this book, there are now numerous immune checkpoint inhibitor molecules (ipilimumab [Yervoy®], pembrolizumab [Keytruda®], nivolumab [Opdivo®], atezolizumab [Tecentriq®], and avelumab [Bavencio®]) that are approved for treating a variety of cancers and many more in the research pipeline. Immunotherapy, once relegated to the back rooms and last days of conferences and spoken about in disbelief that it would ever have the power and promise to treat established cancers, is now front and center in our armamentarium of tools that oncologists use. Now everyone needs to be an immunologist. The cancer treatment paradigm shift is in full swing. While the therapeutic index of these new agents is, in general, excellent, their use comes with a unique range of toxicities that must be recognized and treated effectively for their safe implementation in the community.

The Society for Immunotherapy of Cancer (SITC) was among the first societies to recognize the need for education as well as the identification and management of immune-related adverse events (irAEs), publishing guidelines in the *Journal for ImmunoTherapy of Cancer* in November 2017 (3). SITC representation was involved with the National Comprehensive Cancer Network guidelines as well as the American Society of Clinical Oncology's efforts. And now, SITC has taken the next step in writing this manual for management of immune checkpoint inhibitors.

The first intended use of immune therapy to treat cancer was the intentional use of infection (erysipelas) to treat soft tissue sarcoma in 1868 by the German surgeon Wilhelm Busch and subsequently independently used in 1891 by the American surgeon William Coley (4,5). The 20th century brought the discovery of interferons independently by Yasu-ichi Nagano and Yasuhiko Kojima, and Alick Isaacs and Jean Lindenmann groups (6,7). With the investment from the American Cancer Society, the Finnish Red Cross first commercialized interferons with production of whole cell interferons in the late 1970s and early 1980 (8,9). Many investigators researched the signals involved with T-cell proliferation, leading to Robert Gallo's discovery of T-cell growth factor or IL-2 (10). Over the next few decades, many cytokines were discovered that were involved with activation and regulation of lymphocytes and continue to be explored today as cancer therapeutics. In 1996, Jim Allison and Jim Bluestone's groups demonstrated that blocking the immune regulatory molecule

CTLA-4 with anti-CTLA-4 antibody led to enhanced tumor responses in mice, which ultimately lead to the Food and Drug Administration (FDA) approval of the first checkpoint inhibitor, ipilimumab, 15 years later (2,11,12). Programmed cell death 1 (PD-1) was first described in 1992 by Honjo and his group and in 2000 as an immune checkpoint, setting the stage for FDA approval some 15 years later (13,14). Both Honjo and Allison would share the Nobel Prize for medicine in 2018 for their groundbreaking observation.

SITC's Guide to Managing Immunotherapy Toxicity is intended to be a working guide for clinicians. By understanding immune mechanism of anticancer activity, the clinician is armed with the knowledge to leverage these agents for the benefit of patients. The current empirical evidence for benefit is summarized so that physicians, providers, and patients can make evidence-based decisions regarding care. Finally, this handbook provides an understanding of the adverse events leading to treatment discontinuation or dose-limiting toxicity (grade 3/4) and their management. Clinicians familiar with scoring from the Common Terminology Criteria for Adverse Events (CTCAE) published by the National Cancer Institute, which is skewed to cytotoxic chemotherapy-related acute events used to determine the immediate safety of drugs and drug combinations, will recognize its limitations in the era of immunotherapy.

The use of immune checkpoint inhibitors is increasing across a growing spectrum of cancers, and for both metastatic and adjuvant conditions, SITC has undertaken this effort to provide a concise summary for the clinicians. The use of these agents in an adjuvant setting presents a great challenge in that many of these patients will not ever have recurrent disease so that ethics demand the treatments stay safe. We are cognizant of the cost of these agents and have addressed this concern with a chapter on cost-effective strategies. As data from combination trials with other FDA-approved and experimental immune therapeutics of different classes become available, the full impact of immune therapy will begin to emerge. We will be challenged by the need to contain cost and the desire to use our new knowledge prior to regulatory bodies' acceptance. Thus, engaging patients and their families into the process of choosing a therapy is equally important.

Marc S. Ernstoff, MD

REFERENCES

1. Bretscher PA. A two-step, two-signal model for the primary activation of precursor helper T cells. *Proc Natl Acad Sci USA.* 1999;96:185–190. doi:10.1073/pnas.96.1.185

2. Leach DR, Krummel MF, Allison JP. Enhancement of antitumor immunity by CTLA4 blockade. *Science.* 1996;271:1734–1736. doi:10.1126/science.271.5256.1734

3. Puzanov I, Diab A, Abdallah K, et al. Managing toxicities associated with immune checkpoint inhibitors: consensus recommendations from the Society for Immunotherapy of Cancer (SITC) Toxicity Management Working Group. *J Immunother Cancer.* 2017;5:95–123. doi:10.1186/s40425-017-0300-z

4. Busch W. Berhandlungen artzlicher gesellschaften. *Berl Klin Wochenschr.* 1868;137–138.

5. Coley WB. Contribution to the knowledge of sarcoma. *Ann Surg.* 1891;14:199–220. doi:10.1097/00000658-189112000-00015

6. Nagano Y, Kojima Y. Pouvoir immunisant du virus vaccinal inactive par des rayons ultraviolets. *CR Soc Biol.* 1954;48:1700–1702.

7. Isaacs A, Lindenmann J. Virus interference. I. The interferon. *Proc R Soc Ser B.* 1957;147:258–267. doi:10.1098/rspb.1957.0048

8. Strander H, Cantell K. Production of interferon by human leukocytes in vitro. *Ann Med Exp Biol Fenn.* 1966;44:265–273.

9. Krown SE, Burk MW, Kirkwood JM, et al. Human leukocyte (alpha) interferon in metastatic malignant melanoma: The American Cancer Society Phase II trial. *Cancer Treat Rep.* 1984;68:723–726.

10. Mier JW, Gallo RC. Purification and some characteristics of human T-cell growth factor from phytohemagglutinin-stimulated lymphocyte-conditioned media. *Proc Natl Acad Sci USA.* 1980;77:6134–6138. doi:10.1073/pnas.77.10.6134

11. Walunas TL, Bakker CY, Bluestone JA. CTLA-4 ligation blocks CD28-dependent T cell activation. *J Exp Med.* 1996;183:2541–2550. doi:10.1084/jem.183.6.2541

12. Hodi FS, O'Day SJ, McDermott DF, et al. Improved survival with ipilimumab in patients with metastatic melanoma. *N Engl J Med.* 2010;372:2006–2017. doi:10.1056/NEJMoa1003466

13. Ishida Y, Agata Y, Shibahara K, Honjo T. Induced expression of PD-1, a novel member of the immunoglobulin gene superfamily, upon programmed cell death. *EMBO J.* 1992; 11(11):3887–3895.

14. Freeman GJ, Long AJ, Iwai Y, et al. Engagement of the PD-1 immunoinhibitory receptor by a novel B7 family member leads to negative regulation of lymphocyte activation. *J Exp Med.* 2000;192(7):1027–1034. doi:10.1084/jem.192.7.1027

IMMUNE CHECKPOINT INHIBITORS IN THE CLINIC

CHAPTER 1

OVERVIEW OF ANTI-CTLA-4 AGENTS: IPILIMUMAB AND TREMELIMUMAB

Daniel H. Johnson and Jianjun Gao

INTRODUCTION

T-cell-based immunotherapies have revolutionized the treatment of cancer. Advances in the understanding of T-cell activation and regulation have made possible the development of targeted monoclonal antibodies (mAbs) against regulatory immune checkpoints. A number of intrinsic T-cell immune checkpoint pathways have evolved to regulate the immune system at multiple steps, a process called peripheral tolerance (1). Tumor cells take advantage of these mechanisms developed to limit inflammatory and immune responses to protect themselves from the T-cell attack, a process called adaptive immune resistance (2). There are now six immune checkpoint inhibitors (ICIs) approved by the U.S. Food and Drug Administration (FDA) for use in a variety of malignancies that target two immune checkpoint signaling pathways, cytotoxic T-lymphocyte antigen 4 (CTLA-4) and programmed cell death 1/programmed cell death ligand 1 (PD-1/PD-L1) (3).

Effective activation of the cell-mediated immune system requires both interaction of the T-cell receptor (TCR) with antigen bound MHC molecules and co-stimulatory signals mediated by CD28 on the T-cell surface to B7 proteins (CD80 or CD86) on antigen presenting cells (APCs) (4). These two signals are essential to the antitumor immune response by initiating priming of tumor-specific effector T-cells, proliferation, and migration to disease sites (5). The immune checkpoint molecule CTLA-4 is a homolog of T-cell co-stimulator CD28 but has a higher binding affinity for its ligands (6). This competition between CD28 and CTLA-4 binding to B7 determines whether a T-cell will undergo activation or anergy (7).

IPILIMUMAB

The discovery of CTLA-4 blockade as anticancer therapy was first described by Jim Allison's group in 1995. They demonstrated that anti-CTLA-4 antibodies enhanced rejection of several types of established transplantable tumors in mice (8). These preclinical studies led to the eventual development of ipilimumab, a fully humanized mAb (IgG1) that blocks CTLA-4 to promote antitumor immunity. There were intriguing results from the initial first-in-human pilot trials, where a few patients with massive necrosis of large tumors experienced long-term freedom from progression (9,10). Expanded single arm and

Published by Springer Publishing Company DOI: 10.1891/9780826172150.0001

randomized phase II trials with ipilimumab in patients with metastatic melanoma (MM) re-demonstrated these durable and sometimes complete responses (9,11–14).

Subsequently, a phase III randomized control trial in 676 patients with MM that had progressed on prior standard treatments showed that ipilimumab monotherapy improved overall survival (OS) (15). Patients were assigned to receive either ipilimumab plus gp100 (a glycoprotein 100 peptide vaccine), ipilimumab alone, or gp100 alone. Ipilimumab monotherapy at a dose of 3 mg/kg administered every 3 weeks for up to four treatments improved median OS by 3.7 months compared to gp100 alone (10.1 versus 6.4 months; $p = .003$). There was no added benefit of gp100 vaccine in this trial with median OS 10.0 months in the ipilimumab + gp100 group (HR 1.04; $p = .76$). A significant proportion of a small number of patients in this study who progressed following response to ipilimumab was found to respond to retreatment. This trial led to the approval of ipilimumab by the FDA in March 2011 for the treatment of patients with MM. There was further confirmation of the therapeutic efficacy in melanoma from another phase III clinical trial showing significantly improved OS when adding ipilimumab to standard dacarbazine chemotherapy in patients with MM (16).

The most striking results, though, were from the long-term follow-up analyses of responders from the ipilimumab clinical trials, many of whom were no longer receiving treatment. In 177 patients treated with ipilimumab for MM in three phase II protocols, 5-year survival was 13%, 25%, and 23% (17). In the 15 complete responders from those trials, all but one were ongoing with median follow-up of 71 to 92 months. In a meta-analysis of pooled OS data from 1,861 patients treated with ipilimumab in clinical trials, 3-year OS was 22% (18). In this analysis, most of the clinical trials had more than 5 years of minimum follow up data and three trials observed patients for up to 10 years. A plateau in the pooled Kaplan–Meier curve began at approximately 3 years and extended through 10 years.

Ipilimumab has also improved outcomes in patients with resectable melanoma in the adjuvant setting, where the previous standard interferon provided only modest improvement in recurrence-free survival (RFS) and OS for patients with stage III melanoma (increased 5-year OS from 46.1% to 49.1%) (19). In EORTC 18071, a phase IIItrial in which adjuvant ipilimumab was compared with placebo in patients with resected stage III melanoma, 3-year RFS was significantly improved from 34.8% in the placebo group to 46.5% in the ipilimumab group, leading to FDA approval for this indication being granted in 2015 (20). Results of long-term follow up from this trial revealed a significant OS benefit as well, with a 5-year OS of 65.4% in the ipilimumab group as compared with 54.4% in the placebo group (21). More recently, in a phase III trial among patients undergoing resection of stage IIIB, IIIC, or IV melanoma, adjuvant therapy with nivolumab resulted in significantly longer RFS (medians NR; 12 month RFS 70.5% with nivolumab versus 60.8% with ipilimumab) and a lower rate of grade 3 or 4 adverse events than adjuvant therapy with ipilimumab (25.4% with nivolumab versus 55.2% with ipilimumab) (22).

IMMUNE-RELATED ADVERSE EVENTS

Although the therapeutic efficacy of ipilimumab in melanoma was clear in early trials, there were also dose-related, immune-associated side effects termed immune-related adverse events (irAEs). CTLA-4 ligation antagonizes early T-cell activation, leading to decreased IL-2 production, modulation of TCR signaling, and inhibition of T-cell expansion (1). CTLA-4 deficient mice develop an autoreactive lymphoproliferative disorder and die within 3 to 4 weeks of birth (23). PD-1-deficient mice are also prone to autoimmune disorders, but these reactions are usually targeted to specific organs and take months to develop (24). These findings suggest that CTLA-4 may play a dominant role during self-tolerance throughout the life of T-cells, while PD-1 may only be involved in the maintenance of peripheral tolerance. This theory may explain the differences in the severity, pattern, timing, and incidence rates of irAEs seen with CTLA-4 blockade compared to PD-1/PD-L1 blockade.

Ipilimumab associated irAEs can affect almost any organ system (Table 1.1), but the most common toxicities are skin lesions (rash, pruritus, and vitiligo), colitis, and (less frequently) hepatitis, hypophysitis, and thyroiditis (25). Rare conditions such as uveitis, neuropathy, nephritis, myositis, myocarditis, sarcoidosis, uveitis, Guillain–Barré syndrome, and immune-mediated cytopenias can also occur (25–27). Overall irAEs occur in more than 70% of patients treated with ipilimumab monotherapy with a ~25% incidence of high grade 3–4 events using the Common Terminology Criteria for Adverse Events (CTCAE) scoring system (27,28). Although most irAEs are not severe, rarely these complications can be fatal. In the phase III trial that led to FDA approval of ipilimumab monotherapy for patients with MM, there were 14 deaths related to the study drug (2.1%) (15). The most common affected organs are the skin (40%–68%), gastrointestinal tract (26%–44%), endocrine system (5%–13%), and liver (3%–9%) occurring with characteristic timing and severity (25,28,29). Skin-irAEs can be expected after 2 to 3 weeks of ipilimumab initiation, but are rarely severe. Enterocolitis is the most common severe irAE (grade 3 or 4, 10%–16%) and, along with hepatic AEs, typically occurs 6 to 7 weeks after anti-CTLA4 therapy (28,30). Hypophysitis develops an average of 9 weeks after treatment (28). The diagnosis and management of these specific irAEs will be reviewed in the subsequent chapters.

ASSOCIATION OF TOXICITY AND RESPONSE

Whether the activated immune system in patients experiencing irAEs from anti-CTLA-4 blockade correlates with improved antitumor immunity remains a controversy. In multiple early clinical trials with ipilimumab, there was a significant association between antitumor response and irAEs (31–34). However, in one large retrospective study with ipilimumab, time to treatment failure and OS were similar in patients with and without irAEs (35). Certain irAEs may be more directly related to antitumor efficacy than others. Several studies in patients with melanoma have demonstrated an association between vitiligo and improved CPI response rates,

TABLE 1.1 Incidence of Adverse Events in Patients Treated With Ipilimumab Monotherapy in Clinical Studies (N = 5,632) by Organ System

System organ class	Overall frequency N (%)
Cutaneous	
Pruritus	1,337 (23.74)
Rash	1,237 (21.96)
Vitiligo	88 (1.56)
Gastrointestinal	
Diarrhea	1,490 (26.46)
Nausea	719 (12.77)
Colitis	423 (7.51)
Abdominal pain	271 (4.81)
Pancreatitis	23 (0.41)
Constitutional	
Fatigue	1,261 (22.39)
Decreased appetite	382 (6.78)
Pyrexia	296 (5.26)
Weight loss	201 (3.57)
Asthenia	116 (2.06)
Hepatobiliary	
Alanine aminotransferase Increase	251 (4.46)
Aspartate aminotransferase increase	226 (4.01)
Decreased hepatic function	5 (0.09)
Endocrine	
Hypothyroidism	160 (2.84)
Hypophysitis	157 (2.79)
Adrenal insufficiency	79 (1.4)
Hyperthyroidism	24 (0.43)
Musculoskeletal	
Arthralgia/Arthritis	193 (3.43)
Myalgia	96 (1.71)
Polymyalgia rheumatica	4 (0.04)
Myositis	1 (0.02)
Polymyositis	1 (0.02)
Hematologic	
Anemia	83 (1.47)
Thrombocytopenia	43 (0.76)
Eosinophilia	19 (0.34)
Neutropenia	17 (0.30)
Respiratory	
Dyspnea	78 (1.39)
Cough	73 (1.30)
Pneumonitis	28 (0.50)
Eye	
Conjunctivitis	30 (0.53)
Uveitis	22 (0.39)
Blepharitis	6 (0.11)
Nervous System	
Peripheral neuropathy	42 (0.75)
Guillain–Barré syndrome	2 (0.04)
Myasthenia gravis	2 (0.04)

(continued)

TABLE 1.1 Incidence of Adverse Events in Patients Treated With Ipilimumab Monotherapy in Clinical Studies (N = 5,632) by Organ System (*continued*)

System organ class	Overall frequency N (%)
Renal	
Proteinuria	8 (0.14)
Renal failure	6 (0.11)
Cardiac	
Atrial fibrillation	9 (0.16)
Myocarditis	1 (0.02)

Source: Adapted from Okazaki T, Honjo T. The PD-1–PD-L pathway in immunological tolerance. *Trends Immunol.* 2006;27(4):195–201. doi:10.1016/j.it.2006.02.001

PFS, and OS (36,37). The mechanism underlying this association is intuitive as vitiligo results from an autoimmune reaction against melanosomal antigens presumably shared by melanoma. There have also been associations of ipilimumab clinical activity in melanoma with irAEs in other organs, which lend to the therapy that CTLA-4 plays an essential role in antigen-nonspecific self-tolerance. One single arm ipilimumab study conducted in 198 patients with MM or metastatic renal cell carcinoma (RCC) demonstrated an association between RR and autoimmune toxicity. In this trial, the objective response rate (ORR) for patients with enterocolitis was 36% in MM and 35% in RCC, compared with 11% and 2%, respectively, in patients who did not develop enterocolitis (MM, $p = .0065$; RCC, $p = .0016$) (32). Although small numbers, Blansfield et al. reported eight of 163 (4.9%) patients with MM or RCC treated with ipilimumab who developed hypophysitis. Of the eight, five (62.5%) patients had an objective tumor response (33).

Dose Response

While the approved dose of ipilimumab in the metastatic setting is 3 mg/kg, the approved adjuvant dose for resectable stage III or IV melanoma is 10 mg/kg every 3 weeks for four doses followed by every 3 months for up to 3 years. The 10 mg/kg dose used in EORTC 1807 that lead to this approval was chosen on the basis of phase II data that indicated the potential for improved efficacy with higher doses. In a three-arm study randomizing 221 previously treated melanoma patients receiving ipilimumab at either 0.3, 3, or 10 mg/kg every 3 weeks for four doses, a clear dose response for ORR was observed (ORR: 0%, 4.2%, 11.1%, respectively; $p = .0015$) (38). Improved ORR in this trial came with a cost of more toxicity with rates of Grade 3/4 irAEs of 0%, 12%, and 25% with increasing doses. This dose response for both clinical benefit and autoimmune toxicity was re-demonstrated in a randomized phase III trial, in which ipilimumab 10 mg/kg was associated with significantly longer OS than did ipilimumab 3 mg/kg, but with increased treatment-related adverse events (39). Grade 3/4 irAEs occurred in 37% of patients in the 10 mg/kg group and 18% in the 3 mg/kg group with the most common severe irAEs in this trial being diarrhea and colitis. A large meta-analysis and systematic review of 1,265 patients from 22 clinical trials showed the incidence of all-grade irAEs was 61% (95% CI: 56%–66%) in patients receiving ipilimumab 3 mg/kg and 79% (95% CI: 69%–89%) with ipilimumab 10 mg/kg (27). This dose dependence is also seen when CTLA-4 inhibitors are combined with PD-1 inhibitors. In a phase I safety and efficacy study of the combination of ipilimumab with nivolumab in metastatic RCC, ipilimumab 3 mg/kg + nivolumab 1 mg/kg given every 3 weeks had higher rates of grade 3/4 irAEs compared to ipilimumab 1 mg/kg + nivolumab 3 mg/kg (62% versus 38%) (40).

IPILIMUMAB MONOTHERAPY IN NON-MELANOMA MALIGNANCIES

The only FDA approved indication for ipilimumab use as monotherapy is for patients with melanoma, but ipilimumab monotherapy has activity in other malignancies. In men with castration-resistant prostate cancer with progression after docetaxel chemotherapy, ipilimumab (10 mg/kg every 3 weeks for a total of four doses) versus placebo was added after radiation therapy (41). Although in the intention to treat population statistical improvement in the primary analysis of OS was not met, ipilimumab did improve progression-free survival (PFS). In addition, a selected subset of patients lacking visceral disease with favorable laboratory values did have a significant OS benefit. Another randomized phase III trial with ipilimumab versus placebo in minimally symptomatic patients with chemotherapy-naïve, castration-resistant prostate cancer also did not improve OS but increased PFS and prostate-specific antigen response rates (42). These two studies demonstrated antitumor activity in patient subsets but at a cost of significant grade 3/4 irAEs (26% and 40%, respectively) of which some were fatal (1% and 2%, respectively). Ipilimumab added to chemotherapy (carboplatin and paclitaxel) improved irPFS and PFS in non-small cell lung cancer (43). Single-arm phase II studies have also shown activity of ipilimumab monotherapy in other cancers such as RCC and urothelial carcinoma (32,44–46). However, to date, there have been no phase III data to show the benefit of ipilimumab for non-small cell lung cancer, RCC, and urothelial carcinoma.

Tremelimumab

Tremelimumab is a fully human IgG_2 mAb directed against CTLA-4. Although tremelimumab has produced promising anticancer responses in early clinical trials (47–49), unlike ipilimumab, it has not been FDA approved for any indication (3). A randomized phase III trial of tremelimumab monotherapy versus standard-of-care chemotherapy (dacarbazine or temozolomide) failed to meet the primary endpoint of improved OS (50). Some attribute this negative result to the schedule of tremelimumab administration (15 mg/kg every 3 months) or to expanded-access to ipilimumab in the control arm with subsequent lines of treatment (51). Others suggested that tremelimumab, an IgG_2 immunoglobulin, may have lower affinity binding to CTLA-4 and is less efficacious (52).

Despite not achieving improved OS, tremelimumab did provide clinical benefit in many patients with MM experiencing durable responses in all of these trials.

Tremelimumab has also been tested in other cancers including non-small cell lung cancer, hepatitis C-associated hepatocellular carcinoma, gastroesophageal adenocarcinoma, and metastatic colorectal cancer, though response rates were disappointing (53–56). Results from phase II trials in the treatment of malignant mesothelioma were more promising (57,58), leading to a randomized phase II trial of tremelimumab versus placebo in patients with relapsed mesothelioma. This trial did not meet its primary endpoint as tremelimumab did not significantly prolong OS compared with placebo (59). The toxicity profile of tremelimumab is similar to ipilimumab monotherapy (Table 1.2), though it has a higher incidence of grade 3 adverse events (56%) (59). With disappointing results from tremelimumab monotherapy studies, future investigations have focused on combinatorial approaches. Tremelimumab combined with durvalumab (an anti-PD-L1 inhibitor also developed by AstraZeneca) has been shown to have promising activity in multiple tumor types, and there are currently phase III trials with this combination ongoing in non-small

TABLE 1.2 Summary of Treatment-Emergent Adverse Events of Special Interest in Patients Treated With Tremelimumab Monotherapy in Patients With Mesothelioma (N = 380) by Organ System

System organ class	Overall frequency N (%)	
	Any grade	Grade 3–4
Cutaneous Dermatitis	169 (44.5)	9 (2.4)
Gastrointestinal Diarrhea Colitis Hepatitis Pancreatitis	180 (47.4) 39 (10.3) 24 (6.3) 23 (6.1)	59 (15.5) 26 (6.8) 4 (1.1) 14 (3.7)
Endocrinopathy	32 (8.4)	8 (2.1)
Renal Nephritis	24 (6.3)	4 (1.1)
Allergy Hypersensitivity reaction	11 (2.9)	1 (0.3)
Respiratory Pneumonitis/Interstitial lung disease	3 (0.8)	1 (0.3)
Neurologic Neuropathy/Neuromuscular toxicity	2 (0.5)	2 (0.5)

Source: Adapted from Maio M, Scherpereel A, Calabrò L, et al. Tremelimumab as second-line or third-line treatment in relapsed malignant mesothelioma (DETERMINE): a multicentre, international, randomised, double-blind, placebo-controlled phase 2b trial. *Lancet Oncol.* 2017;18(9): 1261–1273. doi:10.1016/s1470-2045(17)30446-1

cell lung cancer, urothelial carcinoma, head and neck cancer, pancreatic cancer, and sarcoma.

MECHANISMS OF RESISTANCE TO CTLA-4 BLOCKADE

Although ipilimumab therapy results in a significant survival benefit in patients with MM, the majority (~80% of patients are primary refractory. There have been efforts to identify resistance mechanisms, but why most patients do not respond to anti-CTLA-4 monotherapy remains elusive. Mutational burden is a known tumor-intrinsic feature correlated with response to ICIs, presumably by enhanced neoantigen formation from the increased number of nonsynonymous single nucleotide variants (60). Intuitively, alterations in genes encoding components of the antigen presentation machinery (e.g., class I MHC, β2-microglobulin) have been identified as mechanisms of resistance to T-cell-based immunotherapies (61,62).

CTLA-4 blockade enhances T-cell production of interferon (IFN)-γ, which augments tumor antigen presentation along with direct antitumor effects (63). Gao et al. reported nine out of 12 (75%) ipilimumab nonresponders with MM harbored certain genomic defects of the IFN-γ pathway genes (63). Others have confirmed that loss of function mutations in the IFN-γ pathway can lead to acquired resistance to PD-1 inhibitors in melanoma (61). These studies are consistent with the finding that an IFN-γ signature was associated with anti-PD1 clinical responses in patients with metastatic bladder cancer (64). In addition, alternative co-inhibitory immune checkpoints (e.g., TIM-3, LAG-3, VISTA) have been identified, and their expression has been associated with ICI resistance (65–67).

Strategies to evade these resistance mechanisms to improve response rates are being investigated. Promotion of immunogenic tumor cell death (e.g., chemotherapy or radiation) or enhancing antigen presentation by stimulating the innate immune response (e.g., TLR agonists, CD40 agonists, oncolytic viruses) may augment presentation of tumor neoantigens and aid in overcoming anti-CTLA-4 resistance. These combination strategies, along with different ICI combinations, will likely be more effective as compared to anti-CTLA-4 monotherapy based upon early clinical trial data. However, these combination strategies may also be associated with more significant toxicities, which will be reviewed in a separate chapter in this book.

CONCLUSION

The development of anti-CTLA-4 agents began an unprecedented success in immuno-oncologic therapies that has revolutionized the world of oncology. Although these agents have been shown to prolong survival in some cancer patients by providing durable antitumor immune responses, they also lead to autoimmune toxicities known as irAEs. CTLA-4 regulates immune priming at the initial stage of both CD4+ and CD8+ naïve T-cell activation usually in lymph nodes, while PD-1 functions predominantly within peripheral tissues during the effector phase (4,6,8,68). These differences in immune regulatory mechanisms are the reason for the unique antitumor activity, autoimmune toxicity profiles, and synergy between CTLA-4 and PD-1/PD-L1 blockade.

With the emergence of seemingly more efficacious and less toxic PD-1/PD-L1 inhibitors now approved in multiple cancers, the majority of clinical trials with anti-CTLA-4 agents are in combinations (reviewed in Chapter 3). Ipilimumab in combination with nivolumab has already been shown to improve both PFS and OS in patients with untreated MM compared to either agent alone (57). This combination has also been shown to improve PFS over standard of care front-line therapy in RCC (69) and in non-small cell lung cancer with high mutational burden (70). Though there is proven synergy for antitumor activity, there is also synergy for irAEs with anti-CTLA-4/PD-1 inhibitor combinations. In the above-mentioned phase III trial in patients with MM, the incidence of grade 3/4 treatment-related adverse events was 55% with nivolumab-plus-ipilimumab, 27.3% with ipilimumab alone, and 16.3% with nivolumab alone (57). Similar to ipilimumab monotherapy, the most common AEs in patients receiving the combination were dermatitis, enterocolitis, and hepatitis. Although use of CTLA-4 inhibitors as monotherapy may become less relevant, familiarity of oncologists with these agents, their toxicities, and management of toxicities is important as new immuno-oncologic (IO) combinations are developed.

ACKNOWLEDGMENTS

We acknowledge L. Evan Reddick, PhD in Medical Affairs, and his colleagues in Medical Information at AstraZeneca Pharmaceuticals for providing compiled clinical response/toxicity data on tremelimumab used in this manuscript.

REFERENCES

1. Fife BT, Bluestone JA. Control of peripheral T-cell tolerance and autoimmunity via the CTLA-4 and PD-1 pathways. *Immunol Rev.* 2008;224(1):166–182. doi:10.1111/j.1600-065x.2008.00662.x

2. Ribas A. Adaptive immune resistance: how cancer protects from immune attack. *Cancer Discov.* 2015;5(9):915–919. doi:10.1158/2159-8290.cd-15-0563

3. U.S. Food and Drug Administration. Drugs @FDA: FDA approved drug products. 2017; https:// www.accessdata.fda.gov/scripts

4. Lizée G, Overwijk WW, Radvanyi L, et al. Harnessing the power of the immune system to target cancer. *Annu Rev Med.* 2013;64:71–90. doi:10.1146/annurev-med-112311-083918

5. Sharma P, Wagner K, Wolchok JD, et al. Novel cancer immunotherapy agents with survival benefit: recent successes and next steps. *Nat Rev Cancer.* 2011;11(11):805–812. doi:10.1038/nrc3153

6. Krummel MF, Allison JP. CD28 and CTLA-4 have opposing effects on the response of T cells to stimulation. *J Exp Med.* 1995;182(2):459–465. doi:10.1084/jem.182.2.459

7. Poschke I, Mougiakakos D, Kiessling R. Camouflage and sabotage: tumor escape from the immune system. *Cancer Immunol Immunother.* 2011;60(8):1161–1171. doi:10.1007/s00262-011-1012-8

8. Leach DR, Krummel MF, Allison JP. Enhancement of antitumor immunity by CTLA-4 blockade. *Science.* 1996;271(5256):1734–1736. doi:10.1126/science.271.5256.1734

9. Weber J. Ipilimumab: controversies in its development, utility and autoimmune adverse events. *Cancer Immunol Immunother.* 2009;58(5):823. doi:10.1007/s00262-008-0653-8

10. Hodi FS, Mihm MC, Soiffer RJ, et al. Biologic activity of cytotoxic T lymphocyte-associated antigen 4 antibody blockade in previously vaccinated metastatic melanoma and ovarian carcinoma patients. *Proc Natl Acad Sci.* 2003;100(8):4712–4717. doi:10.3410/f.1014595.193929

11. Weber JS, Hersh EM, Yellin M, et al. The efficacy and safety of ipilimumab (MDX-010) in patients with unresectable stage III or stage IV malignant melanoma *J Clin Oncol.* 2007;25(18_suppl):8523–8523.

12. Fischkoff SA, Hersh E, Weber J, et al. Durable responses and long-term progression-free survival observed in a phase II study of MDX-010 alone or in combination with dacarbazine (DTIC) in metastatic melanoma. *J Clin Oncol.* 2005;23(16_suppl):7525–7525. doi:10.1200/jco.2005.23.16_suppl.7525

13. Weber JS, Berman D, Siegel J, et al. Safety and efficacy of ipilimumab with or without prophylactic budesonide in treatment-naive and previously treated patients with advanced melanoma. *J Clin Oncol.* 2008;26(15_suppl):9010–9010. doi:10.1200/jco.2008.26.15_suppl.9010

14. Hamid O, Chin K, Li J, et al. Dose effect of ipilimumab in patients with advanced melanoma: results from a phase II, randomized, dose-ranging study. *J Clin Oncol.* 2008;26(15_suppl):9025–9025. doi:10.1200/jco.2008.26.15_suppl.9025

15. Hodi FS, O'day SJ, McDermott DF, et al. Improved survival with ipilimumab in patients with metastatic melanoma. *N Engl J Med.* 2010;363(8):711–723. doi:10.1056/nejmoa1003466

16. Robert C, Thomas L, Bondarenko I, et al. Ipilimumab plus dacarbazine for previously untreated metastatic melanoma. *N Engl J Med.* 2011;364(26):2517–2526. doi:10.1056/nejmoa1104621

17. Prieto PA, Yang JC, Sherry RM, et al. CTLA-4 blockade with ipilimumab: long-term follow-up of 177 patients with metastatic melanoma. *Clin Cancer Res.* 2012;18(7):2039–2047. doi:10.1158/1078-0432.ccr-11-1823

18. Schadendorf D, Hodi FS, Robert C, et al. Pooled analysis of long-term survival data from phase II and phase III trials of ipilimumab in metastatic or locally advanced, unresectable melanoma. *Eur J Cancer.* 2013;49:S11–S11.

19. Suciu S, Ives N, Eggermont AM, et. al. Predictive importance of ulceration on the efficacy of adjuvant interferon-a (IFN): an individual patient data (IPD) meta-analysis of 15 randomized trials in more than 7,500 melanoma patients (pts). *J Clin Oncol.* 2014;32 (15_suppl):9067–9067.

20. Eggermont AM, Chiarion-Sileni V, Grob JJ, et al. Adjuvant ipilimumab versus placebo after complete resection of high-risk stage III melanoma (EORTC 18071): a randomised, double-blind, phase 3 trial. *Lancet Oncol.* 2015;16:522–530. doi:10.1016/s1470-2045(15)70122-1

21. Eggermont AM, Chiarion-Sileni V, Grob JJ, et al. Prolonged survival in stage III melanoma with ipilimumab adjuvant therapy. *N Engl J Med.* 2016;375(19):1845–1855. doi:10.1056/nejmoa1611299

22. Weber J, Mandala M, Del Vecchio M, et al. Adjuvant nivolumab versus ipilimumab in resected stage III or IV melanoma. *N Engl J Med.* 2017;377(19):1824–1835. doi:10.1056/nejmoa1709030

23. Waterhouse P, Penninger JM, Timms E, et al. Lymphoproliferative disorders with early lethality in mice deficient in Ctla-4. *Science.* 1995;270(5238):985–988. doi:10.1126/science.270.5238.985

24. Okazaki T, Honjo T. The PD-1–PD-L pathway in immunological tolerance. *Trends Immunol.* 2006;27(4):195–201. doi:10.1016/j.it.2006.02.001

25. Investigator's brochure version 20 for ipilimumab (BMS-734016/MDX-010). (March, 2017) Bristol-Myers Squibb.

26. Gao J, He Q, Subudhi S, et al. Review of immune-related adverse events in prostate cancer patients treated with ipilimumab: MD Anderson experience. *Oncogene.* 2015;34(43):5411. doi:10.1038/onc.2015.5

27. Bertrand A, Kostine M, Barnetche T, et al. Immune related adverse events associated with anti-CTLA-4 antibodies: systematic review and meta-analysis. *BMC Med.* 2015;13(1):211. doi:10.1186/s12916-015-0455-8

28. Weber JS, Kähler KC, Hauschild A. Management of immune-related adverse events and kinetics of response with ipilimumab. *J Clin Oncol.* 2012;30(21):2691–2697. doi:10.1200/jco.2012.41.6750

29. Wolchok JD, Hodi FS, Weber JS, et al. Development of ipilimumab: a novel immunotherapeutic approach for the treatment of advanced melanoma. *Ann N Y Acad Sci*. 2013;1291(1):1–13. doi:10.1111/nyas.12180

30. Michot JM, Bigenwald C, Champiat S, et al. Immune-related adverse events with immune checkpoint blockade: a comprehensive review. *Eur J Cancer*. 2016;54:139–148. doi:10.1016/j.ejca.2015.11.016

31. Attia P, Phan GQ, Maker AV, et al. Autoimmunity correlates with tumor regression in patients with metastatic melanoma treated with anti–cytotoxic T-lymphocyte antigen-4. *J Clin Oncol*. 2005;23(25):6043–6053. doi:10.1200/jco.2005.06.205

32. Beck KE, Blansfield JA, Tran KQ, et al. Enterocolitis in patients with cancer after antibody blockade of cytotoxic T-lymphocyte–associated antigen 4. *J Clin Oncol*. 2006;24(15):2283–2289. doi:10.1200/jco.2005.04.5716

33. Blansfield JA, Beck KE, Tran K, et al. Cytotoxic T-lymphocyte–associated antigen-4 blockage can induce autoimmune hypophysitis in patients with metastatic melanoma and renal cancer. *J Immunother*. 2005;28(6):593. doi:10.1097/01.cji.0000178913 .41256.06

34. Downey SG, Klapper JA, Smith FO, et al. Prognostic factors related to clinical response in patients with metastatic melanoma treated by CTL-associated antigen-4 blockade. *Clin Cancer Res*. 2007;13(22):6681–6688. doi:10.1158/1078-0432.ccr-07-0187

35. Horvat TZ, Adel NG, Dang TO, et al. Immune-related adverse events, need for systemic immunosuppression, and effects on survival and time to treatment failure in patients with melanoma treated with ipilimumab at Memorial Sloan Kettering Cancer Center. *J Clin Oncol*. 2015;33(28):3193–3198. doi:10.1200/jco.2015.60.8448

36. Teulings HE, Limpens J, Jansen SN, et al. Vitiligo-like depigmentation in patients with stage III-IV melanoma receiving immunotherapy and its association with survival: a systematic review and meta-analysis. *J Clin Oncol*. 2015;33(7):773–781. doi:10.1200/jco .2014.57.4756

37. Hua C, Boussemart L, Mateus C, et al. Association of vitiligo with tumor response in patients with metastatic melanoma treated with pembrolizumab. *JAMA Dermatol*. 2016;152(1):45–51. doi:10.1001/jamadermatol.2015.2707

38. Wolchok JD, Neyns B, Linette G, et al. Ipilimumab monotherapy in patients with pretreated advanced melanoma: a randomised, double-blind, multicentre, phase 2, dose-ranging study. *Lancet Oncol*. 2010;11:155–164. doi:10.1016/s1470-2045(09)70334-1

39. Ascierto PA, Del Vecchio M, Robert C, et al. Ipilimumab 10 mg/kg versus ipilimumab 3 mg/kg in patients with unresectable or metastatic melanoma: a randomised, double-blind, multicentre, phase 3 trial. *Lancet Oncol*. 2017;18(5):611–622. doi:10.1016/s1470-2045(17)30231-0

40. Hammers HJ, Plimack ER, Infante JR, et al. Safety and efficacy of nivolumab in combination with ipilimumab in metastatic renal cell carcinoma: the CheckMate 016 study. *J Clin Oncol*. 2017;35(34):3851–3858. doi:10.1200/jco.2016.72.1985

41. Kwon ED, Drake CG, Scher HI, et al. Ipilimumab versus placebo after radiotherapy in patients with metastatic castration-resistant prostate cancer that had progressed after docetaxel chemotherapy (CA184-043): a multicentre, randomised, double-blind, phase 3 trial. *Lancet Oncol*. 2014;15(7):700–712. doi:10.1016/s1470-2045(14)70189-5

42. Beer TM, Kwon ED, Drake CG, et al. Randomized, double-blind, phase III trial of ipilimumab versus placebo in asymptomatic or minimally symptomatic patients with metastatic chemotherapy-naive castration-resistant prostate cancer. *J Clin Oncol*. 2016;35(1):40–47. doi:10.1200/jco.2016.69.1584

43. Lynch TJ, Bondarenko I, Luft A, et al. Ipilimumab in combination with paclitaxel and carboplatin as first-line treatment in stage IIIB/IV non–small-cell lung cancer: results from a randomized, double-blind, multicenter phase II study. *J Clin Oncol*. 2012;30(17):2046–2054. doi:10.1200/jco.2011.38.4032

44. Yang JC, Hughes M, Kammula U, et al. Ipilimumab (anti-CTLA4 antibody) causes regression of metastatic renal cell cancer associated with enteritis and hypophysitis. *J Immunother*. 2007;30(8):825. doi:10.1097/cji.0b013e318156e47e

45. Carthon BC, Wolchok JD, Yuan J, et al. Preoperative CTLA-4 blockade: tolerability and immune monitoring in the setting of a presurgical clinical trial. *Clin Cancer Res*. 2010;16(10):2861–2871. doi:10.1158/1078-0432.ccr-10-0569

46. Galsky MD, Hahn NM, Albany C, et al. Phase II trial of gemcitabine+ cisplatin+ ipilimumab in patients with metastatic urothelial cancer. *J Clin Oncol.* 2016;34(2_suppl):357–357. doi:10.1200/jco.2016.34.2_suppl.357

47. Ribas A, Camacho LH, Lopez-Berestein G, et al. Antitumor activity in melanoma and anti-self responses in a phase I trial with the anti-cytotoxic T lymphocyte-associated antigen 4 monoclonal antibody CP-675,206. *J Clin Oncol.* 2005;23(35):8968–8977. doi:10.1200/jco.2005.01.109

48. Camacho LH, Antonia S, Sosman J, et al. Phase I/II trial of tremelimumab in patients with metastatic melanoma. *J Clin Oncol.* 2009;27(7):1075–1081. doi:10.1200/jco.2008.19.2435

49. Kirkwood JM, Lorigan P, Hersey P, et al. Phase II trial of tremelimumab (CP-675,206) in patients with advanced refractory or relapsed melanoma. *Clin Cancer Res.* 2010;16(3):1042–1048. doi:10.1158/1078-0432.ccr-09-2033

50. Ribas A, Kefford R, Marshall MA, et al. Phase III randomized clinical trial comparing tremelimumab with standard-of-care chemotherapy in patients with advanced melanoma. *J Clin Oncol.* 2013;31(5):616–622. doi:10.1200/jco.2012.44.6112

51. Ascierto PA. Is there still a role for tremelimumab in the treatment of cancer?. *Transl Cancer Res.* 2013;2(1):48–50. doi: 10.3978/j.issn.2218-676X.2013.02.02

52. Blank CU, Enk A. Therapeutic use of anti-CTLA-4 antibodies. *Int Immunol.* 2015;27(1):3–10. doi:10.1093/intimm/dxu076

53. Chung KY, Gore I, Fong L, et al. Phase II study of the anti-cytotoxic T-lymphocyte-associated antigen 4 monoclonal antibody, tremelimumab, in patients with refractory metastatic colorectal cancer. *J Clin Oncol.* 2010;28(21):3485–3490. doi:10.1200/jco.2010.28.3994

54. Zatloukal PP, Heo DS, Kang J, et al. Randomized phase II clinical trial comparing tremelimumab (CP-675,206) with best supportive care (BSC) following first-line platinum-based therapy in patients (pts) with advanced non-small cell lung cancer (NSCLC). ASCO Annual Meeting. *J Clin Oncol.* 2009;27(15s suppl) abstr8071.

55. Sangro B, Gomez-Martin C, de la Mata M, et al. A clinical trial of CTLA-4 blockade with tremelimumab in patients with hepatocellular carcinoma and chronic hepatitis C. *J Hepatol.* 2013;59(1):81–88. doi:10.1016/j.jhep.2013.02.022

56. Ralph C, Elkord E, Burt DJ, et al. Modulation of lymphocyte regulation for cancer therapy: a phase II trial of tremelimumab in advanced gastric and esophageal adenocarcinoma. *Clin Cancer Res.* 2010;16(5):1662–1672. doi:10.1158/1078-0432.ccr-09-2870

57. Wolchok JD, Chiarion-Sileni V, Gonzalez R, et al. Overall survival with combined nivolumab and ipilimumab in advanced melanoma. *N Engl J Med.* 2017;377(14):1345–1356. doi:10.1056/nejmoa1709684

58. Calabro L, Morra A, Fonsatti E, et al. Efficacy and safety of an intensified schedule of tremelimumab for chemotherapy-resistant malignant mesothelioma: an open-label, single-arm, phase 2 study. *Lancet Respir Med.* 2015;3(4):301–309. doi:10.1016/s2213-2600(15)00092-2

59. Maio M, Scherpereel A, Calabrò L, et al. Tremelimumab as second-line or third-line treatment in relapsed malignant mesothelioma (DETERMINE): a multicentre, international, randomised, double-blind, placebo-controlled phase 2b trial. *Lancet Oncol.* 2017;18(9):1261–1273. doi:10.1016/s1470-2045(17)30446-1

60. Schumacher TN, Schreiber RD. Neoantigens in cancer immunotherapy. *Science.* 2015;348(6230):69–74. doi:10.1126/science.aaa4971

61. Zaretsky JM, Garcia-Diaz A, Shin DS, et al. Mutations associated with acquired resistance to PD-1 blockade in melanoma. *N Engl J Med.* 2016;375(9):819–829. doi:10.1056/nejmoa1604958

62. Patel SJ, Sanjana NE, Kishton RJ, et al. Identification of essential genes for cancer immunotherapy. *Nature.* 2017;548(7669):537. doi:10.1038/nature23477

63. Gao J, Shi LZ, Zhao H, et al. Loss of IFN-γ pathway genes in tumor cells as a mechanism of resistance to anti-CTLA-4 therapy. *Cell.* 2016;167(2):397–404. doi:10.1016/j.cell.2016.08.069

64. Sharma P, Retz M, Siefker-Radtke A, et al. Nivolumab in metastatic urothelial carcinoma after platinum therapy (CheckMate 275): a multicentre, single-arm, phase 2 trial. *Lancet Oncol.* 2017;18(3):312–322. doi:10.1016/s1470-2045(17)30065-7

65. Thommen DS, Schreiner J, Müller P, et al. Progression of lung cancer is associated with increased dysfunction of T cells defined by coexpression of multiple inhibitory receptors. *Cancer Immunol Res*. 2015;3(12):1344–1355. doi:10.1158/2326-6066.cir-15-0097

66. Koyama S, Akbay EA, Li YY, et al. Adaptive resistance to therapeutic PD-1 blockade is associated with upregulation of alternative immune checkpoints. *Nat Commun*. 2016;7:10501. doi:10.1038/ncomms10501

67. Gao J, Ward JF, Pettaway CA, et al. VISTA is an inhibitory immune checkpoint that is increased after ipilimumab therapy in patients with prostate cancer. *Nat Med*. 2017;23(5):551. doi:10.1038/nm.4308

68. Buchbinder EI, Desai A. CTLA-4 and PD-1 pathways: similarities, differences, and implications of their inhibition. *Am J Clin Oncol*. 2016;39(1):98. doi:10.1097/coc.0000000000000239

69. Motzer RJ, Tannir NM, McDermott DF, et al. Nivolumab plus Ipilimumab versus Sunitinib in Advanced Renal-Cell Carcinoma. *N Engl J Med*. 2018;378(14):1277–1290. doi:10.1056/NEJMoa1712126

70. Hellmann MD, Ciuleanu TE, Pluzanski A, et al. Nivolumab plus ipilimumab in lung cancer with a high tumor mutational burden. *N Engl J Med*. 2018;378(22):2093–2104. doi:10.1056/nejmoa1801946

CHAPTER 2

OVERVIEW OF PD-1 AND PD-L1 INHIBITORS

Nikolaos Andreatos, Shailender Bhatia, and Petros Grivas

INTRODUCTION

The isolation of programmed cell death 1 (PD-1) first took place in the early 1990s (1,2); however, the importance of the PD-1 pathway in T-cell regulation and cancer-related immune evasion was further appreciated with the discovery of programmed cell death ligand 1 (PD-L1 or B7H1/CD274) in 1999 (3,4). Physiologically, the interaction of PD-1 with PD-L1 serves as a molecular "brake/checkpoint" on T-cell-mediated immune responses through a variety of mechanisms, such as promotion of activated T-cell apoptosis and regulatory T-cell function, stimulation of T-cell anergy, and inhibition of T-cell proliferation (5). Interestingly, cancer cells appear to efficiently exploit the PD-1/PD-L1 pathway for the purposes of immune evasion, mainly through aberrant expression of PD-L1 (4,5). In turn, this discovery led to the hypothesis that successful blockade of PD-1/PD-L1 interactions might greatly increase the effectiveness of T-cell-mediated responses against tumor antigens, leading to tumor regression (6). Consequently, the efficacy of PD-1 and PD-L1 inhibitors as immunotherapy agents has attracted considerable scientific and commercial interest (7).

At present (cemiplimab was approved later after the completion of this chapter), two PD-1 inhibitors (pembrolizumab and nivolumab) and three PD-L1 inhibitors (atezolizumab, avelumab, and durvalumab) have been approved by the U.S. Food and Drug Administration (FDA) for the treatment of various cancers, with one of the first approvals granted to pembrolizumab for the treatment of melanoma on September 4, 2014 (7). All three PD-L1 inhibitors are IgG1 monoclonal antibodies; atezolizumab is humanized, while avelumab and durvalumab are fully human (8–10). On the other hand, the two PD-1 inhibitors are IgG4 monoclonal antibodies; pembrolizumab is humanized, while nivolumab is fully human (11,12). Given the rapid expansion of indications for these agents in recent years, we attempt to summarize the most important clinical trials leading to FDA approvals to date (March 2018); however, due to limitations of space the present review is not intended to be an exhaustive account of successful use of these agents in several cancer types.

PD-1 INHIBITORS

Pembrolizumab

Indications

(*summary of indications available at*:
www.accessdata.fda.gov/drugsatfda_docs/label/2017/125514s031lbl.pdf)

Published by Springer Publishing Company DOI: 10.1891/9780826172150.0002

- Unresectable/metastatic melanoma following disease progression after treatment with ipilimumab and a *BRAF* inhibitor if indicated.
- First-line treatment of unresectable/metastatic melanoma irrespective of *BRAF* mutational status.
- Locally advanced/metastatic non-small cell lung cancer (NSCLC) that expresses PD-L1 following progression during or after platinum-based chemotherapy or targeted therapy.
- Metastatic NSCLC without *EGFR* or *ALK* alterations and PD-L1 expression of at least 50%.
- Metastatic NSCLC in combination with pemetrexed and carboplatin.
- Locally advanced or metastatic urothelial carcinoma following progression after platinum-based chemotherapy.
- Locally advanced or metastatic urothelial carcinoma for patients who have not received chemotherapy for advanced disease but are ineligible for cisplatin.
- Recurrent/metastatic squamous cell carcinoma of the head and neck following progression during/after platinum-based chemotherapy.
- Recurrent locally advanced/metastatic gastric/gastroesophageal junction adenocarcinoma with PD-L1 expression and progression after two appropriate systemic therapies.
- Refractory or relapsed classic Hodgkin lymphoma following (a) autologous stem cell transplantation and brentuximab vedotin, (b) salvage chemotherapy and brentuximab vedotin, or (c) autologous stem cell transplantation without brentuximab vedotin.
- Unresectable/metastatic solid tumors with microsatellite instability (MSI-high) or mismatch repair deficiency (MMR-d) that have progressed following prior therapy.

Melanoma

Pembrolizumab was the first PD-1 inhibitor to be approved for use in patients with advanced or unresectable melanoma who progressed following therapy with ipilimumab and/or a *BRAF* inhibitor (September 4, 2014) (7). In turn, this was based on the findings of the KEYNOTE-001 phase I trial, which assessed the efficacy and safety of various doses of pembrolizumab (2 mg/kg or 10 mg/kg every 3 weeks) (12,13). In a cohort of 173 patients (89 treated with 2 mg/kg and 84 with 10 mg/kg) with a median follow-up of 8 months, an overall response rate (ORR) of 26% was noted in both dose groups. Toxicity was relatively mild, with only 15% and 8% of patients developing grade 3/4 treatment-related adverse events (AEs) in the 2 mg/kg and 10 mg/kg groups, respectively (12).

Subsequently, the KEYNOTE-002 phase II trial compared pembrolizumab (2 mg/kg or 10 mg/kg every 3 weeks) versus investigator-choice chemotherapy (paclitaxel plus carboplatin, paclitaxel, carboplatin, dacarbazine, temozolomide) for patients with unresectable stage III/IV melanoma that had progressed following therapy with ipilimumab and/or a *BRAF* inhibitor if indicated (14). A total of 180 patients were randomly assigned to receive pembrolizumab 2 mg/kg, 181 to 10 mg/kg and 179 to investigator-choice chemotherapy. At a median follow-up of 10 months, it was demonstrated that pembrolizumab was associated with significantly improved progression-free survival (PFS) versus investigator-choice chemotherapy [(hazard ratio (HR): 0.57, 95% CI: 0.45–0.73, $p < .0001$) and (HR: 0.50, 95% CI: 0.39–0.64, $p < .0001$) for 2 mg/kg and 10 mg/kg, respectively]. While overall survival (OS) was not shown to differ between study groups, the authors noted that the study was underpowered to confirm the superiority of pembrolizumab in terms of OS. With respect to safety, grade 3/4 treatment-related AEs were more common in the chemotherapy group (26%) than in the 2 mg/kg (11%) and 10 mg/kg (14%) pembrolizumab dose groups.

Lastly, in the KEYNOTE-006 phase III trial, pembrolizumab (10 mg/kg every 2 or every 3 weeks) was compared with ipilimumab (3 mg/kg every 3 weeks for four doses) among patients with unresectable or metastatic melanoma with no more than one prior systemic therapy, irrespective of *BRAF* mutational status (15). A total of 279 patients were randomized to pembrolizumab 10 mg/kg every 2 weeks, 277 every 3 weeks and 278 to ipilimumab. At a median follow-up of 7.9 months, a significantly reduced risk of progression was noted with pembrolizumab [(HR: 0.58, 95% CI: 0.46–0.72, $p < .001$) and (HR: 0.58, 95% CI: 0.47–0.72, $p < .001$) for the 2- and 3-week regimens, respectively, versus ipilimumab]. Similarly, a significantly reduced risk of death was noted in both pembrolizumab arms [(HR: 0.63, 95% CI: 0.47–0.83, $p < .0005$) and (HR: 0.69, 95% CI: 0.52–0.90, $p = .0036$) for the 2- and 3-week regimens, respectively versus ipilimumab]. Grade 3–5 treatment-related AEs were fewer in the two pembrolizumab arms (13.3% and 10.1% for the 2- and 3-week regimens, respectively), versus ipilimumab (19.9%). Given these extremely favorable results, FDA granted an expanded approval to pembrolizumab for first-line treatment of unresectable or metastatic melanoma, irrespective of *BRAF* mutational status (December 18, 2015) (7).

NSCLC

Pembrolizumab first received approval for the treatment of metastatic NSCLC on October 2, 2015, on the basis of the KEYNOTE-001 trial (16–18). This phase I trial assessed the efficacy and safety of varying pembrolizumab doses (2 mg/kg every 3 weeks, 10 mg/kg every 2 or every 3 weeks) among 550 patients with PD-L1 positive, locally advanced/metastatic NSCLC who either progressed after previous platinum-based or targeted therapy (n = 449) or were treatment-naïve ($n = 101$) (18). Efficacy was first assessed in 61 previously treated patients with PD-L1 expression of at least 50%; ORR ranged from 28% (95% CI: 12.1–49.4) to 41.2% (95% CI: 24.7–59.3) for patients treated with 2 mg/kg every 3 weeks to 10 mg/kg every 3 weeks, respectively (17). A subsequent update of the KEYNOTE-001 trial (including results from the treatment-naïve cohort) reported median OS of 22.1 months (95% CI: 17.1–27.2) and 10.6 months (95% CI: 8.6–13.3) for treatment-naïve and previously treated patients, respectively; similarly, 2-year OS rates were 44.5% and 31.3%. Importantly, increased PD-L1 expression was associated with longer OS (18). Interestingly, analysis of 495 patients from the KEYNOTE-001 confirmed the association of PD-L1 expression with treatment response and validated a PD-L1 cut-off of at least 50% as a predictor of higher ORR. The ORR in this cohort was 19.4% (95% CI: 16.0–23.2), with 47 patients experiencing at least a grade 3 AE. Most common immune-mediated AEs were infusion reactions (15 patients), hypothyroidism (34 patients), and pneumonitis (18 patients); a patient with infusion reaction discontinued treatment, while one episode of pneumonitis was fatal (16).

The KEYNOTE-010 phase II/III trial subsequently assessed the safety and efficacy of pembrolizumab (either 2 mg/kg or 10 mg/kg every 3 weeks) versus docetaxel chemotherapy for patients with PD-L1 positive NSCLC that had progressed after platinum-based or targeted therapy (19). A total of 345 patients were randomly allocated to pembrolizumab 2 mg/kg, 346 to pembrolizumab 10 mg/kg, and 343 to docetaxel. After a median follow-up of 13.1 months, a survival advantage was noted for pembrolizumab 2 mg/kg (HR: 0.71, 95% CI: 0.58–0.88, p = .0008) and pembrolizumab 10 mg/kg (HR: 0.61, 95% CI: 0.49–0.75, p < .0001) versus docetaxel, for all included patients. However, PFS was only increased with pembrolizumab among patients with PD-L1 expression of at least 50%. Toxicity was lower with pembrolizumab, with grade 3–5 treatment-related AEs reported in only 13% and 16% of patients treated with pembrolizumab 2 mg/kg and 10 mg/kg, respectively, compared to 35% with docetaxel.

More recently, the KEYNOTE-024 phase III trial examined pembrolizumab (200 mg every 3 weeks) versus platinum-based chemotherapy, as first-line treatment in advanced NSCLC without *EGFR* or *ALK* alterations and with documented PD-L1 expression of at least 50% (20). A total of 154 patients were randomly allocated to pembrolizumab and 151 to chemotherapy. At a median follow-up of 11.2 months, pembrolizumab was associated with significantly lower risk of progression or death (HR: 0.50, 95% CI: 0.37–0.68, p < .001). Toxicity was also less with pembrolizumab, especially for grade 3–5 AEs (26.6% versus 53.3% for pembrolizumab and chemotherapy, respectively). Given these results, the FDA approved pembrolizumab for this indication on October 24, 2016 (7).

Pembrolizumab also recently received approval for use as combination first-line therapy (with pemetrexed/carboplatin) for non-squamous stage IIIB/IV NSCLC without *EGFR* or *ALK* alterations, irrespective of PD-L1 status (May 10, 2017) (7). Specifically, as part of the KEYNOTE-021 phase II trial, 60 patients were randomly assigned to combination chemotherapy with pembrolizumab (200 mg every 3 weeks) and 63 to chemotherapy alone (carboplatin and pemetrexed) (21). After a median follow-up of 10.6 months, combination therapy was shown to significantly increase response rates compared to chemotherapy alone (estimated treatment difference: 26%, 95% CI: 9–42, p = .016); PFS was also improved with combination therapy (HR: 0.53, 95% CI: 0.31–0.91, p = .010). However, OS was not shown to differ between treatment groups. Twenty-three patients on combination therapy had treatment-related AEs of at least grade 3, compared to 16 with chemotherapy. One treatment-related death (sepsis) was noted with combination therapy compared to two with chemotherapy.

Urothelial Carcinoma

On May 18, 2017, pembrolizumab was approved for patients with locally advanced/metastatic urothelial carcinoma as both first-line therapy for cisplatin-ineligible patients (accelerated approval) and as a salvage treatment following progression after platinum-based chemotherapy (regular approval) (7). The first approval was based on the KEYNOTE-052 phase II trial that examined the efficacy and toxicity of pembrolizumab in 370 cisplatin-ineligible patients who had not undergone systemic chemotherapy for advanced disease (22,23). With a median follow-up of 9.5 months, the primary endpoint of ORR was 29% (7% complete response rate). Median time to response was 2 months and median duration of response was not reached. Notably, 82% of responses lasted at least 6 months and 67% of responses were ongoing at data cut-off. Overall, pembrolizumab was well tolerated with 18% of patients experiencing grade 3/4 treatment-related AEs; a treatment-related death in the setting of concurrent myositis, thyroiditis, hepatitis, pneumonia, and myocarditis was noted. Efficacy and safety appeared the same even in the subset of patients with poor performance status and older age (≥ 75 years old), rendering pembrolizumab an attractive option not only in cisplatin-unfit but generally in chemotherapy-unfit patients (24).

Support for the superiority of pembrolizumab as salvage therapy in locally advanced/metastatic urothelial carcinoma was provided by the KEYNOTE-045 phase III trial (25). This trial compared pembrolizumab (200 mg every 3 weeks) versus chemotherapy selected by the investigator (paclitaxel, docetaxel, or vinflunine), with respect to OS and PFS. A total of 542 patients were randomly assigned to pembrolizumab ($n = 270$) and chemotherapy ($n = 272$), respectively. Median follow-up was 14.1 months. While PFS was not significantly different between study arms, patients on pembrolizumab had significantly lower risk of death (HR: 0.73, 95% CI: 0.59–0.91, $p = .002$), as well as improved median and 1-year OS rates (10.3 versus 7.4 months and 43.9% versus 30.7%, respectively). These effects were consistent across all subsets. Treatment-related AEs were less frequent with pembrolizumab versus chemotherapy (60.9% versus 90.2%, and 15.0% versus 49.4%, for all-grade and grade 3–5 AEs, respectively) as was toxicity-related treatment discontinuation (5.6% versus 11.0%). Four treatment-related deaths were reported in each arm.

Squamous Cell Carcinoma of the Head and Neck

Results from the KEYNOTE-012 open label, phase 1b study led to the approval of pembrolizumab for recurrent/metastatic squamous cell carcinoma of the head and neck following progression during/after platinum-based chemotherapy on August 5, 2016 (7,26). Sixty patients with PD-L1 expression of at least 1% were treated with pembrolizumab 10 mg/kg every 2 weeks. Median follow-up was 14 months. ORR was 18% (95% CI: 8–32); median PFS was 2 months and median OS was 13 months. Interestingly, PD-L1 expression was associated with ORR and PFS. Ten patients experienced grade 3/4 treatment-related AEs and no treatment-related deaths were noted.

Gastric Carcinoma

Pembrolizumab was granted accelerated approval for advanced gastric cancer on September 22, 2017, on the basis of the results of the KEYNOTE-059 trial (7,27). This phase II study assessed the efficacy and toxicity of pembrolizumab (200 mg every 3 weeks) in 259 patients with metastatic/recurrent locally advanced gastric cancer that progressed following at least two prior systemic therapies. ORR was 11.2% (95% CI: 7.6–15.7) in the overall cohort. Treatment-related ≥ grade 3 AEs were reported in 43 patients; two treatment-related deaths were noted.

Hodgkin Lymphoma

The KEYNOTE-087 phase II trial examined the efficacy and safety of pembrolizumab (200 mg every 3 weeks) in three separate cohorts with relapsed/refractory classic Hodgkin lymphoma: (a) patients treated with autologous stem cell transplantation and brentuximab vedotin ($n = 69$), (b) patients treated with salvage chemotherapy and brentuximab vedotin ($n = 81$), and (c) patients treated with autologous stem cell transplantation alone without brentuximab vedotin ($n = 60$) (28). After median follow-up of 10.1 months, the combined ORR was 69% (95% CI: 62.3–75.2) for all cohorts. Specifically, cohort (a) showed 73.9% ORR (95% CI: 61.9–83.7), cohort (b) 64.2% ORR (95% CI: 52.8–74.6), and cohort (c) 70% ORR (95% CI: 56.8–81.2). The most frequent grade 3/4 treatment-related AE was neutropenia (2.4%), followed by dyspnea and diarrhea (1%); nine patients discontinued therapy due to treatment-related toxicity. On that basis, pembrolizumab was approved for use for the aforementioned indications on March 15, 2017 (7).

MSI-high/MMR-d Solid Tumors

On May 23, 2017, pembrolizumab became the first antineoplastic agent to be granted approval for solid tumors with specific genomic aberration (MSI-high and/or MMR-d), irrespective of tumor histology and tissue of origin (7). This was based on results from phase II trials reporting encouraging ORR (up to 71%) for patients with MSI-high/MMR-d unresectable/metastatic tumors that had progressed after therapy (29,30). The ongoing KEYNOTE-164 and KEYNOTE-158 global multicenter trials are expected to provide further evidence on the long-term outcomes of patients treated with pembrolizumab for this indication (7).

Nivolumab

Indications

(*summary of indications available at:*
www.accessdata.fda.gov/drugsatfda_docs/label/2018/125554s048s049s050s051s052s061s062s064s065s066lbl.pdf)

- Stage IIIC/IV melanoma following disease progression after treatment with ipilimumab and/or *BRAF* inhibitor if indicated.
- Treatment-naïve, unresectable/metastatic melanoma in combination with ipilimumab.

- Lymph node positive or metastatic melanoma following complete resection.
- Stage IIIB/IV NSCLC following progression after platinum-based chemotherapy.
- Locally advanced or metastatic urothelial carcinoma following progression after platinum-based chemotherapy.
- Advanced renal cell carcinoma with progression on antiangiogenic therapy.
- Recurrent/metastatic squamous cell carcinoma of the head and neck following progression on platinum-based therapy.
- Sorafenib-refractory hepatocellular carcinoma.
- Recurrent/metastatic MSI-high/MMR-d colorectal carcinoma following progression after standard chemotherapy.
- Relapsed/refractory classic Hodgkin lymphoma following autologous stem cell transplantation and brentuximab vedotin.

Melanoma

Nivolumab first received approval (December 22, 2014) for the treatment of stage IIIC/IV melanoma that progressed after treatment with ipilimumab (and *BRAF* inhibitor if indicated) on the basis of the CheckMate 037 phase III trial (7,31). A total of 272 patients were randomly assigned to nivolumab 3 mg/kg every 2 weeks and 133 to investigator-choice chemotherapy (dacarbazine or paclitaxel/carboplatin). At a median follow-up of 8.4 months, ORR was 31.7% (95% CI: 23.5–40.8) with nivolumab versus 10.6% (95% CI: 3.5–23.1) with chemotherapy. An even more pronounced response to nivolumab was noted in patients with PD-L1 positive tumors (43.6%). Overall, 9% of patients on nivolumab versus 31% on chemotherapy experienced grade 3/4 treatment-related AEs.

Subsequently, the CheckMate 069 phase III trial assessed combination therapy with nivolumab/ipilimumab versus ipilimumab alone as first-line treatment for patients with unresectable/metastatic melanoma (32). A total of 142 patients were randomized to combination therapy and ipilimumab monotherapy in a 2:1 ratio. Among patients without *BRAF* V600 mutation, the odds of achieving an objective response were significantly increased in the combination therapy arm (odds ratio: 12.96, 95% CI: 3.91–54.49, $p < .001$); similarly, a decreased risk of progression was noted (HR: 0.40, 95% CI: 0.23–0.68, $p < .001$). Importantly, response to combination therapy was shown to be independent of PD-L1 status. Similar results in terms of efficacy were also noted for the 33 patients with *BRAF* V600 mutations included. Increased toxicity was noted with combination therapy with a reported rate of grade 3/4 AEs of 54.3% versus 23.9% with ipilimumab alone. Three treatment-related deaths were noted with combination therapy, compared to none with ipilimumab alone. On the basis of these findings, the FDA approved nivolumab/ipilimumab combination therapy as first-line treatment for patients with *BRAF* V600 wild-type unresectable/metastatic melanoma on October 1, 2015 (7).

The results of the CheckMate 067 phase III trial were instrumental in the expansion of the indications of nivolumab/ipilimumab first-line therapy to all patients with unresectable/metastatic melanoma, irrespective of *BRAF* mutation status (January 23, 2016) (7,33). A total of 945 previously untreated patients with unresectable stage III/IV disease were randomized in a 1:1:1 ratio to ipilimumab monotherapy, nivolumab monotherapy, or ipilimumab/nivolumab combination therapy; 31.5% of patients were positive for *BRAF* mutation and stratified randomization according to *BRAF* status (in addition to PD-L1 status and metastasis stage) was employed. Importantly, prolonged PFS was noted with combination therapy versus ipilimumab (HR: 0.42, 95% CI: 0.31–0.57, $p < .001$); nivolumab monotherapy was also associated with prolonged PFS versus ipilimumab monotherapy (HR: 0.57, 95% CI: 0.43–0.76, $p < .001$). A trend suggesting longer PFS with combination therapy versus nivolumab monotherapy (HR: 0.74, 95% CI: 0.60–0.92) was also noted; interestingly, the benefit of combination therapy over nivolumab monotherapy appeared to be pronounced among patients with PD-L1 negative tumors (median PFS 11.2 versus 5.3 months for combination therapy and nivolumab monotherapy, respectively, compared to median PFS of 14 months for both arms in patients with PD-L1 positive tumors). Similar results with respect to efficacy were noted regardless of *BRAF* mutation status. As in CheckMate 069, combination therapy was associated with a higher rate of grade 3/4 AEs (55%) compared to nivolumab (16.3%) and ipilimumab (27.3%) monotherapy; nonetheless, no treatment-related deaths were noted with combination therapy, while one occurred each with nivolumab and ipilimumab monotherapy.

On December 20, 2017, nivolumab was also approved as adjuvant therapy following a complete resection of lymph node positive or metastatic melanoma (34). This approval was based on the results of the CheckMate 238 phase III trial, which randomized 906 patients that had undergone complete resection of stage IIIB, IIIC, or IV melanoma to adjuvant therapy with nivolumab (3 mg/kg every 2 weeks) or ipilimumab (10 mg/kg every 3 weeks) in a 1:1 ratio (35). Significantly improved 1-year PFS was noted with nivolumab following a minimum follow-up of 18 months (HR: 0.65, 97.56% CI: 0.51–0.83, $p < .001$). With respect to toxicity, fewer grade 3/4 treatment-related AEs were noted with nivolumab (14.4% versus 45.9%) and a smaller percentage of patients had to discontinue treatment due to AEs (9.7% versus 42.6%). Two treatment-related deaths were noted with ipilimumab versus none with nivolumab.

NSCLC

The CheckMate 017 phase III trial compared the efficacy and safety of nivolumab (3 mg/kg every 2 weeks) versus docetaxel chemotherapy among 272 patients with stage IIIB/IV squamous NSCLC that progressed on platinum-based chemotherapy (36). Importantly, nivolumab monotherapy was associated with significantly decreased risk of death (HR: 0.59, 95% CI: 0.44–0.79, $p < .001$) and/or progression (HR: 0.62, 95% CI: 0.47–0.81, $p < .001$). These findings were independent of PD-L1 expression. Serious toxicity was also far less common on nivolumab with only 7% of patients developing grade 3/4 AEs versus 55% on docetaxel.

Three treatment-related deaths were reported with chemotherapy and none with nivolumab. On the basis of these findings, the FDA approved nivolumab for this indication on March 4, 2015 (7).

Shortly afterwards, the results of the CheckMate 057 phase III trial were instrumental in the expansion of the aforementioned indication to patients with non-squamous NSCLC (October 9, 2015) (7,37). Specifically, 292 patients with stage IIIB/IV non-squamous NSCLC that progressed on platinum-based chemotherapy were randomly allocated to nivolumab 3 mg/kg every 2 weeks and 290 to docetaxel. It was demonstrated that nivolumab therapy led to significantly higher ORR (19% versus 12%, $p = .02$) and decreased risk of death (HR: 0.73, 95% CI: 0.59–0.89, $p = .002$) compared to docetaxel. While a similar trend was noted for PFS, it did not reach statistical significance ($p = .39$). Grade 3–5 AEs were noted in only 10% of patients treated with nivolumab versus 54% with docetaxel.

Urothelial Carcinoma

The CheckMate 275 phase II trial assessed the safety and efficacy of nivolumab in patients with locally advanced or metastatic urothelial carcinoma who progressed after platinum-based chemotherapy (38). A total of 270 patients were treated with nivolumab 3 mg/kg every 2 weeks. ORR was 19.6% (95% CI: 15.0–24.9) in the overall cohort, ranging from 16.1% (95% CI: 10.5–21.3) for patients with PD-L1 expression less than 1% to 28.4% (95% CI: 18.9–39.5) for those with PD-L1 expression of at least 5%. A total of 48 patients experienced grade 3/4 treatment-related AEs with three treatment-related deaths noted. On that basis, FDA provided accelerated approval to nivolumab for this indication on February 2, 2017 (7).

Renal Cell Carcinoma

The efficacy and safety of nivolumab in advanced renal cell carcinoma compared to treatment with everolimus was assessed in the CheckMate 025 phase III trial (39). A total of 821 patients with advanced renal cell carcinoma with clear-cell component that had formerly experienced progression on antiangiogenic therapy were randomized to nivolumab (3 mg/ kg every 2 weeks) or once-daily everolimus in a 1:1 ratio. Importantly, nivolumab was associated with both higher response rates (odds ratio: 5.98, 95% CI: 3.68–9.72, $p < .001$) and significantly reduced risk of death (HR: 0.73, 98.5% CI: 0.57–0.93, $p = .0018$) versus everolimus. Patients treated with nivolumab experienced fewer treatment-related grade 3/4 AEs (19% versus 37%, respectively) and had to discontinue treatment due to toxicity less frequently (8% versus 13%); no treatment-related deaths were noted with nivolumab and two were noted with everolimus. Consequently, the FDA approved nivolumab for this indication on November 23, 2015 (7).

More recently, nivolumab/ipilimumab combination was compared with sunitinib monotherapy in patients with treatment-naïve, advanced renal cell carcinoma in the context of the Checkmate 214 phase III trial (40). Specifically, 1,096 patients were randomized to receive nivolumab/ ipilimumab or sunitinib in a 1:1 ratio; ultimately, 547 patients underwent treatment in the nivolumab/ipilimumab arm and 535 in the sunitinib arm. Of note, significantly improved ORR (42% versus 27%, $p < .001$) and OS (HR: 0.63, 99.8% CI: 0.44–0.89, $p < .001$) were noted with the combination. A trend toward improved PFS was also observed in patients treated with nivolumab/ipilimumab, but failed to reach the predetermined level of statistical significance (HR: 0.82, 99.1% CI: 0.64–1.05, $p = .03$). Grade 3–4 treatment-related AEs were noted in 46% of patients treated with combination versus 63% of those treated with sunitinib; 22% of patients treated with nivolumab/ipilimumab had to discontinue treatment due to toxicity versus 12% of those receiving sunitinib. Eight treatment-related deaths were reported with combination versus four with sunitinib. FDA is assessing (March 2018) whether to approve nivolumab/ipilimumab as first-line treatment for advanced renal cell carcinoma; atezolizumab/bevacizumab combination is also being considered for the same indication as it was reportedly associated with longer PFS versus sunitinib monotherapy in the IMmotion 151 phase III trial (41).

Squamous Cell Carcinoma of the Head and Neck

Nivolumab was assessed for use in patients with recurrent/metastatic squamous cell carcinoma of the head and neck that had progressed after platinum-based therapy in the context of the CheckMate 141 phase III trial (11). A total of 361 patients were randomized in a 2:1 ratio to treatment with nivolumab (3 mg/kg every 2 weeks) or single agent chemotherapy/ systemic therapy (specifically methotrexate, docetaxel, or cetuximab). At a median follow-up of 5.1 months, a significantly decreased risk of death was noted with nivolumab (HR: 0.70, 97.73% CI: 0.51–0.96, $p = .01$); however, PFS was not shown to differ significantly across arms ($p = .32$). Grade 3/4 AEs were less frequent with nivolumab (13.1% versus 35.1%); treatment-related deaths were reported in two patients on nivolumab and one patient on standard therapy. As a result, nivolumab received FDA approval as the first immunotherapy for squamous cell carcinoma of the head and neck on November 10, 2016 (7).

Hepatocellular Carcinoma

The CheckMate 040 phase I/II trial assessed the safety and efficacy of nivolumab among patients with advanced hepatocellular carcinoma refractory to sorafenib (42). A total of 48 patients (dose-escalation phase) were treated with 0.1–10 mg/kg every 2 weeks and 214 received 3 mg/ kg every 2 weeks (dose-expansion phase). ORR was 15% (95% CI: 6–28) in the dose-escalation phase and 20% (95% CI: 15–26) in the dose–expansion phase. Grade 3/4 AEs occurred in 12 patients in the dose-escalation phase. On the basis of these findings, nivolumab received approval for the aforementioned indication on September 22, 2017 (7).

Colorectal Carcinoma

Nivolumab was approved for use in recurrent/metastatic MSI-high and/or MMR-d colorectal carcinoma that progressed after fluoropyrimidine, oxaliplatin, or irinotecan-based chemotherapy on August 1, 2017 (7). This was based on the CheckMate 142 phase II trial, which assigned 74 patients to nivolumab 3 mg/kg every 2 weeks (43). At a median follow-up of 12 months, ORR was 31.1% (95% CI: 20.8–42.9). Fifteen patients experienced grade 3/4 treatment-related AEs; no treatment-related deaths were reported.

Hodgkin Lymphoma

The efficacy and safety of nivolumab for relapsed/refractory classic Hodgkin lymphoma was first assessed in the CheckMate 039 phase I trial; ORR was 87% (95% CI: 66–97) in 23 treated patients and treatment-related AEs of at least grade 3 were noted in five patients (44). Subsequently, the CheckMate 205 phase II trial sought to evaluate the efficacy of nivolumab 3 mg/kg every 2 weeks in patients with relapsed/refractory classic Hodgkin lymphoma following autologous stem cell transplantation and brentux-imab vedotin (45). A total of 80 patients underwent treatment and mean follow-up was 8.9 months. ORR was 66.3% (95% CI: 54.8–76.4); 6-month PFS and OS rates were 76.9% (95% CI: 64.9–85.3) and 98.7% (95% CI: 91.0–99.8). A total of 32 patients experienced at least grade 3 treatment-related AEs. The FDA approved nivolumab for this indication on May 17, 2016 (7).

PD-L1 INHIBITORS

Avelumab

Indications

(*summary of indications available at:*
www.accessdata.fda.gov/drugsatfda_docs/label/2017/761049s00 2lbl.pdf)

- Metastatic Merkel cell carcinoma.
- Locally advanced or metastatic urothelial carcinoma with progression after platinum-based chemotherapy.

Merkel Cell Carcinoma

Avelumab received approval for metastatic Merkel cell carcinoma on March 23, 2017, following the results of JAVELIN Merkel 200, an open-label, single-arm, multi-institutional phase II trial (7,9). In this study, 88 patients with chemotherapy-refractory, stage IV Merkel cell carcinoma were treated with avelumab at 10 mg/kg every 2 weeks. At a median follow-up of 10.4 months, ORR was 31.8% (95.9% CI: 21.9–43.1); 92% (95% CI: 70–98) of responses lasted for at least 6 months. Median PFS was 2.7 months (95% CI: 1.4–6.9) and 40% (29–50) of patients were found to be progression-free at 6 months. Similarly, median OS was 11.3 months (7.5–14.0) and 69% (95% CI: 58–78) of patients were still alive at 6 months. Sixty-two patients (70%) developed AEs due to treatment; fatigue (24%) and infusion-related reactions (17%) were the most common. A total of five grade 3 AEs were reported in four patients (lymphopenia and isolated laboratory abnormalities); only a single grade 3 event was thought to be immune-related (elevated aminotransferases). No grade 4 AEs or treatment-related deaths were noted.

Urothelial Carcinoma

Avelumab received accelerated approval in patients with locally advanced or metastatic urothelial cancer refractory to platinum-based chemotherapy based on the JAVELIN Solid Tumor trial on May 9, 2017 (7,46,47). Early results from the study were reported for a multicenter, single-arm dose-expansion cohort of 44 patients treated with avelumab 10 mg/kg every 2 weeks (46). At a median follow-up of 16.5 months, ORR was 18.2% (95% CI: 8.2–32.7). Median PFS was 11.6 weeks (95% CI: 6.1–17.4) while 19.1% (95% CI: 8.5–32.8) of patients were progression-free at 48 weeks. Median OS was 13.7 months (95% CI: 8.5–not estimable) and 54.3% (95% CI: 37.9–68.1) of patients were alive at 12 months. While 29 out of 44 patients (65.9%) experienced treatment-related AEs, grade 3/4 AEs were noted in only three patients. Nine patients (20.5%) had treatment-related AEs that were potentially immune-mediated, with the most common being hypothyroidism (three patients); no treatment-related deaths were noted.

Updated results from the trial were published in January 2018 (47). In an expanded population of 249 patients with median follow-up of 9.9 months, median PFS was 6.6 weeks (95% CI: 6.1–11.4) and 24% (18–31) of patients were progression-free at 24 weeks. ORR was 17% (95% CI: 11–24) in 161 patients with at least 6 months of follow-up. Median OS was 6.5 months (95% CI: 4.8–9.5) and the 6-month OS rate was 53% (95% CI: 45–60). One hundred and sixty-six patients (67%) experienced treatment-related AEs. However, grade 3 or worse AEs were much rarer (8%); one patient died due to treatment-related pneumonitis.

Durvalumab

Indications

(*summary of indications available at:*
www.accessdata.fda.gov/drugsatfda_docs/label/2018/761069s
002lbl.pdf)

- Unresectable stage III NSCLC following lack of progression after chemoradiotherapy.
- Locally advanced or metastatic urothelial carcinoma with progression after platinum-based chemotherapy.

NSCLC

On February 16 2018, the FDA approved durvalumab for stage III unresectable NSCLC (7). This was based on the PACIFIC Study, a randomized phase III trial that compared consolidation therapy with durvalumab (10 mg/kg every 2 weeks) versus placebo in patients who did not progress after two or more cycles of platinum-based chemoradiotherapy (10). A total of 473 patients were treated with durvalumab and 236 with placebo; median follow-up was 14.5 months. The durvalumab arm had longer median PFS (16.8 versus 5.6 months), superior ORR (28.4% versus 16.0%) and significantly reduced risk of progression or death (HR: 0.52, 95% CI: 0.42–0.65, all $p < .001$) versus placebo. Importantly, results were shown to be unaffected by patient demographic characteristics, stage, histology, previous treatment response, and PD-L1 expression. Median time to death or distant metastasis was also reduced with durvalumab (HR: 0.52, 95% CI: 0.39–0.69, p < .001). The overall frequency of AEs and grade 3/4 AEs (96.8% versus 94.9% and 29.9% versus 26.1% with durvalumab and placebo, respectively) were similar in the two arms.

Urothelial Carcinoma

FDA-accelerated approval for durvalumab in patients with platinum-refractory locally advanced/metastatic urothelial carcinoma was granted on May 1, 2017, on the basis of a phase I/II open label, dose-escalation trial (Study 1108) (7,48,49). Early results from a cohort of 61 patients treated with durvalumab 10 mg/kg every 2 weeks (median follow-up of 4.3 months) demonstrated an acceptable safety profile (three patients developed grade 3 AEs; no grade 4/5 AEs noted) and considerable efficacy, as noted by an ORR of 31% (95% CI: 17.6–47.1) among 42 evaluable patients (48). Interestingly, responses occurred only in patients with PD-L1 positive tumors.

More recent results from an expanded cohort of 191 patients treated in the context of Study 1108 (median follow-up of 5.8 months) continue to support the efficacy and safety of durvalumab in metastatic urothelial carcinoma (49). Specifically, ORR was 17.8% (95% CI: 12.7–24.0) in the overall cohort; median PFS was 1.5 months (95% CI: 1.4–1.9) and 16% (95% CI: 10–23) of patients were progression-free at 12 months. Median OS in the overall cohort was 18.2 months (95% CI: 8.1–not estimable) and 55% (95% CI: 44–65) of patients were alive at 12 months. Importantly, responses were noted in patients with PD-L1 negative tumors. Grade 3/4 treatment-related AEs were relatively rare, occurring in 6.8% of patients. Grade 3/4 immune-mediated AEs were even rarer, affecting only four patients; however, two patients died as a result of severe autoimmune hepatitis and pneumonitis, respectively.

Atezolizumab

Indications

(*summary of indications available at:*
www.accessdata.fda.gov/drugsatfda_docs/label/2018/761034s 005lbl.pdf)

- Metastatic NSCLC with progression during or after platinum-based chemotherapy.
- Locally advanced or metastatic urothelial carcinoma with progression after platinum-based chemotherapy.
- Locally advanced or metastatic urothelial carcinoma for patients who have not received chemotherapy for advanced disease but are ineligible for cisplatin.

NSCLC

The efficacy and safety of atezolizumab versus docetaxel in patients with metastatic NSCLC that progressed during or after platinum-based chemotherapy was assessed in the POPLAR and OAK trials, leading to the approval of atezolizumab for this indication on October 18, 2016 (7,8,50). Specifically, in the context of the POPLAR phase II trial, 144 patients were randomized to atezolizumab (1,200 mg fixed dose every 3 weeks) and 143 to docetaxel (50). Median follow-up was 14.8 months. While PFS was not different between arms (2.7 versus 3.0 months for atezolizumab and docetaxel, respectively; HR: 0.94, 95% CI: 0.72–1.23), atezolizumab was associated with significant OS benefit (12.6 versus 9.7 months for atezolizumab and docetaxel, respectively; HR: 0.73, 95% CI: 0.53–0.99, $p = .04$). Interestingly, increased PD-L1 expression was associated with greater survival benefit with atezolizumab; however, patients with less than 1% PD-L1 expression derived no significant survival benefit from atezolizumab. Grade 3/4 treatment-related AEs were less common with atezolizumab (11%) versus docetaxel (39%); one patient died due to treatment-related AE on atezolizumab versus three on docetaxel.

The findings of POPLAR were largely confirmed by OAK, a phase III trial that compared atezolizumab (1,200 mg fixed dose every 3 weeks) versus docetaxel for patients with stage IIIB/IV NSCLC with progression after platinum-based chemotherapy (8). Each treatment group consisted of 425 patients and median follow-up was 21 months. Treatment with atezolizumab was associated with longer median OS compared to docetaxel (13.8 versus 9.6 months for atezolizumab and docetaxel, respectively; HR: 0.73, 95% CI: 0.62–0.87, $p = .0003$), while PFS was similar across arms (HR: 0.95, 95% CI: 0.82–1.10). Similar to the POPLAR trial, PD-L1 expression was associated with OS benefit with atezolizumab; however, even patients with minimal (<1%) PD-L1 expression were shown to derive survival benefit from atezolizumab treatment (HR: 0.75, 95% CI: 0.59–0.96), in contrast with POPLAR. Grade 3/4 treatment-related AEs were less common with atezolizumab versus docetaxel (15% versus 43%, respectively), as was treatment discontinuation due to AEs (8% versus 19%). A treatment-related death was recorded with docetaxel as a result of respiratory tract infection.

Urothelial Carcinoma

On May 18, 2016, atezolizumab became the first PD-L1 inhibitor to be granted accelerated approval for locally advanced or metastatic urothelial cancer following progression after platinum-based therapy (7). This was based on the cohort 2 of the IMvigor 210 phase II trial, which assessed the efficacy and toxicity of atezolizumab (1,200 mg fixed dose every 3 weeks) in 310 patients, with median follow-up of 11.7 months (51). ORR was 15% (95% CI: 11–19) in the overall cohort, which was superior to the historical response rate of 10% with salvage therapy. Median PFS was 2.1 months and median OS 7.9 months. Of note, higher expression of PD-L1 appeared to correlate with improved ORR and OS; on the contrary, PFS was shown to be independent of PD-L1 expression. Overall, 16% of patients experienced grade 3/4 treatment-related AEs, which were immune-mediated in approximately one-third of cases (5% of patients). However, the confirmatory IMvigor 211 phase III trial comparing atezolizumab to salvage chemotherapy did not detect significant OS advantage in the patient subset with higher PD-L1 expression (IC/2/3), which was the primary endpoint. Atezolizumab did show OS benefit versus chemotherapy in the entire study cohort, but this was an exploratory analysis endpoint. The safety profile for atezolizumab was favorable compared to chemotherapy, while rapid and durable responses were noted consistent with IMvigor 210 trial (52).

On April 17, 2017, the FDA expanded the approved indications of atezolizumab in urothelial cancer to include first-line treatment of locally advanced/metastatic disease among cisplatin-ineligible patients (accelerated approval), based on results from the cohort 1 of the IMvigor 210 trial (7,53). Specifically, 119 cisplatin-ineligible patients were treated with atezolizumab. Following median follow-up of 17.2 months, ORR was 23% (95% CI: 16–31); response rate appeared to correlate with PD-L1 expression. Medial OS was 15.9 months (95% CI: 10.4–not estimable) for the entire cohort. Nineteen patients experienced grade 3/4 treatment-related AEs; in eight patients these AEs were thought to be immune-mediated. A single treatment-related death due to sepsis of unidentified origin was reported.

CONCLUSION

Indications for treatment with PD-1/PD-L1 inhibitors have proliferated rapidly in the relatively short period after the first FDA approval was issued in September 2014 (7). This trend is likely to continue, as anti-PD-1/PD-L1 therapy appears to combine robust efficacy across many different tumor types with a favorable safety profile in comparison with conventional cytotoxic chemotherapy. Nonetheless, a number of important issues remain to be addressed and should be taken into consideration by researchers and clinicians alike.

First of all, as discussed earlier, responses to anti-PD-1/PD-L1 therapy appear to vary significantly. While PD-L1 expression is usually associated with response, techniques/assays for measuring PD-L1 are characterized by significant inter-assay variability and would likely benefit from greater standardization (54). Moreover, PD-L1 expression is an imperfect biomarker and not routinely used in clinical practice with a few exceptions, as discussed in the preceding sections. Additional biomarkers that may aid treatment selection and/or facilitate prognostic assessments (ranging from total mutational burden, DNA repair gene mutations, gene expression profiling, biomarkers of tumor microenvironment, gut microbiome composition, cell-free circulating tumor DNA, etc.) are currently being explored and, upon further validation, may enable clinicians to personalize management in the future (55). Conversely, the identification of biomarkers that predict resistance to treatment remains critical. Moreover, as anti-PD-1/PD-L1 therapy is employed more commonly, the management of treatment toxicity (especially of immune-mediated AEs) is increasingly important, even for non-oncologists. While a number of clinical guidelines were recently published by numerous organizations and authorities providing a solid framework for managing immune-related toxicity, there is still a major need for additional supporting data. In this context, the cumulative experience of multidisciplinary tumor boards, information from multisite registries/databases, and clinical trials focusing on the management of immune-mediated toxicities are also warranted for even more individualized and evidence-based management of AEs (56,57). Furthermore, the applicability of the Response Evaluation Criteria in Solid Tumors (RECIST) 1.1 to patients treated with immunotherapy has been challenged; it remains to be determined whether the newly formulated Immune-related Response Evaluation Criteria in Solid Tumors (iRECIST) will prove to be a superior alternative with universal acceptance even in community oncology practices (58). In addition, the optimal treatment duration for the various anti-PD-1/PD-L1 agents and the presence/extent of cross-resistance between them have not been determined; for example, it is currently unknown whether progression during treatment with one checkpoint inhibitor can be managed by switching to another checkpoint inhibitor of either the same or different class (59). Moreover, a plethora of combination therapies are being tested in various clinical trials. Lastly, given the fact that a large number of current anti-PD-1/PD-L1 therapy indications were the result of accelerated FDA approval and may not be supported by conclusive data from a phase III trial at present, clinicians should use clinical judgment in selecting therapies with the highest level of supporting evidence whenever possible.

In conclusion, immune checkpoint inhibitors have indeed transformed the landscape of cancer management, while novel combinations and biomarker validation may provide further improvements. However, appropriate education on the use and limitations of immunotherapy, as well as early recognition and optimal management of immune-related AEs, are necessary preconditions for promoting effective clinical practice and guiding future research.

REFERENCES

1. Agata Y, Kawasaki A, Nishimura H, et al. Expression of the PD-1 antigen on the surface of stimulated mouse T and B lymphocytes. *Int Immunol.* 1996;8(5):765–772. doi:10.1093/intimm/8.5.765

2. Ishida Y, Agata Y, Shibahara K, et al. Induced expression of PD-1, a novel member of the immunoglobulin gene superfamily, upon programmed cell death. *EMBO J.* 1992;11(11):3887–3895. doi:10.1002/j.1460-2075.1992.tb05481.x

3. Dong H, Zhu G, Tamada K, et al. B7-H1, a third member of the B7 family, co-stimulates T-cell proliferation and interleukin-10 secretion. *Nat Med.* 1999;5(12):1365–1369. doi:10.1038/70932

4. Dong H, Strome SE, Salomao DR, et al. Tumor-associated B7-H1 promotes T-cell apoptosis: a potential mechanism of immune evasion. *Nat Med.* 2002;8(8):793–800. doi:10.1038/nm730

5. He J, Hu Y, Hu M, et al. Development of PD-1/PD-L1 pathway in tumor immune microenvironment and treatment for non-small cell lung cancer. *Sci Rep.* 2015;5:13110. doi:10.1038/srep13110

6. Iwai Y, Ishida M, Tanaka Y, et al. Involvement of PD-L1 on tumor cells in the escape from host immune system and tumor immunotherapy by PD-L1 blockade. *Proc Natl Acad Sci USA.* 2002;99(19):12293–12297. doi:10.1073/pnas.192461099

7. Gong J, Chehrazi-Raffle A, Reddi S, et al. Development of PD-1 and PD-L1 inhibitors as a form of cancer immunotherapy: a comprehensive review of registration trials and future considerations. *J Immunother Cancer*. 2018;6(1):8. doi:10.1186/s40425-018-0316-z

8. Rittmeyer A, Barlesi F, Waterkamp D, et al. Atezolizumab versus docetaxel in patients with previously treated non-small-cell lung cancer (OAK): a phase 3, open-label, multicentre randomised controlled trial. *Lancet*. 2017;389(10066):255–265. doi:10.1016/s0140-6736(16)32517-x

9. Kaufman HL, Russell J, Hamid O, et al. Avelumab in patients with chemotherapy-refractory metastatic Merkel cell carcinoma: a multicentre, single-group, open-label, phase 2 trial. *Lancet Oncol*. 2016;17(10):1374–1385. doi:10.1016/s1470-2045(16)30364-3

10. Antonia SJ, Villegas A, Daniel D, et al. Durvalumab after chemoradiotherapy in stage III non-small-cell lung cancer. *N Engl J Med*. 2017;377(20):1919–1929. doi:10.1056/nejmoa1709937

11. Ferris RL, Blumenschein G Jr, Fayette J, et al. Nivolumab for recurrent squamous-cell carcinoma of the head and neck. *N Engl J Med*. 2016;375(19):1856–1867. doi:10.1056/nejmoa1602252

12. Robert C, Ribas A, Wolchok JD, et al. Anti-programmed-death-receptor-1 treatment with pembrolizumab in ipilimumab-refractory advanced melanoma: a randomised dose-comparison cohort of a phase 1 trial. *Lancet*. 2014;384(9948):1109–1117. doi:10.1016/s0140-6736(14)60958-2

13. Hamid O, Robert C, Daud A, et al. Safety and tumor responses with lambrolizumab (anti-PD-1) in melanoma. *N Engl J Med*. 2013;369(2):134–144. doi:10.1056/nejmoa1305133

14. Ribas A, Puzanov I, Dummer R, et al. Pembrolizumab versus investigator-choice chemotherapy for ipilimumab-refractory melanoma (KEYNOTE-002): a randomised, controlled, phase 2 trial. *Lancet Oncol*. 2015;16(8):908–918. doi:10.1016/s1470-2045(15)00083-2

15. Robert C, Schachter J, Long GV, et al. Pembrolizumab versus ipilimumab in advanced melanoma. *N Engl J Med*. 2015;372(26):2521–2532. doi:10.1056/nejmoa1503093

16. Garon EB, Rizvi NA, Hui R, et al. Pembrolizumab for the treatment of non-small-cell lung cancer. *N Engl J Med*. 2015;372(21):2018–2028. doi:10.1056/nejmoa1501824

17. Sul J, Blumenthal GM, Jiang X, et al. FDA approval summary: pembrolizumab for the treatment of patients with metastatic non-small cell lung cancer whose tumors express programmed death-ligand 1. *Oncologist*. 2016;21(5):643–650. doi:10.1634/theoncologist.2015-0498

18. Ramalingam S, Hui R, Gandhi L, et al. P2.39: Long-term OS for patients with advanced NSCLC enrolled in the KEYNOTE-001 study of pembrolizumab: track: immunotherapy. *J Thorac Oncol*. 2016;11(10S):S241–S242. doi:10.1016/j.jtho.2016.08.110

19. Herbst RS, Baas P, Kim DW, et al. Pembrolizumab versus docetaxel for previously treated, PD-L1-positive, advanced non-small-cell lung cancer (KEYNOTE-010): a randomised controlled trial. *Lancet*. 2016;387(10027):1540–1550. doi:10.1016/s0140-6736(15)01281-7

20. Reck M, Rodriguez-Abreu D, Robinson AG, et al. Pembrolizumab versus chemotherapy for PD-L1-positive non-small-cell lung cancer. *N Engl J Med*. 2016;375(19):1823–1833. doi:10.1056/nejmoa1606774

21. Langer CJ, Gadgeel SM, Borghaei H, et al. Carboplatin and pemetrexed with or without pembrolizumab for advanced, non-squamous non-small-cell lung cancer: a randomised, phase 2 cohort of the open-label KEYNOTE-021 study. *Lancet Oncol*. 2016;17(11):1497–1508. doi:10.1016/s1470-2045(16)30498-3

22. Balar AV, Castellano D, O'Donnell PH, et al. First-line pembrolizumab in cisplatin-ineligible patients with locally advanced and unresectable or metastatic urothelial cancer (KEYNOTE-052): a multicentre, single-arm, phase 2 study. *Lancet Oncol*. 2017;18(11):1483–1492. doi:10.1016/s1470-2045(17)30616-2

23. O'Donnell PH, Grivas P, Balar AV, et al. Biomarker findings and mature clinical results from KEYNOTE-052: first-line pembrolizumab (pembro) in cisplatin-ineligible advanced urothelial cancer (UC). *J Clin Oncol*. 2017;35(15_suppl):4502–4502. doi:10.1200/jco.2017.35.15_suppl.4502

24. Grivas P, Plimack ER, Balar AV, et al. Pembrolizumab (pembro) as first-line therapy in cisplatin-ineligible advanced urothelial cancer (UC): outcomes from KEYNOTE-052 in senior patients (pts) with poor performance status. *Ann Oncol*. 2017;28(suppl_5):301. doi:10.1093/annonc/mdx371.011

25. Bellmunt J, de Wit R, Vaughn DJ, et al. Pembrolizumab as second-line therapy for advanced urothelial carcinoma. *N Engl J Med*. 2017;376(11):1015–1026. doi:10.1056/nejmoa1613683

26. Seiwert TY, Burtness B, Mehra R, et al. Safety and clinical activity of pembrolizumab for treatment of recurrent or metastatic squamous cell carcinoma of the head and neck (KEYNOTE-012): an open-label, multicentre, phase 1b trial. *Lancet Oncol*. 2016;17(7):956–965. doi:10.1016/s1470-2045(16)30066-3

27. Fuchs CS, Doi T, Jang RW-J, et al. KEYNOTE-059 cohort 1: efficacy and safety of pembrolizumab (pembro) monotherapy in patients with previously treated advanced gastric cancer. *J Clin Oncol*. 2017;35(15_suppl):4003–4003. doi:10.1200/jco.2017.35.15_suppl.4003

28. Chen R, Zinzani PL, Fanale MA, et al. Phase II study of the efficacy and safety of pembrolizumab for relapsed/refractory classic Hodgkin lymphoma. *J Clin Oncol*. 2017;35(19):2125–2132. doi:10.1200/jco.2016.72.1316

29. Le DT, Uram JN, Wang H, et al. PD-1 blockade in tumors with mismatch-repair deficiency. *N Engl J Med*. 2015;372(26):2509–2520. doi:10.1056/NEJMoa1500596

30. Le DT, Durham JN, Smith KN, et al. Mismatch repair deficiency predicts response of solid tumors to PD-1 blockade. *Science*. 2017;357(6349):409–413. doi:10.1126/science.aan6733

31. Weber JS, D'Angelo SP, Minor D, et al. Nivolumab versus chemotherapy in patients with advanced melanoma who progressed after anti-CTLA-4 treatment (CheckMate 037): a randomised, controlled, open-label, phase 3 trial. *Lancet Oncol*. 2015;16(4):375–384. doi:10.1016/s1470-2045(15)70076-8

32. Postow MA, Chesney J, Pavlick AC, et al. Nivolumab and ipilimumab versus ipilimumab in untreated melanoma. *N Engl J Med*. 2015;372(21):2006–2017. doi:10.1056/nejmoa1414428

33. Larkin J, Chiarion-Sileni V, Gonzalez R, et al. Combined nivolumab and ipilimumab or monotherapy in untreated melanoma. *N Engl J Med*. 2015;373(1):23–34. doi:10.1056/nejmoa1504030

34. U.S. Food & Drug Administration. FDA grants regular approval to nivolumab for adjuvant treatment of melanoma. https://www.fda.gov/Drugs/InformationOnDrugs/ApprovedDrugs/ucm590004.htm

35. Weber J, Mandala M, Del Vecchio M, et al. Adjuvant nivolumab versus ipilimumab in resected stage III or IV melanoma. *N Engl J Med*. 2017;377(19):1824–1835. doi:10.1056/nejmoa1709030

36. Brahmer J, Reckamp KL, Baas P, et al. Nivolumab versus docetaxel in advanced squamous-cell non-small-cell lung cancer. *N Engl J Med*. 2015;373(2):123–135. doi:10.1056/nejmoa1504627

37. Borghaei H, Paz-Ares L, Horn L, et al. Nivolumab versus docetaxel in advanced non-squamous non-small-cell lung cancer. *N Engl J Med*. 2015;373(17):1627–1639. doi:10.1056/nejmoa1507643

38. Sharma P, Retz M, Siefker-Radtke A, et al. Nivolumab in metastatic urothelial carcinoma after platinum therapy (CheckMate 275): a multicentre, single-arm, phase 2 trial. *Lancet Oncol*. 2017;18(3):312–322. doi:10.1016/s1470-2045(17)30065-7

39. Motzer RJ, Escudier B, McDermott DF, et al. Nivolumab versus everolimus in advanced renal-cell carcinoma. *N Engl J Med*. 2015;373(19):1803–1813. doi:10.1056/nejmoa1510665

40. Motzer RJ, Tannir NM, McDermott DF, et al. Nivolumab plus ipilimumab versus sunitinib in advanced renal-cell carcinoma. *N Engl J Med*. 2018;378(14):1277–1290. doi:10.1056/NEJMoa1712126

41. Motzer RJ, Powles T, Atkins MB, et al. IMmotion151: a randomized phase III study of atezolizumab plus bevacizumab vs sunitinib in untreated metastatic renal cell carcinoma (mRCC). *J Clin Oncol*. 2018;36(6_suppl):578–578. doi:10.1200/jco.2018.36.6_suppl.578

42. El-Khoueiry AB, Sangro B, Yau T, et al. Nivolumab in patients with advanced hepatocellular carcinoma (CheckMate 040): an open-label, non-comparative, phase 1/2 dose escalation and expansion trial. *Lancet*. 2017;389(10088):2492–2502. doi:10.1016/s0140-6736(17)31046-2

43. Overman MJ, McDermott R, Leach JL, et al. Nivolumab in patients with metastatic DNA mismatch repair-deficient or microsatellite instability-high colorectal cancer (CheckMate 142): an open-label, multicentre, phase 2 study. *Lancet Oncol*. 2017;18(9):1182–1191. doi:10.1016/s1470-2045(17)30422-9

44. Ansell SM, Lesokhin AM, Borrello I, et al. PD-1 blockade with nivolumab in relapsed or refractory Hodgkin's lymphoma. *N Engl J Med.* 2015;372(4):311–319. doi:10.1056/nejmoa1411087

45. Younes A, Santoro A, Shipp M, et al. Nivolumab for classical Hodgkin's lymphoma after failure of both autologous stem-cell transplantation and brentuximab vedotin: a multicentre, multicohort, single-arm phase 2 trial. *Lancet Oncol.* 2016;17(9):1283–1294. doi:10.1016/s1470-2045(16)30167-x

46. Apolo AB, Infante JR, Balmanoukian A, et al. Avelumab, an anti-programmed death-ligand 1 antibody, in patients with refractory metastatic urothelial carcinoma: results from a multicenter, phase Ib study. *J Clin Oncol.* 2017;35(19):2117–2124. doi:10.1200/jco.2016.71.6795

47. Patel MR, Ellerton J, Infante JR, et al. Avelumab in metastatic urothelial carcinoma after platinum failure (JAVELIN Solid Tumor): pooled results from two expansion cohorts of an open-label, phase 1 trial. *Lancet Oncol.* 2018;19(1):51–64. doi:10.1016/s1470-2045(17)30900-2

48. Massard C, Gordon MS, Sharma S, et al. Safety and efficacy of durvalumab (MEDI4736), an anti-programmed cell death ligand-1 immune checkpoint inhibitor, in patients with advanced urothelial bladder cancer. *J Clin Oncol.* 2016;34(26):3119–3125. doi:10.1200/jco.2016.67.9761

49. Powles T, O'Donnell PH, Massard C, et al. Efficacy and safety of durvalumab in locally advanced or metastatic urothelial carcinoma: updated results from a phase 1/2 open-label study. *JAMA Oncol.* 2017;3(9):e172411. doi:10.1001/jamaoncol.2017.2411

50. Fehrenbacher L, Spira A, Ballinger M, et al. Atezolizumab versus docetaxel for patients with previously treated non-small-cell lung cancer (POPLAR): a multicentre, open-label, phase 2 randomised controlled trial. *Lancet.* 2016;387(10030):1837–1846. doi:10.1016/s0140-6736(16)00587-0

51. Rosenberg JE, Hoffman-Censits J, Powles T, et al. Atezolizumab in patients with locally advanced and metastatic urothelial carcinoma who have progressed following treatment with platinum-based chemotherapy: a single-arm, multicentre, phase 2 trial. *Lancet.* 2016;387(10031):1909–1920. doi: 10.1016/S0140-6736(16)00561-4

52. Powles T, Duran I, van der Heijden MS, et al. Atezolizumab versus chemotherapy in patients with platinum-treated locally advanced or metastatic urothelial carcinoma (IMvigor211): a multicentre, open-label, phase 3 randomised controlled trial. *Lancet.* 2018;391(10122):748–757. doi:10.1016/s0140-6736(17)33297-x

53. Balar AV, Galsky MD, Rosenberg JE, et al. Atezolizumab as first-line treatment in cisplatin-ineligible patients with locally advanced and metastatic urothelial carcinoma: a single-arm, multicentre, phase 2 trial. *Lancet.* 2017;389(10064):67–76. doi:10.1016/s0140-6736(16)32455-2

54. Hirsch FR, McElhinny A, Stanforth D, et al. PD-L1 Immunohistochemistry assays for lung cancer: results from phase 1 of the blueprint PD-L1 IHC assay comparison project. *J Thorac Oncol.* 2017;12(2):208–222. doi:10.1016/j.jtho.2016.11.2228

55. Dijkstra KK, Voabil P, Schumacher TN, Voest EE. Genomics- and transcriptomics-based patient selection for cancer treatment with immune checkpoint inhibitors: a review. *JAMA Oncol.* 2016;2(11):1490–1495. doi:10.1001/jamaoncol.2016.2214

56. Puzanov I, Diab A, Abdallah K, et al. Managing toxicities associated with immune checkpoint inhibitors: consensus recommendations from the Society for Immunotherapy of Cancer (SITC) Toxicity Management Working Group. *J Immunother Cancer.* 2017;5(1):95. doi:10.1186/s40425-017-0300-z

57. Brahmer JR, Lacchetti C, Schneider BJ, et al. Management of immune-related adverse events in patients treated with immune checkpoint inhibitor therapy: American Society of Clinical Oncology Clinical Practice Guideline. *J Clin Oncol.* 2018;36(17):1714–1768. doi:10.1200/JCO.2017.77.6385

58. Seymour L, Bogaerts J, Perrone A, et al. iRECIST: guidelines for response criteria for use in trials testing immunotherapeutics. *Lancet Oncol.* 2017;18(3):e143–e152. doi:10.1016/s1470-2045(17)30074-8

59. Martini DJ, Lalani AA, Bosse D, et al. Response to single agent PD-1 inhibitor after progression on previous PD-1/PD-L1 inhibitors: a case series. *J Immunother Cancer.* 2017;5(1):66. doi:10.1186/s40425-017-0273-y

CHAPTER 3

INDICATIONS AND TOXICITIES OF IMMUNE CHECKPOINT INHIBITOR COMBINATIONS

Lavinia Spain, Michael A. Postow, James Larkin, and Jeffrey Weber

INTRODUCTION

The advent of immune checkpoint inhibition as a therapeutic strategy has significantly improved survival in patients with metastatic melanoma and renal, lung, and bladder cancers, among others. This approach releases the constraints placed within the tumor microenvironment on the host's own immune response at the so-called "checkpoints" of the immune system (e.g., cytotoxic T-lymphocyte antigen 4 [CTLA-4] and programmed cell death 1 [PD-1]) and overcomes strategies developed by tumors to evade and avoid immune attack. Concurrent blockade of two checkpoints involved in nonredundant pathways (PD-1 and CTLA-4) has recently demonstrated remarkable clinical efficacy.

To date, the backbone of immune checkpoint inhibitor (ICI) combination treatment has been an anti-CTLA-4 antibody (e.g., ipilimumab or tremelimumab) with an anti-PD-1 (e.g., nivolumab or pembrolizumab) or anti-programmed cell death ligand 1 (PD-L1) (e.g., durvalumab, avelumab, or atezolizumab) antibody. All of these agents have activity as monotherapies, however response rates may favor their use in combination and in the case of ipilimumab combined with nivolumab (ipi+nivo) overall survival (OS) outcomes in melanoma are also improved compared to single agent ipilimumab. The key disadvantage of combination ICI therapy is the higher rate of moderate-to-severe immune-related adverse events (irAEs), including an increased risk of multiple irAEs and more rapid onset. Nonetheless, with early detection and appropriate treatment, the majority of these resolve (1).

In this chapter, we discuss the established indication for combination ipi+nivo in melanoma, recent evidence supporting use of ipi+nivo in renal cancer and touch upon the emerging evidence for ipi+nivo and durvalumab and tremelimumab (durva+treme) in lung cancer and mesothelioma. We also review the rates and timing of onset of various irAEs with combination ICIs, describe particular management issues and discuss the impact of toxicity on disease outcomes and subsequent choice of therapy.

Published by Springer Publishing Company DOI: 10.1891/9780826172150.0003

INDICATIONS IN ADVANCED DISEASE

Melanoma

In untreated unresectable stage III or stage IV melanoma, ipilimumab 3 mg/kg combined with nivolumab 1 mg/kg for four cycles every 3 weeks, followed by nivolumab 3 mg/kg every other week as maintenance, is a first-line treatment option in fit patients (regardless of their *BRAF* mutation status) that is approved by the U.S. Food and Drug Administration (FDA). It is superior to ipilimumab in response rate (58% versus 19%, $p <$ .001) and overall survival (OS; median not reached versus 20 months, HR, 0.55, $p <$ .001) (2–4). While ipi+nivo has demonstrated a better response rate than nivolumab monotherapy (58% versus 44%), and an improved median progression-free survival (PFS) in the subgroup of patients with tumors expressing less than 1% PD-L1 (PD-L1 negative) (11.2 versus 5.3 months), the phase III Checkmate 067 trial was not powered to compare ipi+nivo to nivolumab monotherapy (2,4). At the 3 year mark within this trial, 58% of patients treated with ipi+nivo were alive compared with 52% treated initially with nivolumab and 34% treated initially with ipilimumab monotherapy. The benefit of ipi+nivo over nivolumab alone in PFS and OS appears to be in the subgroup tumor expression of less than 1% PD-L1 (3), however the use of PD-L1 as a reliable biomarker remains indeterminate.

Renal Cancer

Recently, the combination of lower dose ipilimumab (1 mg/kg) with nivolumab (3 mg/kg) for four cycles every 3 weeks, followed by nivolumab 3 mg/kg every other week maintenance, was compared with sunitinib in untreated metastatic clear cell renal cell carcinoma (RCC) (CM-214 (5). Ipi+nivo significantly improved the response rate (42% versus 27%, $p <$ .0001), PFS (11.6 versus 8.4 months, $p =$ .0331) and OS (not reached versus 26 months) in the population of patients with intermediate and poor risk disease. Interestingly, the ipi+nivo combination was inferior to sunitinib in those with good risk disease using the International Metastatic Renal Cell Carcinoma Database Consortium (IMDC) score (response rate 29% versus 52%, PFS 15.3 versus 25.1 months, OS not reported). These results are likely to be practice-changing in the group of patients with poor risk RCC.

Lung Cancer and Mesothelioma

In non-small cell lung cancer (NSCLC), both ipi+nivo and treme+durva have been evaluated in first and subsequent lines of therapy. The phase I trial of ipi+nivo in NSCLC (6) enrolled 78 patients and evaluated the safety of three combination dosing regimens (nivolumab 3 mg/kg with an ipi dose of 1 mg/kg every 6 or 12 weeks and nivolumab 1 mg/kg every 2 weeks with ipi 1 mg/kg every 6 weeks). Objective response rates of 38% and 47% in the two dose regimens were deemed tolerable. The phase III, four-arm Checkmate-227 study (NCT02477826) compares ipi+nivo with nivolumab monotherapy, platinum-based chemotherapy, and chemotherapy combined with nivolumab and is currently recruiting. While the phase Ib study of treme+durva demonstrated promising clinical activity in immunotherapy-naïve patients with NSCLC (7), the interim analysis of the three-arm phase III study of treme+durva versus durvalumab monotherapy versus standard of care cytotoxic chemotherapy in the first-line setting did not show a benefit in PFS with treme+durva over cytotoxic chemotherapy (NCT02453282) (8) and was not powered for a comparison of treme+durva with durvalumab alone. The OS results remain immature. The two-arm NEPTUNE phase III trial (NCT02542293) is also evaluating first-line treme+durva compared to chemotherapy and continues to recruit patients.

The combination of ipi+nivo in small cell lung cancer (SCLC) was also explored in the Phase 1/2 Checkmate 032 trial, enrolling 216 patients who had progressed on prior platinum therapy (9). In this challenging population, an objective response rate of approximately 20% was noted, with some durable responses. In mesothelioma, trials are in progress evaluating treme+durva in the first and second line settings (NCT03075527 and NCT02588131).

TOXICITIES

Combination ipi+nivo and durva+treme are associated with higher rates of irAEs than with monotherapy involving their components. This section will focus on the evidence from studies evaluating ipi+nivo in melanoma, where toxicity data using the Common Terminology Criteria for Adverse Events (CTCAE) criteria are available from large phase II and III studies with long follow-up. It is not possible to draw firm conclusions about the differences in the toxicity profile of durva+treme in comparison to ipi+nivo from the available published literature due to differences in patient populations between trials and differences in the dosing and schedule of agents. There is generally an earlier onset of irAEs with ipi+nivo compared to ICI monotherapy and 30% of patients develop irAEs that affect more than one organ system (1), as opposed to 5% with single agent nivolumab (2,4). Clinicians need to be aware that any organ system may be impacted (see Figure 3.1) and presentations may be atypical. Patient education to enable early recognition of irAEs, along with open pathways of communication with the treating team, is essential to mitigate the impact of toxicity associated with combination regimens.

Rates of irAEs and Their Timing of Onset

In a pooled analysis of 448 patients who received ipi+nivo across phase I, II, and III trials for melanoma (1), 94% of patients reported treatment-related adverse events (AEs) and 55% experienced a grade 3 or 4 AE. The most common AEs overall were diarrhea (44%), fatigue (37%), pruritus (35%), and rash (35%). The most common grade 3/4 AEs were hepatitis (17%), diarrhea (9.8%), colitis (8.7%), and increased lipase (8.5%). Of note, all-grade hypophysitis occurred in 8.5%, pneumonitis in 6.9%, and renal

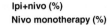

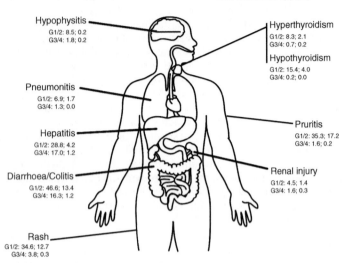

Percentages taken from treatment-related select adverse event rates in References 1, 10, and 11
Figure original to authors

FIGURE 3.1 Differences in the rates of immune-related adverse events across organ systems between combination ipilimumab with nivolumab and nivolumab monotherapy in melanoma.

toxicity in 4.5%. By comparison, in a pooled analysis of nivolumab monotherapy incorporating 576 patients, 49% reported a select immune-related AE and only 4% experienced a grade 3/4 AE (10,11). Fatigue (25%), pruritis (17%), and diarrhea and rash (both 13%) were the most common all-grade AEs and hepatitis (1%), colitis (0.7%), diarrhea (0.5%), and rash (0.3%) were the most common grade 3/4 adverse events. Figure 3.1 describes these differences in more detail.

Different dosing regimens of ipi+nivo appear to impact the rate of irAEs. In the renal Checkmate-214 study (5) using the lower ipilimumab dose (1 mg/kg), the total rate of AEs was 93%, with 46% experiencing AEs at grade 3/4 severity. This regimen was less toxic than sunitinib, an anti-vascular endothelial growth factor (VEGF) tyrosine kinase inhibitor and a current standard of care, where 63% reported grade 3–5 AEs, most commonly hypertension (16%), palmar-plantar erythema (9%), fatigue (9%), and diarrhea (5%). Comparing the two trials, overall rates of all-grade toxicity were similar in the Checkmate-067 study (2,4) in melanoma with 100% of patients reporting an AE, but a larger proportion of patients (69%) experiencing a grade 3/4 event. With the exception of thyroid dysfunction, most irAEs appear more common in the Checkmate-067 trial in melanoma, likely due to the dose of ipilimumab at 3 mg/kg as opposed to 1 mg/kg (see Table 3.1). Results from the phase 1b study of standard-dose pembrolizumab 2 mg/kg in combination with

TABLE 3.1 Rates of Immune-Related Adverse Events Associated With a Combination of Ipilimumab and Nivolumab in Key Melanoma and Renal Cancer Trials

| | Melanoma (CM-067) Ipi 3 mg/kg + Nivo 1 mg/kg | | Renal (CM-214) Ipi 1 mg/kg + Nivo 3 mg/kg | |
	All grade (%)	Grade 3/4 (%)	All grade (%)	Grade 3/4 (%)
Rash	40	5	17	3
Diarrhea/colitis	44/12	9/8	10	5
Hepatitis	30	19	7	6
Renal	NR	NR	5	2
Pneumonitis	6	1	4	2
Infusion reaction	NR	NR	1	0
Hypothyroidism	15	0	19	<1
Hyperthyroidism	10	1	12	<1
Adrenal insufficiency	NR	NR	8	3
Hypophysitis	8	2	5	3
Thyroiditis	NR	NR	3	<1
Diabetes mellitus	NR	NR	3	1

NR, not reported; CM-067, Checkmate 067; CM-214, Checkmate 214.

reduced-dose ipilimumab 1 mg/kg (pembro+ipi) support the notion that most toxicity is associated with the use of ipilimumab (12). In this study, the rate of irAEs was 60%, with grade 3/4 irAEs experienced in only 27% and the ORR of 61% was comparable to that of ipi+nivo in Checkmate-067 (58%). Data are awaited from a direct comparison of ipi 1 mg/kg + nivo 3 mg/kg versus ipi 3 mg/kg + nivo 1 mg/kg in a cohort of patients with advanced melanoma in the Checkmate-515 trial (NCT02714218).

Although the majority of irAEs attributed to ipi+nivo occur within the first 3 to 4 months on treatment, they may also occur later, including after treatment cessation. When categorized by organ system, the earliest onset of AEs involved the skin (cycle 1, median 2 weeks), followed by the gastrointestinal (GI) system (cycle 2, median 5 weeks), and liver (cycle 2–3, median 6 weeks) (1). The timing of onset of grade 3/4 AEs by these categories is summarized in Figure 3.2. It is worth noting that skin, GI, and hepatic toxicities have been shown to occur up to 11 months after the commencement of treatment.

While diarrhea, colitis, hepatitis, skin, and endocrine irAEs have been studied in detail, less recognized irAEs that appear to be more common with combination regimens than single agent treatment include pneumonitis, renal dysfunction, and cardiac toxicity (1,13). Neurological toxicity has been described in association with ipi+nivo (14) and, in a single institution series, occurred more frequently with ipi+nivo than with ICI

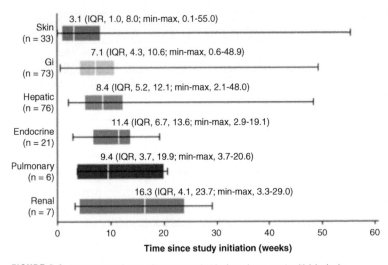

FIGURE 3.2 Time to onset of grade 3/4 treatment related select adverse events with ipi+nivo in melanoma.

Source: From Sznol M, Ferrucci PF, Hogg D, et al. Pooled analysis safety profile of nivolumab and ipilimumab combination therapy in patients with advanced melanoma. *J Clin Oncol.* 2017;35:3815–3822. doi:10.1200/JCO.2016.72.1167; Figure 3, page 6.

monotherapies (14% versus 3% for anti-PD-1 and 1% for ipilimumab), albeit with a small number of ipi+nivo treated patients (15). Neurological irAEs may result in significant morbidity and mortality, so a low threshold for investigation and neurology consultation is advised.

Long-term data are also reassuring regarding the safety of ipi+nivo. After a 3-year minimum follow-up, no change in the safety profile of ipi+nivo was noted in the Checkmate-067 trial (3). Only four treatment-related deaths (<1%) were noted in the large pooled analysis of over 448 patients (1).

Symptoms and Management of irAEs

Specific symptoms of irAEs due to combination ICIs are the same as for monotherapy-related irAEs. As 23% of patients are noted to experience two irAEs and 6% develop three irAEs with ipi+nivo, patients require close monitoring, especially during the weaning of corticosteroids. Clinicians should also be aware of unusual presentations, for example, neurological toxicity involving the diaphragm that may present with dyspnea. Some presentations may be fulminant, such as type 1 diabetes presenting with ketoacidosis (16) or myocarditis presenting with decompensated cardiac failure with cardiac conduction abnormalities (13).

The approach to management of irAEs from combination ICI is the same as for single agent ICI. Corticosteroids (prednisolone 1 mg/kg or methylprednisolone 1–2 mg/kg) should generally be initiated for any grade 3/4 irAE, and nonresolving grade 2 events. Additional immunomodulating medications (IMMs), such as infliximab or myco-phenolate mofetil, are more commonly required in patients who develop toxicity on ipi+nivo compared to monotherapy. The combination group is therefore at a greater risk of iatrogenic complications related to cor-ticosteroids and immunosuppression such as opportunistic infections (17). Guidance on the management of irAEs is included in the product information for ipilimumab and nivolumab, as well as being the subject of several review articles (18–22). There is no good evidence to suggest that use of IMMs to treat irAEs resulting from combination checkpoint inhibition compromises patient outcomes. In a subanalysis of the impact of infliximab use in the Checkmate-067 population (23), and in a large retrospective review of patients on ipilimumab receiving corticosteroids (24), no clear detriment was shown.

With the exception of endocrine irAEs warranting permanent hor-mone replacement, 79% of grade 3 and 4 irAEs due to ipi+nivo within clinical trials resolved within 4 to 5 weeks when proper management fol-lowing established treatment paradigms was used (1). The median time to resolution for all-grade select irAEs were: skin, 2 weeks; GI, 5.0 weeks; hepatitis, 6.1 weeks; endocrine, 7.4 weeks; renal dysfunction, 10.2 weeks; and pneumonitis 10.6 weeks (see Figure 3.3).

Outcomes and Treatment Subsequent to Toxicity

The question of whether toxicity as a surrogate marker for immune activation is predictive and/or prognostic of ICI treatment benefit remains unanswered. In the large pooled analysis of ipi+nivo treated patients, a higher response rate was noted in the patients who devel-oped toxicity (63% versus 21%); however, the group who did not expe-rience any irAEs had a relatively greater proportion of poor prognostic features such as M1c disease and an elevated lactate dehydrogenase (LDH), and a time-delay bias may complicate such an analysis. Given that these patients probably progressed earlier, reducing their treat-ment exposure and chance of developing toxicity, this information is too confounded to reliably support an association between toxicity and response (1).

Reassuringly, the outcomes of patients who discontinue ipi+nivo due to toxicity within the first 3 months of treatment do not appear to be compromised when compared to patients who continue treatment for a longer period. In the Checkmate-067 trial, 36% of patients treated with ipi+nivo stopped therapy due to toxicity compared with 8% receiving nivolumab (2,4). A pooled analysis of the Checkmate-067 and Phase II Checkmate-069 trial cohorts (patients receiving ipi+nivo) revealed that discontinuation of treatment was most common during the induction phase (first 3 months) and prior to the fourth planned cycle of ipi+nivo (23). Response rates (58% versus 50%), median PFS (8.4 versus 10.8 months), and OS (not reached in either group) were similar in those who ceased treatment due to toxicity and in those who did not. There is a sug-gestion that survival may actually be superior in patients who develop immune-related gastrointestinal toxicity due to ipi+nivo versus those

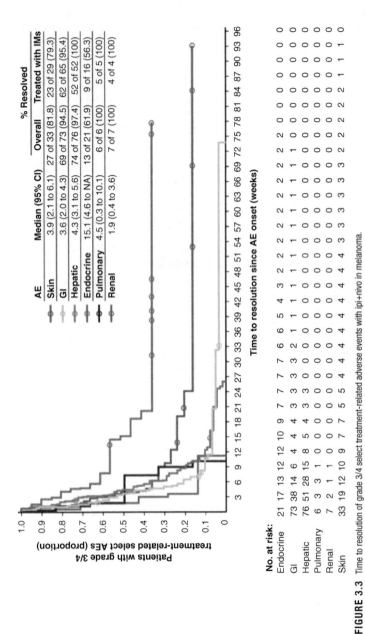

FIGURE 3.3 Time to resolution of grade 3/4 select treatment-related adverse events with ipi+nivo in melanoma.

Source: From Sznol M, Ferrucci PF, Hogg D, et al. Pooled analysis safety profile of nivolumab and ipilimumab combination therapy in patients with advanced melanoma. *J Clin Oncol.* 2017;35:3815–3822. doi:10.1200/JCO.2016.72.1167; Figure 4, page 6.

who do not (71% versus 64% alive at 2 years) (10,11). Despite the notably higher rates of treatment complications, health-related quality of life was not compromised in the ipi+nivo arm of Checkmate-067 (25).

In a smaller retrospective series of 64 patients treated with ipi+nivo at a single institution (26), there was no difference in time to treatment failure between those who did and did not hold, delay, or discontinue treatment due to toxicity. Only 39% of patients completed four cycles of combination treatment. Ninety-one percent experienced clinically significant AEs (defined as grade ≥2 toxicity or any toxicity requiring systemic steroids), 50% presented to an emergency department, and 36% were admitted to a hospital.

Strong evidence to guide treatment decisions after cessation of combination ICIs due to irAEs is lacking. One multi-institution retrospective series described the outcomes of 80 patients with metastatic melanoma who resumed anti-PD-1 therapy after experiencing significant irAEs attributed to ipi+nivo (27). The majority of patients (81%) resumed nivolumab as maintenance therapy and 16% resumed for disease progression, at a median of 58 days (range 14–395). Grade 3–5 toxicities were experienced by 18% of patients upon resumption of anti-PD-1, with one death due to Stevens–Johnson syndrome (that patient had a prior grade 2 rash from combination ipi+nivo). While hepatitis recurred in 17%, colitis only recurred in 6% of patients. Patients still on corticosteroids for management of the ipi+nivo-related AE were more likely to experience toxicity than patients who had weaned off corticosteroids. This study provides some useful insights and suggests that resumption of maintenance nivolumab is reasonable, though not without risk. However, observing patients until such time that they progress and then re-instituting treatment is arguably the safest approach. At this point, consideration could be given to a targeted therapy if available, such as dabrafenib and trametinib or vemurafenib and cobimetinib in *BRAF*-mutant melanoma patients, rather than re-challenge with an ICI.

Although adequate safety data are lacking to make any firm recommendations regarding re-challenge with combination ipi+nivo in those who experience toxicity, or the safety of ipi+nivo after severe toxicity with ICI monotherapy, the nature and severity of the irAE should be taken into account. For example, ipi+nivo commencement or re-challenge after manageable skin or endocrine toxicity is arguably less risky than administration of ipi+nivo after myocarditis, colitis, or a severe neurological event.

CONCLUSION

Combination ICIs have shown improved response rates and survival in advanced melanoma and RCC compared to monotherapy. Novel combinations of ICIs with other immune-oncology and epigenetic agents including indoleamine 2,3-deoxygenase (IDO) inhibitors, genetically modified viral oncolysates (e.g., Talimogene laherparepvec), other immune checkpoint targets, and entinostat are being investigated. Despite evidence of clinical activity, the role of combination ICI therapy in lung cancer is not yet defined, although trials are ongoing. Combination

ICI regimens are also being evaluated in head and neck and urothelial cancers, among other malignancies. Established immune checkpoint antibodies, such as pembrolizumab and durvalumab, are being combined with epacadostat, an IDO inhibitor, in melanoma (NCT02752074), RCC (NCT03260894), NSCLC, and other tumor types (NCT02318277). Inhibitory antibodies to immune checkpoints such as LAG-3 (NCT01968109) and TIM-3 (NCT03099109) are also being used in combination strategies for advanced tumors. In the neoadjuvant and adjuvant settings ipi+nivo is being investigated in melanoma (NCT03068455 and NCT02977052, respectively) and an adjuvant study including durva+treme is due to open for renal cell cancer (NCT03288532).

Given the benefit seen with combination immune checkpoint strategies, and the number of combinations under investigation, it is important for clinicians to be mindful of the associated toxicities observed with these regimens. Although the evidence to date suggests that the majority of irAEs resolve with appropriate management, the majority of safety information comes from large, randomized studies in melanoma and patients who would not have met inclusion criteria for these trials; for example, due to performance status, pre-existing autoimmune disorders or underlying organ dysfunction are likely to be more vulnerable to adverse events. In these cases, multidisciplinary input and management in a center experienced in delivering combination ICIs may help optimize patient outcomes.

REFERENCES

1. Sznol M, Ferrucci PF, Hogg D, et al. Pooled analysis safety profile of nivolumab and ipilimumab combination therapy in patients with advanced melanoma. *J Clin Oncol.* 2017;35(34):3815–3822. doi:10.1200/JCO.2016.72.1167

2. Larkin J, Chiarion-Sileni V, Gonzalez R, et al. Combined nivolumab and ipilimumab or monotherapy in untreated melanoma. *N Engl J Med.* 2015;373(1):23–34. doi:10.1056/NEJMoa1504030

3. Wolchok JD, Chiarion-Sileni V, Gonzalez R, et al. Overall survival with combined nivolumab and ipilimumab in advanced melanoma. *N Engl J Med.* 2017;377(14):1345–1356. doi:10.1056/NEJMoa1709684

4. Larkin J, Chiarion-Sileni V, Gonzalez R, et al. Efficacy and safety in key patient subgroups of nivolumab (NIVO) alone or combined with ipilimumab (IPI) versus IPI alone in treatment-naïve patients with advanced melanoma (MEL) (CheckMate 067). Paper presented at the European Cancer Congress, Vienna. *Eur J Cancer.* 2015;51:S664–S665. doi:10.1016/s0959-8049(16)31822-6

5. Escudier B, Tannir N, McDermott DF, et al. CheckMate 214: efficacy and safety of nivolumab + ipilimumab (N+I) v sunitinib (S) for treatment-naïve advanced or metastatic renal cell carcinoma (mRCC), including IMDC risk and PD-L1 expression subgroups. Paper presented at the ESMO, Madrid. *Ann Oncol.* 2017;28(suppl_5). doi:10.1093/annonc/mdx440.029

6. Hellmann MD, Rizvi NA, Goldman JW, et al. Nivolumab plus ipilimumab as first-line treatment for advanced non-small-cell lung cancer (CheckMate 012): results of an open-label, phase 1, multicohort study. *Lancet Oncol.* 2017;18(1):31–41. doi:10.1016/S1470-2045(16)30624-6

7. Antonia S, Goldberg SB, Balmanoukian A, et al. Safety and antitumour activity of durvalumab plus tremelimumab in non-small cell lung cancer: a multicentre, phase 1b study. *Lancet Oncol.* 2016;17(3):299–308. doi:10.1016/S1470-2045(15)00544-6

8. AstraZeneca. (2017). https://www.astrazeneca.com/media-centre/press-releases/2017/astrazeneca-reports-initial-results-from-the-ongoing-mystic-trial-in-stage-iv-lung-cancer-27072017.html

9. Antonia SJ, Lopez-Martin JA, Bendell J, et al. Nivolumab alone and nivolumab plus ipilimumab in recurrent small-cell lung cancer (CheckMate 032): a multicentre, open-label, phase 1/2 trial. *Lancet Oncol.* 2016;17(7):883–895. doi:10.1016/S1470-2045(16)30098-5

10. Weber JS, Hodi FS, Wolchok JD, et al. Safety profile of nivolumab monotherapy: a pooled analysis of patients with advanced melanoma. *J Clin Oncol.* 2017;35(7):785–792. doi:10.1200/JCO.2015.66.1389

11. Weber JS, Larkin JMG, Schadendorf D, et al. Management of gastrointestinal (GI) toxicity associated with nivolumab (NIVO) plus ipilimumab (IPI) or IPI alone in phase II and III trials in advanced melanoma (MEL). *J Clin Oncol.* 2017;35(15_suppl):9523–9523. doi:10.1200/JCO.2017.35.15_suppl.9523

12. Long GV, Atkinson V, Cebon JS, et al. Standard-dose pembrolizumab in combination with reduced-dose ipilimumab for patients with advanced melanoma (KEYNOTE-029): an open-label, phase 1b trial. *Lancet Oncol.* 2017;18(9):1202–1210. doi:10.1016/S1470-2045(17)30428-X

13. Johnson DB, Balko JM, Compton ML, et al. Fulminant myocarditis with combination immune checkpoint blockade. *N Engl J Med.* 2016;375(18):1749–1755. doi:10.1056/NEJMoa1609214

14. Larkin J, Chmielowski B, Lao CD, et al. Neurologic serious adverse events associated with nivolumab plus ipilimumab or nivolumab alone in advanced melanoma, including a case series of encephalitis. *Oncologist.* 2017;22(6):709–718. doi:10.1634/theoncologist.2016-0487

15. Spain L, Walls G, Julve M, et al. Neurotoxicity from immune-checkpoint inhibition in the treatment of melanoma: a single centre experience and review of the literature. *Ann Oncol.* 2017;28(2):377–385. doi:10.1093/annonc/mdw558

16. Lowe JR, Perry DJ, Salama AK, et al. Genetic risk analysis of a patient with fulminant autoimmune type 1 diabetes mellitus secondary to combination ipilimumab and nivolumab immunotherapy. *J Immunother Cancer.* 2016;4:89. doi:10.1186/s40425-016-0196-z

17. Del Castillo M, Romero FA, Arguello E, et al. The spectrum of serious infections among patients receiving immune checkpoint blockade for the treatment of melanoma. *Clin Infect Dis.* 2016;63(11):1490–1493. doi:10.1093/cid/ciw539

18. Friedman CF, Proverbs-Singh TA, Postow MA. Treatment of the immune-related adverse effects of immune checkpoint inhibitors: a review. *JAMA Oncol.* 2016;2(10):1346–1353. doi:10.1001/jamaoncol.2016.1051

19. Haanen J, Carbonnel F, Robert C, et al. Management of toxicities from immunotherapy: ESMO Clinical Practice Guidelines for diagnosis, treatment and follow-up. *Ann Oncol.* 2017;28(suppl_4):iv119–iv142. doi:10.1093/annonc/mdx225

20. Hassel JC, Heinzerling L, Aberle J, et al. Combined immune checkpoint blockade (anti-PD-1/anti-CTLA-4): Evaluation and management of adverse drug reactions. *Cancer Treat Rev.* 2017;57:36–49. doi:10.1016/j.ctrv.2017.05.003

21. Puzanov I, Diab A, Abdallah K, et al. Managing toxicities associated with immune checkpoint inhibitors: consensus recommendations from the Society for Immunotherapy of Cancer (SITC) Toxicity Management Working Group. *J Immunother Cancer.* 2017;5(1):95. doi:10.1186/s40425-017-0300-z

22. Spain L, Diem S, Larkin J. Management of toxicities of immune checkpoint inhibitors. *Cancer Treat Rev.* 2016;44:51–60. doi:10.1016/j.ctrv.2016.02.001

23. Schadendorf D, Wolchok JD, Hodi FS, et al. Efficacy and safety outcomes in patients with advanced melanoma who discontinued treatment with nivolumab and ipilimumab because of adverse events: a pooled analysis of randomized phase II and III trials. *J Clin Oncol.* 2017;35(34):3807–3814. doi:10.1200/JCO.2017.73.2289

24. Horvat TZ, Adel NG, Dang TO, et al. Immune-related adverse events, need for systemic immunosuppression, and effects on survival and time to treatment failure in patients with melanoma treated with ipilimumab at Memorial Sloan Kettering Cancer Center. *J Clin Oncol.* 2015;33(28):3193–3198. doi:10.1200/JCO.2015.60.8448

25. Schadendorf D, Larkin J, Wolchok J, et al. Health-related quality of life results from the phase III CheckMate 067 study. *Eur J Cancer.* 2017;82:80–91. doi:10.1016/j.ejca.2017.05.031

26. Shoushtari AN, Friedman CF, Navid-Azarbaijani P, et al. Measuring toxic effects and time to treatment failure for nivolumab plus ipilimumab in melanoma. *JAMA Oncol.* 2017;4(1):98. doi:10.1001/jamaoncol.2017.2391

27. Pollack MH, Betof A, Dearden H, et al. Safety of resuming anti-PD-1 in patients with immune-related adverse events (irAEs) during combined anti-CTLA-4 and anti-PD1 in metastatic melanoma. *Ann Oncol.* 2017;29(1):250–255. doi:10.1093/annonc/mdx642

PART II

SPECIFIC IMMUNE CHECKPOINT INHIBITOR TOXICITIES

CHAPTER 4

GENERAL PRINCIPLES OF IMMUNE-RELATED TOXICITIES

Osama E. Rahma and Patrick A. Ott

INTRODUCTION

With the rapid pace and development of immune checkpoint inhibitors (ICIs) and their wide use and expanded indications in many malignancies, it is important to understand the variety of toxicity patterns associated with these agents and to identify suitable patients based on these safety profiles. Unlike chemotherapy or targeted therapy, ICIs do not aim directly at cancer cells but rather counteract inhibitory pathways thereby inducing or invigorating immune responses directed against specific antigens on the cancer cells. Unleashing the immune system against cancer is a double-edged sword because activated T-cells can have cross-reactivity to host antigens, which may induce immune-related adverse events (irAEs).

It can be argued that the actual "drugs" that mediate both clinical efficacy and toxicity of ICIs are not the antibodies that disinhibit regulatory pathways (cytotoxic T-lymphocyte antigen 4 [CTLA-4], programmed cell death 1 [PD-1], and others), but the T-effector cells and other immune cells that are unleashed by this disinhibition. Several key features of ICIs include the potential durability of treatment responses, the delayed and to some extent unpredictable onset of both antitumor responses and immune-related toxicities, and the lack of a strict time correlation between administration of ICI therapy and its effect are better understood when bearing these basic concepts in mind. While the pathogenesis underlying ICI-mediated irAEs is incompletely understood, it is likely that a break in peripheral T-cell tolerance plays a critical role. ICIs likely lead to activation and increased frequencies of preexisting organ-specific T-cells—once this process reaches a critical threshold, organ damage ensues.

Although most irAEs are mild-to-moderate, serious life-threatening irAEs have been reported, especially with the combination of ICIs, leading to death in up to 2% of patients treated (1). These irAEs could affect any organ, with the most commonly affected sites being skin, thyroid, pituitary and adrenal glands, gastrointestinal tract, musculoskeletal, and lungs, while renal, cardiovascular, and neurological sites are affected less frequently (Figure 4.1). Severe irAEs that can be life-threatening include toxic epidermal necrolysis, encephalitis, myocarditis, pneumonitis, colitis, and type I diabetes leading to diabetic ketoacidosis (2). It is notable that simultaneous occurrence of irAEs in multiple different organs of an individual patient is relatively uncommon. The irAEs occur late after starting the treatment (usually within 4–8 weeks) and unlike chemotherapy they last for weeks to months and can even occur months after ICIs discontinuation (3,4).

Published by Springer Publishing Company DOI: 10.1891/9780826172150.0004

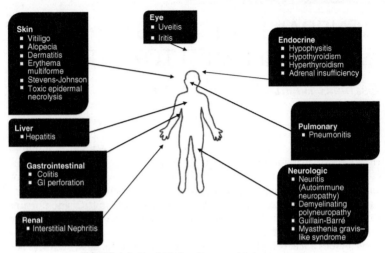

FIGURE 4.1 The distribution of immune-related adverse events.

CLINICAL PRESENTATION AND EPIDEMIOLOGY

The incidence and patterns of irAEs vary between CTLA-4 and PD-1/programmed cell death ligand 1 (PD-L1) targeted agents (Table 4.1, Figure 4.1). irAEs have been reported in up to 75% of patients (43% grade (G)3/4) treated with ipilimumab (5) and up to 30% in patients treated with PD-1/PD-L1 targeted agents (20% G3/4) (6) while in patients treated with the combination of anti-PD-1 (nivolumab) and anti-CTLA-4 (ipilimumab) the incidence has been reported as 99.5% (55% G3/4) (7). Dermatitis can occur with both CTLA-4 and PD-1/PD-L1 targeted therapies (11%–28%), colitis and hepatitis are more common with CTLA-4 inhibition (10% and

TABLE 4.1 Immune-Related Adverse Events With Different ICIs (anti-PD-1/PD-L1, anti-CTLA-4, or Combination anti-CTLA-4/PD-1)

	Dermatitis	Colitis	Hepatitis	Endocrinopathy	Pneumonitis
	% all grades (% grade 3/4)				
Ipilimumab	14.5 (12)	10 (7)	5 (2)	10 (3)	<1%
Ipi+Nivo	30 (3)	26 (16)	13 (6)	35 (4)	6 (2.2)
Nivolumab	28 (1.5)	2.9 (0.7)	1.8 (0.7)	12 (0)	3.1 (1.1)
Pembrolizumab	20 (0.5)	1.7 (1.1)	0.7 (0.4)	12.5 (.3)	3.4 (1.3)
Atezolizumab	17 (0.8)	1 (<1)	1.3 (<1)	5.9 (<1)	2.6 (<1)
Avelumab	15 (0.4)	1.5 (0.4)	0.9 (.7)	6.5 (0.3)	1.2 (0.5)
Durvalumab	11 (1)	1.3 (0.3)	1.1 (.6)	16.2 (0.1)	2.3 (0.5)

CTLA-4, cytotoxic T-lymphocyte antigen 4; ICIs, immune checkpoint inhibitors; PD-1, programmed cell death 1; PD-L1, programmed cell death ligand 1.

5%, respectively) (8) compared to PD-1/PD-L1 targeted therapies (up to 3% and 2%, respectively) (9–13), while pneumonitis is rarely seen with CTLA-4 inhibition but occurs with anti-PD-1/PD-L1 treatment in up to 5% of patients (14). Indeed, the mechanisms by which these agent-specific irAEs are mediated are not fully known. It has been speculated that pneumonitis induced by anti-PD-1 therapy is related to PD-L2 expression in the lung; however, blocking PD-L1 selectively with anti-PD-L1 was not associated with lower incidence of pneumonitis (11). Hypophysitis has been reported in 4% of patients receiving anti-CTLA-4 and has been attributed to the development of antibodies against the pituitary gland correlating with expression of CTLA-4 on prolactin- and thyrotropin-secreting cells (15); nevertheless, anti-PD-1 and PD-L1 can also induce hypophysitis (<1%) (9–13). Accordingly, further studies to understand the mechanisms leading to the development of individual organ specific immune-related toxicities are needed.

Single-Agent ICI Therapy

While a correlation between dose and toxicity has not been clearly established with ICIs, consistent with experience with other immunotherapies including cancer vaccines (16), there may be differences among different ICIs. Adverse events (AEs) induced by CTLA-4 inhibitors have been reported to be dose-related in a phase I study of ipilimumab 10 mg/kg versus 3 mg/kg (17) and in a large meta-analysis that included 22 clinical trials (5). A similar correlation has not been established with PD-1/PD-L1-directed therapies. Although a meta-analysis reported that AEs related to treatment with pembrolizumab correlated with increased doses (18), the data set excluded a large number of relevant studies and did not specifically evaluate immune-related events.

ICI Combination Therapy

Different toxicity profiles were identified with various doses and schedules of nivolumab plus ipilimumab combination therapy. The combination of nivolumab (1 or 3 mg/kg) and ipilimumab (1 or 3 mg/kg) given every 3 weeks followed by nivolumab 3 mg/kg every 2 weeks resulted in poor tolerability with 50% to 55% of patients having grade 3/4 irAEs (19,20). On the other hand, the regimen of nivolumab 3 mg/kg every 2 weeks plus ipilimumab 1 mg/kg given either every 12 weeks or every 6 weeks was better tolerated with grade 3/4 treatment-related toxicity occurring in 37% patients in the every-12-weeks cohort and in 33% in the every-6-weeks cohort (21). The current phase IIIb/IV, randomized, double-blinded, study of nivolumab 3 mg/kg in combination with ipilimumab 1 mg/kg versus nivolumab 1 mg/kg in combination with ipilimumab 3 mg/kg is designed to address the dosing questions in advanced melanoma (NCT02714218). Interestingly, the high discontinuation rate (36%) due to the toxicity of the combination regimen did not appear to have a detrimental effect on its efficacy in the CheckMate 069 study that investigated the combination of nivolumab 1 mg/kg plus ipilimumab

3 mg/kg or ipilimumab 3 mg/kg plus placebo, every 3 weeks for four doses followed by nivolumab 3 mg/kg every 2 weeks in the nivolumab arm (22).

Duration of ICI Therapy

Another important question is whether longer exposure of ICIs can lead to cumulative toxicities and higher incidence of irAEs. This issue is relevant given the uncertainty regarding the optimal duration of ICI treatment for maximal clinical efficacy while minimizing toxicity (22). There seems to be an association between development of irAEs and clinical benefit with ICIs, at least in some patients. For example, the development of vitiligo has been reported to correlate with tumor response in patients with metastatic melanoma treated with pembrolizumab (23). Large retrospective and prospective studies are needed to assess the potential correlation between other irAEs and response rate to ICIs or survival.

BIOMARKERS

There are many ongoing efforts to identify biomarkers related to patient characteristics as well as inflammatory, genetic, and environmental composition of tumor and other tissues that could predict the development of irAEs. A review of the FDA Adverse Event Reporting System (FAERS) for AEs associated with the use of CTLA-4, PD-1, and PD-L1 inhibitors suggested that older patients are more likely to develop irAEs and are more prone to be hospitalized because of irAEs (24).

Microbiome

Gut microbiota have recently been identified as a potential predictor for response to PD-1 inhibitors, and the use of antibiotics was found to negatively impact the efficacy of PD-1/PD-L1 inhibitors by changing the diversity of the gut microbiome (25). Whether similar effects of the microbiota diversity could be observed in relation to irAEs remains to be determined.

Cytokines and Chemokines

Cytokines and chemokines orchestrate the recruitment, survival, expansion, effector function, and contraction of lymphocytes mediating autoimmunity. IL-17 levels at pre-treatment and during treatment with ipilimumab were found to correlate with the incidence of grade-3 diarrhea/colitis in melanoma in two reports (26,27) while patients with lower pre-treatment IL-6 levels were at higher risk to develop grade 3/4 toxicities related to ipilimumab in another report (28). The effects of other inflammatory cytokines on the development of irAEs should also be studied.

Organ Specificity

The toxicity profile of ICIs appears to be largely consistent across trials investigating these agents in different tumors; however, the rate of organ-specific irAEs may vary depending on the primary tumor type or the site of the metastases. For example, the incidence of grade 3 or higher immune-related pneumonitis resulting from treatment with PD-1 inhibitors was higher in non-small cell lung cancer compared with melanoma in a retrospective analysis (14). Whether there is variability across tumor types with other organ-specific irAEs such as colitis and hepatitis is currently under investigation.

Genomic Expression Signatures

Immune-related gene expression signatures related to T-cell cytotoxic function, antigen presentation, and interferon (IFN-γ) signaling have been associated with response to PD-1 therapy across multiple tumor types (29). It would be interesting to explore similar signatures that could be associated with the development irAEs and may predict which patients are at higher risk of developing irAEs upon treatment with ICIs.

PREEXISTING AUTOIMMUNITY

There is limited data regarding the use of ICIs in patients with a history of autoimmune disease. The largest dataset available to date is a retrospective report of 30 melanoma patients with preexisting autoimmune diseases treated with ipilimumab (30). Interestingly, autoimmune conditions were exacerbated in 27% of these patients while 33% developed grade 3–5 irAEs, which were treated successfully, while no immune-related symptoms or exacerbation of autoimmune conditions was observed in the remaining 50% of these patients. Data informing on the risk of recurrence or exacerbation of irAEs in patients with prior ICIs exposure are also scarce. This question was investigated in a retrospective study of 119 melanoma patients with preexisting autoimmune disorders or major toxicity with ipilimumab who were subsequently treated with PD-1 inhibitors (31). Fifty-four percent of the patients with rheumatoid arthritis had exacerbation while none of the patients with inflammatory bowel diseases experienced flares. Interestingly, only two (3%) of the 67 patients with irAEs due to ipilimumab that required immune suppression had a recurrence of ipilimumab-related irAEs and 23 patients (34%) developed new irAEs with 21% grade 3/4 and 12% discontinued treatment (31). Given the rising number of FDA approvals for ICIs resulting in rapidly increasing use of ICIs in a wide spectrum of solid and hematological malignancies, it is expected that the number of patients who develop irAEs due to ICIs will increase. We therefore expect more data in the future regarding the true incidence of irAEs when these patients go on to receive further therapy with ICIs. In addition, many novel targets are currently investigated as single agents or in combinations, and there is much more to be learned regarding their toxicity profiles. In the era of ICIs, treating oncologists should be vigilant and cautious when using ICIs in patients with preexisting autoimmune disease or irAEs due to prior therapy, and they should weigh the risk of exacerbating the preexisting autoimmunity with the potential benefit of these agents. Nonetheless, the toxicities of ICIs should be studied prospectively in cancer patients with preexisting autoimmune conditions in order to truly identify the risks and benefits of these agents.

Patients With Immune Deficiency

Furthermore, the safety of ICIs has been recently reported in 17 patients with HIV prospectively treated with pembrolizumab (32). The trial included three cohorts of cancer patients based on CD4+ counts (100–199, 200–350, and >350 cells/uL). Patients were required to be on antiretroviral therapy and to have HIV viral load of less than 200 copies/mL. The safety profile was comparable between cohorts with most side effects being grade 1/2 and consistent with pembrolizumab safety profile. Anti-PD-1 therapy did not affect CD4+ counts or viral load. Accordingly, HIV patients with cancer should be considered for anti-PD-1 therapy and not be excluded from participation in clinical trials.

COMBINATION OF ICIs AND CHEMOTHERAPY, TARGETED THERAPY, AND RADIATION THERAPY

Many clinical trials are currently investigating the combination of ICIs and standard of care chemotherapy, targeted therapy, and radiation therapy, potentially taking advantage of synergies that could result, for example, from immunogenic cell death induced by cytotoxic therapy or the immune modulation effect of targeted therapies such as anti-angiogenesis, among many other mechanisms. These studies have so far reported a similar safety profile to what is expected of these treatment modalities with no exacerbated irAEs (33,34).

NO ROLE FOR ICI DOSE MODIFICATION IN MANAGING irAEs

For the practicing clinician who treats cancer patients with ICIs, it is important to understand the basic mechanisms by which these therapies lead to: antitumor activity and immune-related toxicities. Because the T-cell response directed against the host's organ is an active process—and to some extent uncoupled from treatment with ICIs—in general, "active" treatment with immune suppressive agents is needed to control moderate or severe irAEs, while simply holding or even continuing ICIs is generally reserved for low-grade irAEs not involving vital organs. Because there appears to be an association between the dose/schedule of CTLA-4 inhibition and the rate of irAEs while no clear relationship between the dose or schedule of PD-1/PD-L1 and the frequency of irAEs has been established to date, intra-patient dose modification, a common practice for the management of toxicities resulting from chemotherapy or targeted therapy, has no role in the management of ICI-related toxicities.

MANAGEMENT OF irAEs

An important lesson from the experience with ICIs to date has been that the vast majority of irAEs can be managed effectively if they are recognized and addressed early. Successful mitigation of toxicities from ICIs therefore requires:

- Well-trained teams of oncologists, nurses, and pharmacists.
- Education of oncology providers and patients.
- Systematic laboratory testing in all patients to ascertain structured assessment and early detection of irAEs.
- Early involvement of multidisciplinary teams where oncology care providers work closely with disease specialists (gastroenterologists, pulmonologists, rheumatologists, etc.) to establish and execute workflows of diagnostic workup and treatment of challenging cases of irAEs.

Corticosteroids are the mainstay of treatment for moderate-to-severe irAEs and are effective for the majority of toxicities resulting from ICIs. General principles of managing irAEs across different affected organs include:

- Holding drug for grade 2 or higher toxicities.
- Initiate corticosteroids and permanently discontinue ICIs for grade 3 or higher events.
- Consideration of infliximab (if gastrointestinal toxicity) or mycophenolate (if hepatotoxicity) if steroids do not resolve symptoms.

More specific guidance adapted for the respective affected organs will be given in the following chapters. It should be recognized that existing treatment recommendations are largely empiric because systematic or randomized data on optimal doses, schedules, or duration of tapers are lacking.

Corticosteroids

While retrospective analyses suggest that patients with irAEs who are treated with corticosteroids do not have inferior outcomes, the balance between steroid-mediated immune suppression and potentially stronger tumor-directed immune responses (mediated by ICIs) and its relative impact on outcome cannot be distinguished in individual patients (4,35). Given the known inhibition of T-effector cells and stimulation of Treg development mediated by corticosteroids (36), steroids-sparing agents (with less damaging impact on T-cell responses) used in the first line may lead to improved efficacy outcomes and should be tested in clinical trials. Patients receiving long-term corticosteroids are at increased risk of developing opportunistic infections such as pneumocystis pneumonia and should be covered with prophylactic antibiotics. Other known risks of high dose and long-term corticosteroids are diabetes mellitus and osteoporosis, among others. Accordingly, patients should have their blood glucose monitored closely and should receive vitamin D and calcium supplements while on corticosteroids.

CONCLUSION

In summary, the administration of ICIs is associated with unique AEs that are in line with their mechanism of action targeting the effector immune cells rather than directly targeting the cancer cells. The rates of those AEs range from 20% to 30% for single agents to over 90% for the combinations, and from mild-grade 1/2 dermatitis, colitis, or hepatitis that can resolve by holding the ICIs agent to severe-grade 3/4 colitis or pneumonitis that requires hospitalization, high dose corticosteroids, and other immune suppressive agents such as infliximab.

Although a clear pattern of toxicities associated with specific ICIs (i.e., CTLA-4 or PD-1/PD-L1 directed monotherapy and combined CTLA-4/PD-1/PD-L1) has emerged, predictive markers that could help anticipate timing or organs at risk for the development of irAEs have been largely elusive. With the rapid pace of drug development involving the combinations of PD-1/PD-L1 and CTLA-4 with other novel ICIs, immune co-stimulatory molecules, and non-immune modulating agents, much will be learned regarding their toxicity profiles. Nonetheless, future studies should prospectively study the factors that may predict the development and severity of ICIs-induced irAEs and how to prevent those irAEs while maintaining the efficacy of these agents.

REFERENCES

1. Puzanov I, Diab A, Abdallah K, et al. Managing toxicities associated with immune checkpoint inhibitors: consensus recommendations from the Society for Immunotherapy of Cancer (SITC) Toxicity Management Working Group. *J Immunother Cancer*. 2017;5:95. doi:10.1186/s40425-017-0300-z

2. Michot JM, Bigenwald C, Champiat S, et al. Immune-related adverse events with immune checkpoint blockade: a comprehensive review. *Eur J Cancer*. 2016;54:139–148. doi:10.1016/j.ejca.2015.11.016

3. Weber JS, Kahler KC, Hauschild A. Management of immune-related adverse events and kinetics of response with ipilimumab. *J Clin Oncol*. 2012;30:2691–2697. doi:10.1016/j.ejca.2015.11.016

4. Weber JS, Hodi FS, Wolchok JD, et al. Safety profile of nivolumab monotherapy: a pooled analysis of patients with advanced melanoma. *J Clin Oncol*. 2017;35:785–792. doi:10.1200/jco.2015.66.1389

5. Bertrand A, Kostine M, Barnetche T, et al. Immune related adverse events associated with anti-CTLA-4 antibodies: systematic review and meta-analysis. *BMC Medicine*. 2015;13:211. doi:10.1186/s12916-015-0455-8

6. Maughan BL, Bailey E, Gill DM, et al. Incidence of immune-related adverse events with program death receptor-1- and program death receptor-1 ligand-directed therapies in genitourinary cancers. *Front Oncol*. 2017;7:56. doi:10.3389/fonc.2017.00056

7. Wolchok JD, Chiarion-Sileni V, Gonzalez R, et al. Overall survival with combined nivolumab and ipilimumab in advanced melanoma. *N Engl J Med*. 2017;377:1345–1356. doi:10.1056/nejmoa1709684

8. Ipilimumab(Yervoy)HighlightsofPrescribingInformation.2017.https://www.accessdata.fda.gov/drugsatfda_docs/label/2015/125377s073lbl.pdf

9. Nivolumab (Opdivo) Highlights of Prescribing Information. 2017. https://packageinserts.bms.com/pi/pi_opdivo.pdf

10. Pembrolizumab (Keytruda) Highlights of Prescribing Information 2017. https://www.merck.com/product/usa/pi_circulars/k/keytruda/keytruda_pi.pdf

11. Atezolizumab (Tecentriq) Highlights of Prescribing Information 2017. https://www.gene.com/download/pdf/tecentriq_prescribing.pdf

12. Durvalumab (Imfinzi) Highlights of Prescribing Information. 2017. https://www.accessdata.fda.gov/drugsatfda_docs/label/2017/761069s000lbl.pdf

13. Avelumab(Bavencio)HighlightsofPrescribingInformation.2017.https://www.bavencio.com/en_US/document/Prescribing-Information.pdf

14. Nishino M, Giobbie-Hurder A, Hatabu H, et al. Incidence of programmed cell death 1 inhibitor-related pneumonitis in patients with advanced cancer: a systematic review and meta-analysis. *JAMA Oncol.* 2016;2:1607–1616. doi:10.1001/jamaoncol.2016.2453

15. Iwama S, De Remigis A, Callahan MK, et al. Pituitary expression of ctla-4 mediates hypophysitis secondary to administration of ctla-4 blocking antibody. *Sci Transl Med.* 2014;6:230ra45. doi:10.1126/scitranslmed.3008002

16. Rahma OE, Gammoh E, Simon RM, et al. Is the "3+3" dose-escalation phase I clinical trial design suitable for therapeutic cancer vaccine development? A recommendation for alternative design. *Clin Cancer Res.* 2014;20:4758–4767. doi:10.1158/1078-0432.ccr-13-2671

17. Ascierto PA, Del Vecchio M, Robert C, et al. Ipilimumab 10 mg/kg versus ipilimumab 3 mg/kg in patients with unresectable or metastatic melanoma: a randomised, double-blind, multicentre, phase 3 trial. *Lancet Oncol.* 2017;18:611–622. doi:10.1016/s1470-2045(17)30231-0

18. Lin Z, Chen X, Li Z, et al. PD-1 Antibody monotherapy for malignant melanoma: a systematic review and meta-analysis. *PloS One.* 2016;11:e0160485.

19. Sznol M, Ferrucci PF, Hogg D, et al. Pooled analysis safety profile of nivolumab and ipilimumab combination therapy in patients with advanced melanoma. *J Clin Oncol.* 2017;35:3815–3822. doi:10.1200/jco.2016.72.1167

20. Wolchok JD, Kluger H, Callahan MK, et al. Nivolumab plus ipilimumab in advanced melanoma. *N Engl J Med.* 2013;369:122–133. doi:10.1056/nejmoa1302369

21. Hellmann MD, Rizvi NA, Goldman JW, et al. Nivolumab plus ipilimumab as first-line treatment for advanced non-small-cell lung cancer (CheckMate 012): results of an open-label, phase 1, multicohort study. *Lancet Oncol.* 2017;18:31–41. doi:10.1016/s1470-2045(16)30624-6

22. Schadendorf D, Wolchok JD, Hodi FS, et al. Efficacy and safety outcomes in patients with advanced melanoma who discontinued treatment with nivolumab and ipilimumab because of adverse events: a pooled analysis of randomized phase II and III trials. *J Clin Oncol.* 2017;35:3807–3814. doi:10.1200/jco.2017.73.2289

23. Hua C, Boussemart L, Mateus C, et al. Association of vitiligo with tumor response in patients with metastatic melanoma treated with pembrolizumab. *JAMA Dermatol.* 2016;152:45–51. doi:10.1001/jamadermatol.2015.2707

24. Elias R, Rider J, Tan X, et al. Single agent and combination checkpoint inhibitors therapy: a post marketing safety analysis. *J Clin Oncol.* 2017;35(15_suppl):4125–4125. doi:10.1200/jco.2017.35.15_suppl.4125

25. Routy B, Le Chatelier E, Derosa L, et al. Gut microbiome influences efficacy of PD-1-based immunotherapy against epithelial tumors. *Science.* 2018;359:91–97. doi:10.1126/science.aan3706

26. Tarhini AA, Zahoor H, Lin Y, et al. Baseline circulating IL-17 predicts toxicity while TGF-beta1 and IL-10 are prognostic of relapse in ipilimumab neoadjuvant therapy of melanoma. *J Immunother Cancer.* 2015;3:39. doi:10.1186/s40425-015-0081-1

27. Callahan MK, Yang A, Tandon S, et al. Evaluation of serum IL-17 levels during ipilimumab therapy: Correlation with colitis. *J Clin Oncol.* 2011;29(15_suppl):2505–2505. doi:10.1200/jco.2011.29.15_suppl.2505

28. Valpione S, Pasquali S, Campana L, et al. Predictors of toxicity for metastatic melanoma patients treated with ipilimumab. *Immunother Cancer.* 2015;3:247. doi:10.1186/2051-1426-3-s2-p247

29. Ayers M, Lunceford J, Nebozhyn M, et al. Relationship between immune gene signatures and clinical response to PD-1 blockade with pembrolizumab (MK-3475) in patients with advanced solid tumors. *J Immunother Cancer.* 2015;3(Suppl 2):1. doi:10.1186/2051-1426-3-s2-p80

30. Johnson DB, Sullivan RJ, Ott PA, et al. Ipilimumab therapy in patients with advanced melanoma and preexisting autoimmune disorders. *JAMA Oncol.* 2016;2:234–240. doi:10.1001/jamaoncol.2015.4368

31. Menzies AM, Johnson DB, Ramanujam S, et al. Anti-PD-1 therapy in patients with advanced melanoma and preexisting autoimmune disorders or major toxicity with ipilimumab. *Ann Oncol.* 2017;28:368–376. doi:10.1093/annonc/mdw443

32. Uldrick TS, Ison G, Rudek MA, et al. Modernizing clinical trial eligibility criteria: recommendations of the American Society of Clinical Oncology-Friends of Cancer Research HIV Working Group. *J Clin Oncol.* 2017;35:3774–3780. doi:10.1200/jco.2017.73.7338

33. Langer CJ, Gadgeel SM, Borghaei H, et al. Carboplatin and pemetrexed with or without pembrolizumab for advanced, non-squamous non-small-cell lung cancer: a randomised, phase 2 cohort of the open-label KEYNOTE-021 study. *Lancet Oncol.* 2016;17:1497–1508. doi:10.1016/s1470-2045(16)30498-3

34. Katz MH, Varadhachary GR, Bauer TW, et al. Preliminary safety data from a randomized multicenter phase Ib/II study of neoadjuvant chemoradiation therapy (CRT) alone or in combination with pembrolizumab in patients with resectable or borderline resectable pancreatic cancer. *J Clin Oncol.* 2017;35(15_suppl):4125–4125. doi:10.1200/jco.2017.35.15_suppl.4125

35. Horvat TZ, Adel NG, Dang TO, et al. Immune-related adverse events, need for systemic immunosuppression, and effects on survival and time to treatment failure in patients with melanoma treated with ipilimumab at Memorial Sloan Kettering Cancer Center. *J Clin Oncol.* 2015;33:3193–3198. doi:10.1200/jco.2015.60.8448

36. Libert C, Dejager L. How steroids steer T cells. *Cell Reports.* 2014;7:938–939. doi:10.1016/j.celrep.2014.04.041

CHAPTER 5

DERMATOLOGIC TOXICITIES: RASH, MUCOSAL IRRITATION, AND PRURITUS

Jennifer Wu and Mario E. Lacouture

INTRODUCTION

Dermatologic adverse events (AEs) are among the most frequent immune-related adverse events (irAEs) and are usually the first to appear, within the first few weeks after initiation of immunotherapy (1,2). Moreover, the development of dermatologic irAE including rash and vitiligo has been correlated with increased progression-free survival and overall survival, underscoring the importance of managing these events (3–6).

POSSIBLE MECHANISMS OF DERMATOLOGIC irAEs

The pathomechanisms underlying dermatologic irAEs remain unclear but maybe related to the interruption of immunological homeostasis by immune checkpoint inhibitors (ICIs). Cytotoxic T-lymphocyte antigen 4 (CTLA-4) inhibits an immune response by attenuating T-cell activation at the priming phase in lymph nodes; while programmed cell death 1 (PD-1) inhibits T-cells at the effector phase of the immune response in peripheral tissues. The differences in treatment efficacy and toxicity profiles of anti-CTLA-4 and anti-PD-1/programmed cell death ligand 1 (PD-L1) checkpoint blockade reflect the distinct functions of CTLA-4 and PD-1 (7–10).

- The incidence and severity of dermatologic irAEs to anti-CTLA-4 therapy are generally higher than anti-PD-1/PD-L1 (11).
- Certain dermatologic irAEs have been reported to be class-specific AEs, for example, bullous pemphigoid and lichenoid rashes are more common with anti-PD-1/PD-L1 agents (12). It seems that in addition to T-cell-mediated cellular immunity, anti–PD-1/PD-L1 treatment also affects humoral immunity.
- Autoreactive T-cells and/or autoantibodies may contribute to different irAEs to a variable extent.

Four possible mechanisms of irAEs have been proposed that may also be applicable for dermatologic irAEs:

- Increasing T-cell activity against common antigens in both tumors and normal tissue. For example, vitiligo frequently seen in patients with melanoma treated with ICIs is hypothesized to result from cross-reactivity of T-cells against melanoma and melanocytes in normal tissue.
- Increasing levels of autoantibodies, for example, anti-BP180/ BP-230 in bullous pemphigoid.

Published by Springer Publishing Company DOI: 10.1891/9780826172150.0005

- Increasing levels of inflammatory cytokines (e.g., interleukin-6 level reported in patients with nivolumab-associated psoriasiform dermatitis) (13).
- Enhancing complement-mediated inflammation due to direct binding of an anti-CTLA-4 antibody with CTLA-4 expressed on normal tissue (7).

INCIDENCES AND CLINICAL MANIFESTATIONS OF DERMATOLOGIC irAEs

Dermatologic irAEs are a spectrum of conditions associated with immune checkpoint blockade with anti-CTLA-4 and anti-PD-1/PD-L1 monoclonal antibodies. Dermatologic AEs related to anti-CTLA-4 or anti-PD-1/PD-L1 may differ.

- Dermatologic toxicities are more frequent in patients receiving anti-CTLA-4 therapy, with a 44% to 68% reported incidence compared to those treated with anti-PD-1/PD-L1 therapy (incidence 37%–42%) (1,8,9,14).
- Up to 58% to 71% of patients treated with anti-CTLA-4 plus anti-PD-1 combination therapy developed dermatologic irAEs (9).
- Severe dermatologic irAEs related to anti-PD-L1 occur in less than 5% of patients (15,16).

Pruritus and rash are the most common reported dermatologic irAEs, occurring in up to 47% and 55% of patients receiving ICIs (anti-CTLA-4, anti-PD1, or combination therapy), respectively. Vitiligo is more frequently seen in patients with melanoma compared to other solid tumors. The incidences of common dermatologic irAEs associated with different ICIs are summarized in Table 5.1 (1,7–9,11).

Other dermatologic AEs include lichenoid dermatitis, bullous pemphigoid, psoriasis or psoriasiform dermatitis, alopecia areata, xerosis, dermatomysitis, Sweets' syndrome, scleroderma, mucositis, xerostomia, sarcoidosis, Grover's disease, eruptive keratoacanthoma, and granuloma annulare, etc. Common dermatologic AEs associated with ICIs are shown in Figure 5.1.

- Severe cutaneous adverse reactions (SCARs) such as erythema multiforme (EM), Stevens–Johnson syndrome (SJS), toxic epidermal necrosis (TEN), and drug rash with eosinophilia and systemic symptoms (DRESS) syndrome have been rarely reported (8,11,12,15,17–22).

Pruritus (Itching)

Pruritus is an irAE that can negatively impact a patient's quality of life (23–26). Pruritus is frequently reported with anti-CTLA-4 and anti-PD-1 agents, affecting 24% to 36% of patients treated with ipilimumab, 14% to 21% with anti-PD-1, and as high as 33% to 47% with combination therapy (1,9,27). The incidence of high-grade pruritus is usually less than 1% (1,9,27).

TABLE 5.1 Incidences of Immune-Related Dermatologic AEs

Dermatologic irAEs All grade % (grade 3%)	Ipilimumab	Nivolumab	Pembrolizumab	Ipi+Nivo	Atezolizumab	Durvalumab	Avelumab
Pruritus	24–36 (1)	17–18.8 (0.5)	14.1–20.7 (1)	33.2–47 (2)	10 (<1)	7.1 (<1)	4.5 (0)
Rash	14.5–26.1 (2)	15–21.7 (0.5)	13.4–20.7 (2)	28.4–55 (5)	7 (<1)	6.6 (<1)	6.8 (0)
Maculopapular rash	2.7–17.4 (0.4)	2.5–4.2 (0.3)	1.5–3.6 (0.4)	11.8–16 (3)	NA	2 (<1)	5.7 (0)
Vitiligo	1.6–8.7 (0)	7–10.7 (0.3)	8.9–11 (0)	6.7–11 (0)	0	0	0

AEs, adverse events.

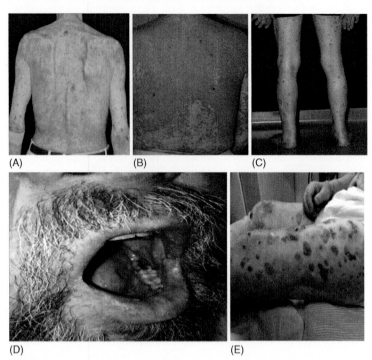

(A)   (B)   (C)

(D)   (E)

FIGURE 5.1 Common dermatologic adverse events associated with ICIs. (A) Maculopapular rash, (B) Psoriasiform rash, (C) Lichenoid rash, (D) Lichenoid mucositis, and (E) Bullous pemphigoid.

ICIs, immune checkpoint inhibitors.

- Pruritus can develop alone or accompany a skin rash, either early within weeks after the initiation of immunotherapy or late after months or years.

Rash

The incidence of all-grade skin rash ranges from 15% to 26% with anti-CTLA-4 therapy, 14% to 22% with anti-PD-1 agents, 28% to 55% with combination treatment, and 6% to 7% with anti-PD-L1 agents (1,7–9,11). The rashes reported in the literature as dermatologic irAEs are nonspecific, and may include majorly maculopapular rash and other types, which will be discussed separately in the following sections.

Maculopapular Rash

Maculopapular rash is the predominant type of rash induced by ICIs, occurring in 3% to 17% of patients treated with anti-CTLA-4 antibody and 11% to 16% of combination therapy, and is less commonly reported in anti-PD-1/PD-L1 therapy (9).

- Maculopapular rash usually develops rapidly after the first doses, but can progress after subsequent treatment cycles.
- Lesions usually manifest as erythematous macules and/or papules, discrete or confluent, with or without scaling or itching; mainly distributed on the trunk and extremities, usually sparing the face (1,8,9).
- Wheal-like, urticarial rashes can also occur with anti-PD-1/PD-L1 therapies which differ from maculopapular rash.

Severe Cutaneous Adverse Reactions

Maculopapular rash may be the initial presentation of SCARs such as SJS/TEN or DRESS syndrome, which need special precaution.

- Although very rare, SJS/TEN has been reported in patients treated with ipilimumab, nivolumab, and pembrolizumab and DRESS syndrome in patients receiving ipilimumab (21,28–30).
- Signs/symptoms suspicious of potentially life-threatening skin reactions include targetoid lesions, blister formation, Nikolsky sign, mucosal lesions, skin pain, and fever (31–33).

Lichenoid Rash/Dermatitis

Lichenoid rash/dermatitis is also seen in patients receiving anti-PD-1/PD-L1 therapy and is probably underestimated.

- The onset may be relatively delayed, until months after the initiation of immunotherapy, compared to that of maculopapular rash (18).
- Lichenoid rash usually locates mainly on the trunk, occasionally on the extremities, with either discrete or multiple scattered violaceous polygonal papules/plaques. Pruritus and oral involvement may accompany the rash (9,15,18).

Psoriasis

New onset or flare of psoriasis and development of psoriasiform rash have been reported in patients treated with anti-CTLA-4 and anti-PD-1/PD-L1 agents.

- Lesions manifest as pruritic or asymptomatic, scaly, sharply demarcated, erythematous papules/plaques on the trunk and extremities.
- Palmoplantar psoriasis or inverse psoriasis involving major skin folds and anogenital area can be seen (9,15).

Vitiligo

The development of vitiligo is a well-known dermatologic irAE most commonly seen in melanoma patients, affecting 2% to 11% of patients receiving ICIs.

- Lesions induced by ICIs usually appear as scattered, flecked, depigmented macules on photo-exposed areas without Koebner phenomenon, compared to symmetric-distributed, well-circumscribed white macules of idiopathic vitiligo.

- Vitiligo usually develops after months of treatment.
- The occurrence of vitiligo has been related to favorable cancer outcomes in patients with melanoma treated with pembrolizumab or nivolumab (1,9,19,21,34).

MUCOSAL INVOLVEMENT

Mucosal manifestations of dermatologic AEs include xerostomia (dry mouth), nonspecific stomatitis or mucositis, and lichenoid mucositis, and other skin disorders with oral involvement have been sporadically reported with both anti-PD-1 and PD-L1 therapy.

- Lichenoid mucositis presents as whitish confluent papules with characteristic Wickham's striae (white reticular streaks) on the tongue, lips, gingiva, hard palate, or buccal mucosae, and the anogenital mucosa can also be involved.
- Dysgueusia and xerostomia have been reported in around 5% of patients receiving ICIs.
- Oral candidiasis must be excluded, and autoimmune survey such as antinuclear antibodies (ANA), and SSA (anti-Ro)/SSB (anti-LA) screen for Sjögren's syndrome should be considered (15,18).

ASSESSMENT AND MANAGEMENT OF DERMATOLOGIC AEs

Pre-treatment patient counseling, proper prophylactic skin care, early recognition, and intervention are essential for the management of dermatologic AEs, which may help maintain the patients on immunotherapy and their quality of life, and eventually may benefit the cancer outcomes.

DIAGNOSTIC EVALUATION

- Initial assessment of a dermatologic AE using the Common Terminology Criteria for Adverse Events (CTCAEs) grading system should be performed (35).
  - Classification of dermatologic AEs based on CTCAE has limitations, which may be, in part, reflected by high reported incidence of rash and/or nonspecific maculopapular rash in the literature. Immune-related dermatologic AEs should be categorized accurately to optimize supportive care interventions.
  - CTCAE currently still serves as a useful initial evaluation tool for multidiscipline communication.
- Patients should receive comprehensive skin and mucosal examination.
  - Imaging with photography or sketching is recommended to assist the documentation of the morphology, distribution, and body surface area (BSA) involvement when a dermatologic AE first appears or changes during the treatment course (36,37).
  - This may facilitate prompt dermatology consultation, accurate diagnosis, monitoring, and later analyzing of the dermatologic AEs when necessary (36).

- Dermatologic evaluation is recommended for pati
  of immune-related skin disorders such as psorias
  pemphigoid, or lupus (36).

WHEN TO REFER

- Dermatology referral is recommended for any
  CTCAE grade ≥2.
  - Rashes with unclear diagnosis, rashes suspicious of erythema multiforme (EM), blistering disorders of any BSA, psoriasis, lichenoid dermatitis, or any rash not responsive to topical intervention.
- Any grade 3 dermatologic toxicity warrants the same-day dermatology consultation.
  - Blisters or skin detachment covering ≥1% BSA, a rash accompanied by mucosal lesions, any rash with ≥30% involvement of BSA, and rash with skin pain with or without blisters (excluding varicella zoster).
- A skin biopsy for pathology and immunofluorescence study may be beneficial for selected patients.
- Patients with suspected SJS/TEN, DRESS syndrome, autoimmune bullous dermatosis, or severe mucocutaneous reactions with ≥10% epidermal necrosis or detachment, or any complications should be hospitalized immediately and evaluated by a dermatologist for further management (36).

GENERAL MANAGEMENT STRATEGY OF DERMATOLOGIC AEs

The initial approach for dermatologic AEs is supportive with topical or oral agents. Prophylactic strategy with gentle skin care, including fragrance-free detergents and soaps, moisturizers, and sun protection, is recommended.

- Management usually starts from topical antipruritic agents and topical corticosteroids for grades 1/2 dermatologic AEs.
- Oral antihistamines can be added for grade 2 dermatologic AEs that are not responsive to topical treatments.
- Systemic treatments including oral antihistamine, GABA agonist (gabapentin, pregabalin), doxepin, antidepressants, neurokinin-1 (NK-1) receptor antagonist (aprepitant), or corticosteroids are options for grade 3 or intolerable grade 2 pruritus (21,38–42).
- Systemic immune suppressors or immune-modulating agents such as systemic corticosteroids, biologics, mycophenolate mofetil, and so on should be considered for other grade 3 or intolerable grade 2 dermatologic AEs based on the specific dermatologic diagnosis to achieve the optimal treatment response and minimal side effects.
- Interruption of ICIs with reassessment is necessary for any dermatologic AEs of grade 3 or intolerable grade 2 (1,36,43,44).

sal AEs can be managed with supportive care such as oral rinses n topical corticosteroids, viscous lidocaine hydrochloride, and good oral hygiene. Oral medications such as saliva stimulants (e.g., cevimeline or pilocarpine chlorhydrate) may improve the symptoms of xerostomia (11).

The proposed treatment algorithms are summarized in Figure 5.2.

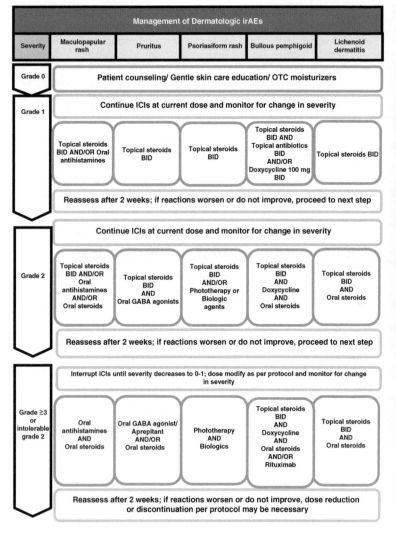

FIGURE 5.2 Management of immune-related dermatologic adverse events.
ICIs, immune checkpoint inhibitors; irAEs, immune-related adverse events; OTC, over the counter.

DISCUSSION

Pruritus and rash are the most frequently reported irAEs and the earliest to occur after initiation of ICIs. However, it is possible that these toxicities are reported earlier than other organ irAEs because they are more visible and noticeable as compared, for example, to GI or thyroid irAEs. Vitiligo is another well-known irAEs, primarily seen in melanoma patients after treatment with ICI. Although the exact immune biology is not fully understood for all skin irAEs, vitiligo is thought to be mediated through distinct immune response that resemble more antitumor immune response. Several other less common and more severe dermatologic irAEs have been reported. Of note, the occurrence of dermatologic irAEs such as rash and vitiligo has been found to correlate with a positive response to ICIs in melanoma patients. Therefore, meticulous evaluation and management of those toxicities is necessary without the need to interrupt or discontinue ICI therapy unless indicated as per the SITC guidelines.

REFERENCES

1. Belum VR, Benhuri B, Postow MA, et al. Characterisation and management of dermatologic adverse events to agents targeting the PD-1 receptor. *Eur J Cancer.* 2016;60:12–25. doi:10.1016/j.ejca.2016.02.010

2. Weber JS, Yang JC, Atkins MB, et al. Toxicities of immunotherapy for the practitioner. *J Clin Oncol.* 2015;33(18):2092–2099. doi:10.1200/jco.2014.60.0379

3. Freeman-Keller M, Kim Y, Cronin H, et al. Nivolumab in resected and unresectable metastatic melanoma: characteristics of Immune-Related Adverse Events and Association with Outcomes. *Clin Cancer Res.* 2016;22(4):886–894. doi:10.1158/1078-0432.ccr-15-1136

4. Hua C, Boussemart L, Mateus C, et al. Association of vitiligo with tumor response in patients with metastatic melanoma treated with pembrolizumab. *JAMA Dermatol.* 2016;152(1):45–51. doi:10.1001/jamadermatol.2015.2707

5. Weber JS, O'Day S, Urba W, et al. Phase I/II study of ipilimumab for patients with metastatic melanoma. *J Clin Oncol.* 2008;26(36):5950–5956. doi:10.1200/jco.2008.16.1927

6. Teulings HE, Limpens J, Jansen SN, et al. Vitiligo-like depigmentation in patients with stage III-IV melanoma receiving immunotherapy and its association with survival: a systematic review and meta-analysis. *J Clin Oncol.* 2015;33(7):773–781. doi:10.1200/jco.2014.57.4756

7. Postow MA, Sidlow R, Hellmann MD. Immune-related adverse events associated with immune checkpoint blockade. *N Engl J Med.* 2018;378(2):158–168. doi:10.1056/nejmra1703481

8. Curry JL, Tetzlaff MT, Nagarajan P, et al. Diverse types of dermatologic toxicities from immune checkpoint blockade therapy. *J Cutan Pathol.* 2017;44(2):158–176. doi:10.1111/cup.12858

9. Sibaud V, Meyer N, Lamant L, et al. Dermatologic complications of anti-PD-1/PD-L1 immune checkpoint antibodies. *Curr Opin Oncol.* 2016;28(4):254–263. doi:10.1097/cco.0000000000000290

10. Hoos A. Development of immuno-oncology drugs—from CTLA4 to PD1 to the next generations. *Nat Rev Drug Discov.* 2016;15(4):235–247. doi:10.1038/nrd.2015.35

11. Michot JM, Bigenwald C, Champiat S, et al. Immune-related adverse events with immune checkpoint blockade: a comprehensive review. *Eur J Cancer.* 2016;54:139–148. doi:10.1016/j.ejca.2015.11.016

12. Naidoo J, Schindler K, Querfeld C, et al. Autoimmune bullous skin disorders with Immune Checkpoint Inhibitors Targeting PD-1 and PD-L1. *Cancer Immunol Res.* 2016;4(5):383–389. doi:10.1158/2326-6066.cir-15-0123

13. Tanaka R, Okiyama N, Okune M, et al. Serum level of interleukin-6 is increased in nivolumab-associated psoriasiform dermatitis and tumor necrosis factor-alpha is a biomarker of nivolumab recativity. *J Dermatol Sci.* 2017;86(1):71–73. doi:10.1016/j.jdermsci.2016.12.019

14. Minkis K, Garden BC, Wu S, et al. The risk of rash associated with ipilimumab in patients with cancer: a systematic review of the literature and meta-analysis. *J Am Acad Dermatol.* 2013;69(3):e121–e128. doi:10.1016/j.jaad.2012.12.963

15. Sibaud V, Eid C, Belum VR, et al. Oral lichenoid reactions associated with anti-PD-1/PD-L1 therapies: clinicopathological findings. *J Eur Acad Dermatol Venereol.* 2017;31(10):e464–e469. doi:10.1111/jdv.14284

16. Kroschinsky F, Stolzel F, von Bonin S, et al. New drugs, new toxicities: severe side effects of modern targeted and immunotherapy of cancer and their management. *Crit Care.* 2017;21(1):89. doi:10.1186/s13054-017-1678-1

17. Zarbo A, Belum VR, Sibaud V, et al. Immune-related alopecia (areata and universalis) in cancer patients receiving immune checkpoint inhibitors. *Br J Dermatol.* 2017;176(6):1649–1652. doi:10.1111/bjd.15237

18. Tetzlaff MT, Nagarajan P, Chon S, et al. Lichenoid dermatologic toxicity from immune checkpoint blockade therapy: a detailed examination of the clinicopathologic features. *Am J Dermatopathol.* 2017;39(2):121–129. doi:10.1097/dad.0000000000000688

19. Larsabal M, Marti A, Jacquemin C, et al. Vitiligo-like lesions occurring in patients receiving anti-programmed cell death-1 therapies are clinically and biologically distinct from vitiligo. *J Am Acad Dermatol.* 2017;76(5):863–870. doi:10.1016/j.jaad.2016.10.044

20. Freites-Martinez A, Kwong BY, Rieger KE, et al. Eruptive keratoacanthomas associated with pembrolizumab therapy. *JAMA Dermatol.* 2017;153(7):694. doi:10.1001/jamadermatol.2017.0989

21. Collins LK, Chapman MS, Carter JB, Samie FH. Cutaneous adverse effects of the immune checkpoint inhibitors. *Curr Probl Cancer.* 2017;41(2):125–128. doi:10.1016/j.currproblcancer.2016.12.001

22. Wu J, Kwong BY, Martires KJ, et al. Granuloma annulare associated with immune checkpoint inhibitors. *J Eur Acad Dermatol Venereol.* 2017;32(4):e124–e126. doi:10.1111/jdv.14617

23. Lacouture ME, Wolchok JD, Yosipovitch G, et al. Ipilimumab in patients with cancer and the management of dermatologic adverse events. *J Am Acad Dermatol.* 2014;71(1):161–169. doi:10.1016/j.jaad.2014.02.035

24. Rosen AC, Case EC, Dusza SW, et al. Impact of dermatologic adverse events on quality of life in 283 cancer patients: a questionnaire study in a dermatology referral clinic. *Am J Clin Dermatol.* 2013;14(4):327–333. doi:10.1007/s40257-013-0021-0

25. Ensslin CJ, Rosen AC, Wu S, et al. Pruritus in patients treated with targeted cancer therapies: systematic review and meta-analysis. *J Am Acad Dermatol.* 2013;69(5):708–720. doi:10.1016/j.jaad.2013.06.038

26. Kini SP, DeLong LK, Veledar E, et al. The impact of pruritus on quality of life: the skin equivalent of pain. *Arch Dermatol.* 2011;147(10):1153–1156. doi:10.1001/archdermatol.2011.178

27. Weber JS, Dummer R, de Pril V, et al. Patterns of onset and resolution of immune-related adverse events of special interest with ipilimumab: detailed safety analysis from a phase 3 trial in patients with advanced melanoma. *Cancer.* 2013;119(9):1675–1682. doi:10.1002/cncr.27969

28. Nayar N, Briscoe K, Fernandez Penas P. Toxic epidermal necrolysis-like reaction with severe satellite cell necrosis associated with nivolumab in a patient with ipilimumab refractory metastatic melanoma. *J Immunother.* 2016;39(3):149–152. doi:10.1097/cji.0000000000000112

29. Goldinger SM, Stieger P, Meier B, et al. Cytotoxic cutaneous adverse drug reactions during anti-pd-1 therapy. *Clin Cancer Res.* 2016;22(16):4023–4029. doi:10.1158/1078-0432.ccr-15-2872

30. Weber JS, Kahler KC, Hauschild A. Management of immune-related adverse events and kinetics of response with ipilimumab. *J Clin Oncol.* 2012;30(21):2691–2697. doi:10.1200/jco.2012.41.6750

31. Chung WH, Wang CW, Dao RL. Severe cutaneous adverse drug reactions. *J Dermatol.* 2016;43(7):758–766. doi:10.1111/1346-8138.13430

32. Wu J, Lee YY, Su SC, et al. Stevens-Johnson syndrome and toxic epidermal necrolysis in patients with malignancies. *Br J Dermatol*. 2015;173(5):1224–1231. doi:10.1111/bjd.14052

33. Bastuji-Garin S, Fouchard N, Bertocchi M, et al. SCORTEN: a severity-of-illness score for toxic epidermal necrolysis. *J Invest Dermatol*. 2000;115(2):149–153. doi:10.1046/j.1523-1747.2000.00061.x

34. Mochel MC, Ming ME, Imadojemu S, et al. Cutaneous autoimmune effects in the setting of therapeutic immune checkpoint inhibition for metastatic melanoma. *J Cutan Pathol*. 2016;43(9):787–791. doi:10.1111/cup.12735

35. U.S. Department of Health and Human Services. Common Terminology Criteria for Adverse Events (CTCAE) Version 4.03. Bethesda, MD: National Institutes of Health. National Cancer Institute; 2010.

36. Puzanov I, Diab A, Abdallah K, et al. Managing toxicities associated with immune checkpoint inhibitors: consensus recommendations from the Society for Immunotherapy of Cancer (SITC) Toxicity Management Working Group. *J Immunother Cancer*. 2017;5(1). doi:10.1186/s40425-017-0300-z

37. Brahmer JR, Lacchetti C, Schneider BJ, et al. Management of immune-related adverse events in patients treated with immune checkpoint inhibitor therapy: American Society of Clinical Oncology Clinical Practice Guideline. *J Clin Oncol*. 2018;36(17):1714–1768.

38. Lacouture ME, Anadkat MJ, Bensadoun RJ, et al. Clinical practice guidelines for the prevention and treatment of EGFR inhibitor-associated dermatologic toxicities. *Support Care Cancer*. 2011;19(8):1079–1095. doi:10.1007/s00520-011-1197-6

39. de Golian E, Kwong BY, Swetter SM, et al. Cutaneous complications of targeted melanoma therapy. *Curr Treat Options Oncol*. 2016;17(11):57. doi:10.1007/s11864-016-0434-0

40. Melosky B, Leighl NB, Rothenstein J, et al. Management of egfr tki-induced dermatologic adverse events. *Curr Oncol*. 2015;22(2):123–132. doi:10.3747/co.22.2430

41. Bergman H, Walton T, Del Bel R, et al. Managing skin toxicities related to panitumumab. *J Am Acad Dermatol*. 2014;71(4):754–759. doi:10.1016/j.jaad.2014.06.011

42. Fischer A, Rosen AC, Ensslin CJ, et al. Pruritus to anticancer agents targeting the EGFR, BRAF, and CTLA-4. *Dermatol Ther*. 2013;26(2):135–148. doi:10.1111/dth.12027

43. Spain L, Diem S, Larkin J. Management of toxicities of immune checkpoint inhibitors. *Cancer Treat Rev*. 2016;44:51–60. doi:10.1016/j.ctrv.2016.02.001

44. Friedman CF, Proverbs-Singh TA, Postow MA. Treatment of the immune-related adverse effects of immune checkpoint inhibitors: a review. *JAMA Oncol*. 2016;2(10):1346–1353. doi:10.1001/jamaoncol.2016.1051

CHAPTER 6

MUSCULOSKELETAL AND RHEUMATOLOGIC TOXICITIES

Noha Abdel-Wahab, Clifton O. Bingham III, and Maria E. Suarez-Almazor

INTRODUCTION

Musculoskeletal and rheumatologic immune-related adverse events (irAEs) are increasingly being considered as potential adverse consequences from the use of immune checkpoint inhibitors (ICIs) in the treatment of cancer (1). Lack of recognition of these irAEs can represent a major challenge leading to a delay in their diagnosis and treatment (2,3). Hence, these events may significantly impact a patient's function and daily living activities, become chronic, and potentially result in irreversible end organ damage. Moreover, these events may require prolonged therapy with high-dose corticosteroids and other immunosuppressive therapies with the concern of dampening antitumor immunity (4). In order to prevent these harms, it is crucial for providers to promptly recognize the broad range of potential presenting symptoms, identify patients at increased risk, and adequately monitor and treat musculoskeletal and rheumatologic irAEs (1,5–7).

In this chapter, we will briefly review the epidemiology, known pathogenic mechanisms, clinical presentation, and management of the most common musculoskeletal and rheumatologic irAEs that occur in patients receiving ICI therapy. These include arthralgia, inflammatory arthritis, myositis, and polymyalgia-like syndromes. We will also highlight other rare rheumatologic and musculoskeletal irAEs that have been documented thus far in the literature. Finally, we will summarize the evidence on irAEs and worsening of underlying autoimmune conditions in those patients with preexisting rheumatologic diseases who receive ICI.

EPIDEMIOLOGY

Arthralgia is the most common musculoskeletal and rheumatologic irAE reported in 1% to 43% of patients across ICI clinical trials. Inflammatory arthritis is not as frequent, reported in 1% to 7% of participants in trials. Myalgia is the second most common musculoskeletal irAE reported in 2% to 21% of the clinical trial population (1). Inflammatory myopathies, including polymyositis, dermatomyositis, and necrotizing myositis, have been recently reported in small series and from the pharmacovigilance data of the U.S. Food and Drug Administration Adverse Events Reporting System (8,9). These irAEs have been more frequently reported in patients receiving anti–programmed cell death 1 (PD-1)/programmed cell death ligand 1 (PD-L1) agents and when nivolumab is given in combination with ipilimumab (2,8–11). Other rheumatologic events of interest that

Published by Springer Publishing Company DOI: 10.1891/9780826172150.0006

have been described include polymyalgia rheumatica, giant cell arteritis, vasculitis, Sjögren's syndrome with sicca symptoms and parotitis, lupus nephritis, sarcoidosis, and scleroderma, to name a few (6,12).

Of note, the true incidence of musculoskeletal and rheumatologic irAEs may be higher than what has been published as these events are likely to be underreported in oncology clinical trials, and usually there is no detailed description of the associated clinical, laboratory, and imaging data to truly determine the presence of inflammatory arthritis or other rheumatic irAEs. The Common Terminology Criteria for Adverse Events (CTCAE) v.4.03 that is currently used does not accurately characterize the myriad of rheumatic manifestations that can occur in patients developing irAEs (3). For instance, a swollen joint can be coded either as arthritis, joint effusion, joint pain, or joint function, and myopathy can be coded as myalgia, muscle weakness, or change in lower extremity function. Most often, only events of grade 3 or higher toxicity are reported in clinical trials. Moreover, rheumatic manifestations may not be perceived as severe because physicians may be more immediately concerned about life-threatening events rather than the more insidious effects on quality of life. Interestingly, musculoskeletal and rheumatologic irAEs are typically coded as grade 2 if they require corticosteroids, other immunomodulatory therapies, or limit instrumental activities of daily living (ADL) such as preparing meals, shopping, managing money, or using a telephone or transportation (13). However, from a rheumatology perspective, these adverse events (AEs) would be coded as grade 3 according to the Rheumatology Common Toxicity Criteria v.2.0, as they are considered to result in substantial functional limitations, affecting quality of life (14).

PATHOPHYSIOLOGY

The pathogenic mechanisms of irAEs in patients receiving ICI therapy are not completely understood. Treatment with ICI enhance T helper 1 (Th1) and T helper 17 (Th17) responses with augmented production of pro-inflammatory cytokines such as interleukin (IL)-1, IL-6, IL-8, IL-12, IL-17, tumor necrosis factor-α (TNFα), and interferon-γ (IFNγ) (15,16). While Th1 and CD8+ T-cells are instrumental in antitumor immunity, Th17 pathways are more complex and have paradoxical effects, and likely contribute to the inflammatory and autoimmune events arising from ICI therapy (17). Notably, an altered regulatory T-cell (Treg)/Th17 axis plays a role in the development of several autoimmune diseases (18–23), and also in ICI-induced colitis (24). T-cell dysregulation and subsequent augmented production of IL-6 and other pro-inflammatory cytokines might contribute to the development of irAEs in patients receiving ICI therapy. Patients with ICI-induced inflammatory arthritis have disease patterns similar to those observed in rheumatoid arthritis (RA) or spondyloarthropathies, diseases with Th17 cell upregulation (2,10,25). IL-6 stimulates induction of Th17, and IL-6 inhibition could re-balance the altered Treg/Th17 axis without inhibiting Th1-CD8+ T-cell subsets (20,26). Tocilizumab, an anti-IL-6 receptor antibody, has been used in a few patients with ICI-induced inflammatory arthritis leading to a significant improvement (10,27).

Similarly, anti-TNFα therapies have also been effective for ICI arthritis, possibly through a direct mechanism of action on Th1 responses, or indirectly by decreasing IL-6 and subsequent Th17 activation (25). The role of B cells on ICI-induced rheumatic AEs has not been well defined, but some patients have developed autoantibodies such as rheumatoid factor (RF), antinuclear antibodies (ANAs), anti-SSA, or SSB (10,25).

The genetic background of patients receiving ICI therapy may play a role in susceptibility to irAEs. Many patients develop profound multisystem inflammatory and irAEs, while others develop irAE limited to one organ, or may never develop toxicity despite continuous checkpoint inhibition (28). Mutations in cytotoxic T-lymphocyte antigen 4 (CTLA-4) and PD-1 have been previously linked to a number of autoimmune diseases. Mice with a genetically engineered CTLA-4 deletion on Tregs die from massive T-lymphocyte proliferation and inflammation (29). On the other hand, PD-1/PD-L1 knockout mice have higher risk of developing inflammatory and autoimmune diseases but are less likely to die (30). In humans, single nucleotide polymorphisms in certain CTLA-4 and PD-1 alleles have been identified as susceptibility genetic markers for various rheumatic autoimmune diseases including RA, ankylosing spondylitis, and systemic lupus erythematosus (31–38). Nevertheless, the functional consequences of associated genes in these diseases are not fully understood. With respect to ICI-induced inflammatory arthritis, some patients present with typical seropositive RA, suggesting a prior pre-RA status that manifests clinically after receiving ICI (39). Retrospective evaluation of serum samples collected in these patients before starting ICI revealed positive antibodies against citric citrullinated peptide (anti-CCP) in two out of three patients, although none had preexisting clinical symptoms before treatment. Another patient with ICI-induced polymyositis associated with myasthenia gravis was found to have preexisting positive anti-acetylcholine receptor antibodies detected in a sample collected before starting ICI (40). Similar observations have been reported in patients with cryoglobulinemic vasculitis, Sjögren's syndrome, and a few other autoimmune diseases that manifested clinically after initiation of ICI therapy (41–45).

INFLAMMATORY ARTHRITIS

Clinical Presentation

Patients may initially complain of arthralgia (joint pain) with or without joint stiffness that can rapidly progress to overt synovitis. Joint stiffness typically occurs in the morning or after a period of rest or inactivity, lasts a minimum of 30 to 60 minutes, and improves with activity. Physical examination shows joint tenderness and swelling, and can present with erythema and warmth in surrounding soft tissues and limitation in the range of motion. Inflammation along adjacent tendons and at tendinous insertions into bone (enthesitis) may also be seen. Inflammatory arthritis can occur at any time after initiation of ICI. A few of the reported patients developed arthritis immediately after the first dose, while others developed arthritis as a late effect, in one case after 44 months of treatment initiation (10). Arthritis may be the sole irAE, but is often associated with other irAEs (2,10,46). It may persist after discontinuation of ICI, significantly limiting patients' function and quality of life. Persistence of arthritis for up to two years, requiring ongoing immunomodulatory therapy, has been reported (7).

Several patterns of ICI-induced inflammatory arthritis have been reported (10,46) (Table 6.1).

- Seronegative oligoarthritis/polyarthritis of medium-to-large joints. These patients present with arthritis of larger joints such as knees, ankles, or wrists, in some cases resembling reactive arthritis. The arthritis can present in a symmetric or asymmetric distribution. RF and anti-CCP are generally negative. Some patients may have positive ANA. At presentation, most cases will have normal radiographs, but persistent inflammation can result in erosive disease. Occasionally, patients may develop extra-articular features of reactive arthritis such as conjunctivitis or urethritis.
- Seronegative spondyloarthropathy. In addition to oligo/polyarthritis, some patients present with inflammatory back pain or cervical pain. These patients can develop enthesitis with pain and tenderness in areas such as the heel or iliac crest. Patients with primary spondyloarthritis often carry human leukocyte antigen (HLA) B27 alleles; however, the few patients that have been tested with ICI-induced arthritis were B27 negative.
- RA-like. Patients may present with symmetrical polyarthritis, predominantly involving small joints of the hands and wrists, along with larger joints. RF, anti-CCP antibodies, and/or ANA may be present in their sera. This pattern of arthritis is potentially erosive, leading to permanent joint damage.

Evaluation and Management

At presentation, clinicians should confirm that symptoms started after receiving ICI therapy and exclude any preexisting rheumatic condition that could account for similar symptoms (5). Differential diagnoses include other joint diseases such as osteoarthritis, crystal-induced arthropathy, soft tissue regional syndromes, and metastatic disease within adjacent bone or joint structures (47). Septic arthritis needs to be excluded in patients with monoarthritis, especially if there are accompanying risk factors such as infection in other organs, fever, or neutrophilia.

The Society for Immunotherapy of Cancer (SITC) Toxicity Management Working Group (3) and the American Society of Clinical Oncology (ASCO) have published recommendations for managing ICI-induced inflammatory arthritis according to the CTCAE grade, which are summarized in the following Diagnostic Evaluation and Treatment sections(48). Erosive and irreversible joint damage have been reported in few patients with ICI-induced inflammatory arthritis within a few weeks of symptoms onset, and therefore a rheumatology consult is

TABLE 6.1 Reported Cases of Muscle and Joint Toxicity After Immune Checkpoint Inhibitor Use

Toxicity	Clinical presentation	Diagnostic evaluation	Treatment
Inflammatory Arthritis	Seronegative oligoarthritis/ polyarthritis (Rheumatoid factor and anti-CCP are generally negative) Seronegative spondyloarthropathy Rheumatoid arthritis-like (RF, anti-CCP antibodies, and/or ANA may be positive)	Structure: Radiography, musculoskeletal ultrasound, MRI Inflammation: ESR, CRP Autoimmune: ANA, RF, anti-CCP Seronegative spondyloarthropathy: HLA-B27	Grade 1: Continue ICI therapy. Analgesia: acetaminophen/NSAIDs Grade 2: Hold ICI therapy. Oral prednisone or equivalent: 10 to 20 mg/day for 4 weeks Arthrocentesis and intra-articular injection of corticosteroids if ≤ 2 large joints. Resume ICI after resolution of symptoms while on prednisone ≤ 10 mg/day. Grade 3 & 4: Hold ICI therapy. Oral prednisone or equivalent: 0.5 to 1 mg/kg/day for 4 weeks. Synthetic DMARDs: MTX, sulfasalazine, hydroxychloroquine, leflunomide. Biologic DMARDs: infliximab, anti-TNF antibody, or tocilizumab (not with colitis).
Inflammatory Myositis	Myositis alone is the most common, occasionally severe necrotizing myositis with rhabdomyolysis. Dermatomyositis with skin rash, including Gottron's papules	CK AST, ALT, LDH also elevated Inflammatory markers: ESR, CRP Troponin Myositis autoimmune pane EMG, nerve conduction MRI Muscle biopsy Echocardiogram	Grade 1: Continue ICI therapy. Analgesia: acetaminophen/NSAIDs Grade 2: Hold ICI therapy. Acetaminophen/NSAIDs. Oral prednisone or equivalent: 0.5 to 1 mg/kg/day if CK level 3x higher than normal. Resume ICI after resolution of symptoms and normalization of CK level while on prednisone ≤ 10 mg/day. May discontinue ICI permanently with elevated enzymes, abnormal muscle findings in EMG, MRI, or muscle biopsy. Discontinue ICI permanently if there is myocardial involvement. Grade 3 & 4: Hold ICI therapy. Oral prednisone or equivalent: 1 mg/ kg/day. Intravenous pulse methylprednisolone: 1 to 2 mg/kg. IVIG. Synthetic DMARDs: MTX, azathioprine, or mycophenolate mofetil. Biologic DMARDs: Rituximab, anti-CD20 chimeric antibody. Resume ICI if symptoms improve to grade 1. Discontinue ICI permanently if there is myocardial involvement. Hospitalization for severe weakness and life-threatening complications.

(continued)

TABLE 6.1 Reported Cases of Muscle and Joint Toxicity After Immune Checkpoint Inhibitor Use (*continued*)

Toxicity	Clinical presentation	Diagnostic evaluation	Treatment
Polymyalgia Rheumatica-like Syndrome	Physical examination: normal muscle strength, only limited by pain, typically without joint swelling. Some may have effusions in proximal large joints, which can be seen by ultrasound or MRI. Inflammatory markers are highly elevated with negative RF and anti-CCP antibodies, and normal CK levels.	CK Inflammatory markers: ESR, CRP Autoimmune: ANA, RF, anti-CCP Referral to ophthalmology if the patient complains of headache or visual disturbances, and consider temporal artery biopsy.	Grade 1: Continue ICI therapy. Analgesia: acetaminophen/NSAIDs Grade 2: Hold ICI therapy. Oral prednisone or equivalent: 20 mg/day. Resume ICI after resolution of symptoms while on prednisone ≤10 mg/day. Grade 3 & 4: Hold ICI therapy. Oral prednisone or equivalent: 20 mg/day. Synthetic DMARDs: MTX. Biologic DMARDs: Tocilizumab. Consider hospital admission for pain management in severe cases.

ALT, alanine transaminase; ANA, antinuclear antibodies; AST, aspartate transaminase; CCP, citric citrullinated peptide; CK, creatine-kinase; CRP, C-reactive protein; DMARDs, disease-modifying anti-rheumatic drugs; EMG, electromyography; ESR, erythrocyte sedimentation rate; ICI, immune checkpoint inhibitors; IVIG, Intravenous immunoglobulin; LDH, lactate dehydrogenase; MTX, methotrexate; NSAIDs, nonsteroidal anti-inflammatory drugs; RF, rheumatoid factor; TNF, tumor necrosis factor.

recommended if arthritis ≥ grade 2, joint pain persists more than 4 weeks, there is evidence of joint swelling (synovitis), or if the patient has not been able to taper corticosteroids to less than 10 mg/day within 4 weeks. A rheumatology consult early on is essential to confirm the diagnosis of inflammatory arthritis, exclude other rheumatic disorders, identify early signs of joint damage, assess the need for arthrocentesis and intra-articular injection of corticosteroids, and evaluate the need for initiation and optimal dosing of disease-modifying anti-rheumatic drugs (DMARDs).

Diagnostic Evaluation

All patients should undergo complete rheumatologic history, physical examination (including peripheral and axial joints and the spine), and functional assessment (Table 6.1).

- Imaging can be performed to clarify diagnoses and to assess structural involvement. Radiographs of the affected joints can evaluate joint damage, especially erosions and joint space narrowing. Musculoskeletal ultrasound and/or MRI are more sensitive than plain radiography in detecting synovitis, inflammatory signals, tendinopathies and enthesitis, and erosions.
- Laboratory testing should include:
  - Markers of inflammation: Erythrocyte sedimentation rate (ESR) and C-reactive protein (CRP) if inflammatory symptoms persist.
  - Autoimmune panel: ANA, RF, and anti-CCP if inflammatory symptoms persist.
  - HLA-B27 if the pattern of arthritis mimics seronegative spondyloarthropathy or reactive arthritis.

Early referral to rheumatology is recommended. The course of arthritis should be monitored with periodic clinical assessments every 2 to 4 weeks until resolution, and including joint examination and evaluation of inflammatory markers (ESR and/or CRP). Patients should be tested for hepatitis B and C, HIV, and tuberculosis, as they may require immunosuppressive therapy that can reactivate latent infectious diseases.

Treatment

Grade 1: Mild joint pain with signs of inflammation, erythema, or joint swelling. No functional impact on ADL (Table 6.1).

- Continue ICI therapy.
- Analgesia: acetaminophen or nonsteroidal anti-inflammatory drugs (NSAIDs) if there are no contraindications.
- Escalate to grade 2 management if there is no improvement within 4 weeks.

Grade 2: Moderate joint pain with signs of inflammation, erythema, or joint swelling. Functional limitations in ADL, not interfering with self-care.

- Hold ICI therapy.
- Oral prednisone or equivalent: 10 to 20 mg/day for 4 weeks, and taper slowly over 4 to 6 weeks if symptoms improved.

- May offer arthrocentesis and intra-articular injection of corticosteroids if ≤ 2 large joints are involved.
- Resume ICI after resolution of symptoms, while on prednisone ≤ 10 mg/day.
- Escalate to grade 3 management if there is no improvement after 4 to 6 weeks, or unable to withdraw prednisone to 10 mg/day after 3 months.

Grade 3/4: Severe joint pain with signs of inflammation, erythema, or joint swelling. Functional limitations in self-care ADL. Imaging can show joint damage.

- Hold ICI therapy.
- Oral prednisone or equivalent: 0.5 to 1 mg/kg/day for 4 weeks, and taper slowly over 4 to 6 weeks if symptoms improved.
- Add DMARDs: If there is no improvement after 4 weeks or worsening of the symptoms in the meantime.
  - Synthetic DMARDs: oral low-dose methotrexate (MTX) is most commonly used at a dose between 15 and 25 mg once a week plus folic acid supplementation daily. Subcutaneous or intramuscular weekly MTX can also be considered. Other synthetic DMARDs that may be used include: sulfasalazine, hydroxychloroquine, or leflunomide.
  - Biological DMARDs: infliximab, an anti-TNF monoclonal antibody, has been used for many other irAEs such as colitis, pneumonitis, or ocular toxicity. Unlike colitis, which resolves quickly with infliximab, inflammatory arthritis may require prolonged anti-TNF therapy and it is unclear whether long-term therapy may dampen ICI antitumor immunity (4). Tocilizumab is another treatment option, but it might not be the most appropriate agent in patients with colitis or gastrointestinal disease given the potential risk of intestinal perforation, although isolated case reports have not shown complications in patients receiving ICI and tocilizumab for irAEs, and who also had colitis or inflammatory bowel disease (27,49) To date, there is no experience with the use of other targeted biological agents for ICI-induced arthritis.

Treatment with ICI can be resumed if arthritis improves to grade 1. If there is no improvement of arthritis with treatment after 4 to 6 weeks, ICI should be discontinued permanently.

INFLAMMATORY MYOSITIS

Clinical Presentation

Myositis is a rare complication of ICI therapy that can be severe and occasionally fatal. It generally occurs early after starting treatment, and has been primarily reported in patients receiving anti-PD1 agents or combination therapy. Patients complain of weakness, occasionally with myalgia, and have difficulty lifting their arms above their head, standing up, and walking; if severe, they may develop dysphagia, hoarseness, and difficulty breathing. Severe myositis can cause myocarditis, a potentially fatal complication, associated in a few cases with third degree atrioventricular heart block. Acute rhabdomyolysis has also been reported. On physical examination, patients have primarily proximal muscle weakness of the upper and lower extremities and neck flexor weakness. Resolution of myositis with treatment has been reported, but myositis leading to death has also been reported (9,50–55). ICI-induced inflammatory myositis typically occur as one of the following patterns (Table 6.1):

- Myositis alone is the most common pattern seen in clinical practice, only affecting muscle, without accompanying rash and can occasionally present as severe necrotizing myositis with rhabdomyolysis.
- Dermatomyositis has been also reported in a few cases either as a reactivation of preexisting paraneoplastic disease (9) or as a de novo irAE (56). In those patients, muscle weakness was associated with skin rash including Gottron's papules over the dorsal aspects of the metacarpophalangeal and interphalangeal joints, ragged cuticles and abnormal nailfolds, heliotropic rash and edema of the upper eyelids, facial erythema crossing the nasolabial folds, erythema of the neck and upper chest (V-neck sign) or the upper back (shawl sign), or lateral thighs (holster sign).

Evaluation and Management

Clinicians should confirm that symptoms started after receiving ICI therapy and exclude any preexisting rheumatic condition that can cause similar symptoms, such as prior paraneoplastic myositis (5). Differential diagnosis includes other causes of muscle weakness such as muscular dystrophy, drug-induced myopathy (e.g., prior use of statin or corticosteroids), neurological syndromes, and hormonal disorders such as hypothyroidism or adrenal insufficiency, which can also occur as irAE. Myositis causes primarily muscle weakness and should be differentiated from diseases associated predominantly with myalgia or muscle pain, such as fibromyalgia or polymyalgia rheumatica. A summary of the ASCO guidelines for managing ICI-induced myositis follows (48).

Because myositis can be a life-threatening irAE, an early rheumatology or neurology consult is needed promptly for any patient receiving ICI in whom myositis is suspected.

Diagnostic Evaluation

All patients should undergo a thorough history and physical examination, including assessment of muscle strength for major muscle groups, neurological examination, and skin inspection for dermatomyositis rash (Table 6.1).

- Laboratory testing should include:
  - Creatine-kinase (CK). Aldolase, aspartate transaminase (AST), alanine transaminase (ALT), and lactate dehydrogenase (LDH) are also typically elevated, but CK is the most common laboratory test used to monitor disease activity.
  - Markers of inflammation: ESR and CRP.

- ○ Troponin: To evaluate myocardial involvement.
- ○ Myositis autoimmune panel can help determine whether the patient may have a paraneoplastic myositis. However, it is not clear that commonly tested specific autoantibodies associated with primary or paraneoplastic myositis have a role in ICI-induced myositis.
- ○ Other paraneoplastic autoantibodies to evaluate neurological disorders such as myasthenia-like syndromes, which can occur as irAE or as a paraneoplastic disease.
- Electromyography (EMG) and nerve conduction studies can be conducted to differentiate between muscular and neurological causes of weakness. Muscle fibrillation is a typical finding in myopathy.
- Imaging with MRI can be performed in cases where diagnosis is unclear, or when a biopsy is needed to locate areas with inflammatory changes. Affected areas show edema and increased intensity.
- Muscle biopsy may not be necessary for management but could be useful in cases with diagnostic uncertainty, especially if the CK is only mildly elevated, as this can be seen with neurological syndromes.
- Echocardiogram should be performed if myocarditis is suspected.

The course of myositis should be monitored according to severity, and until resolution, every 2 to 4 weeks, with clinical and laboratory evaluations including muscle strength, CK, and inflammatory markers such as ESR and CRP. As for arthritis, patients should be screened for hepatitis B, C, HIV, and tuberculosis before initiating immunosuppression.

Treatment

Grade 1: Mild weakness with or without pain (Table 6.1).

- Continue ICI therapy.
- Analgesia with acetaminophen or NSAIDs as needed if there is no contraindication.
- Escalate to grade 2 management if the patient has muscle weakness with elevated CK.

Grade 2: Moderate weakness with or without pain, and limitation in instrumental ADL.

- Hold ICI therapy.
- Acetaminophen or NSAIDs for muscle pain as needed.
- Oral prednisone or equivalent: 0.5 to 1 mg/kg/day if CK level is elevated three times higher than normal.
- Resume ICI after resolution of symptoms and normalization of CK level, while on prednisone ≤ 10 mg/day.
- May discontinue ICI permanently in patients with elevated enzymes, abnormal muscle findings in EMG, MRI, or muscle biopsy.
- Discontinue ICI permanently if there is myocardial involvement.
- Escalate to grade 3 management if there is no improvement.

Grade 3/4: Severe muscle pain and weakness, with limitation in self-care ADL.

- Hospitalization for severe weakness and life-threatening complications.
- Hold ICI therapy.
- Oral prednisone or equivalent: 1 mg/kg/day until symptoms improve to grade 1, and then slowly taper over 4 to 6 weeks.
- Intravenous pulse methylprednisolone: 1 to 2 mg/kg or higher-dose bolus if the patient has dysphagia, cardiac, respiratory, or severe muscle weakness, limiting mobility.
- Plasmapheresis can be considered if there is no adequate response to corticosteroids and patient presents with life-threatening complications.
- Intravenous immunoglobulin (IVIG) therapy may be considered.
- DMARDs may be considered if there is no improvement after 4 to 6 weeks or worsening of the symptoms and laboratory findings in the meantime, but their onset of action is slower that plasmapheresis or IVIG therapy.
  - Synthetic DMARDs: MTX, azathioprine, or mycophenolate mofetil.
  - Biological DMARDs: Rituximab, an anti-CD20 chimeric monoclonal antibody, is typically used for primary polymyositis or dermatomyositis. However, caution is recommended in patients with cancer receiving ICI therapy because of its long biological duration.
- Resume ICI if symptoms improve to grade 1 and the patient is weaned off immunosuppressive therapies.
- Discontinue ICI permanently if there is myocardial involvement.

POLYMYALGIA RHEUMATICA-LIKE SYNDROME

Clinical Presentation

Patients present with symptoms typical of polymyalgia rheumatica with marked myalgia in the proximal muscles of the upper and lower extremities, arthralgia, morning stiffness, and fatigue (39,57–59). Physical examination shows normal muscle strength, only limited by pain, and typically without joint swelling (Table 6.1). Some patients may have effusions in proximal large joints (shoulders and/or hips), which can be seen by ultrasound or MRI. Inflammatory markers are highly elevated, with negative RF and anti-CCP antibodies, and normal CK levels. No evidence of muscle inflammation or myopathy is found in MRI, EMG, or histology.

Evaluation and Management

Patients with polymyalgia-like symptoms complain primarily of pain, do not have objective weakness, and their CK is normal, which distinguishes them from patients with myositis. Other causes of myalgia should be excluded such as fibromyalgia, statin-induced myopathy, and other possible causes of arthritis and soft tissue rheumatism causing widespread proximal pain. A prompt rheumatology consultation is recommended to evaluate differential diagnoses, especially myositis. If a patient complains of temporal headache, visual disturbance, or jaw claudication, then giant cell arteritis, a condition associated with polymyalgia rheumatica needs to be considered, as this has been previously reported in patients receiving ipilimumab (60). These patients will require urgent ophthalmological examination and temporal artery biopsy, as this form of vasculitis can result in permanent blindness, which can rapidly develop. Recommendations by ASCO for managing ICI-induced, polymyalgia-like syndromes according to CTCAE grade are summarized in the following Diagnostice Evaluation and Treatment sections (48).

Diagnostic Evaluation

Patients should undergo a thorough rheumatologic examination, including assessment of muscle strength (Table 6.1).

- Laboratory testing should include: CK to evaluate possible myositis, inflammatory markers (ESR and CRP), and RF, anti-CCP, and ANA to evaluate other rheumatic differential diagnoses.
- Referral to ophthalmology if the patient complains of headache or visual disturbances, and consider temporal artery biopsy.

Imaging, EMG, and muscle biopsy are generally not needed unless there is diagnostic uncertainty.

Patients should be evaluated every 4 weeks until symptoms improve, monitoring therapeutic response with serial testing of inflammatory markers.

Treatment

Grade 1: Mild muscle pain and stiffness, no weakness (Table 6.1).

- Continue ICI therapy.
- Analgesia: acetaminophen or NSAIDs if there is no contraindication.

Grade 2: Moderate muscle pain and stiffness, no weakness. Limitation in instrumental ADL.

- Hold ICI therapy.
- Oral prednisone or equivalent: 20 mg/day until symptoms improve, and then slowly taper after 3 to 4 weeks.
- Resume ICI after resolution of symptoms, while on prednisone ≤ 10 mg.
- Escalate to grade 3 management if there is no improvement or requirement of higher dose of prednisone after 4 weeks.

Grade 3/4: Severe muscle pain and stiffness, but no weakness. Limitation in self-care ADL.

- Hold ICI therapy.
- Oral prednisone or equivalent: 20 mg/day until symptoms improve, and then slowly taper after 3 to 4 weeks.
- DMARDs may be considered as steroid-sparing drugs: If no improvement or required higher doses of prednisone for prolonged time.
  - Synthetic DMARDs: MTX.
  - Biological DMARDs: Tocilizumab is an effective treatment for giant cell arteritis, a condition associated with polymyalgia rheumatica.

Although there is no experience in polymyalgia-like irAE, and it is not approved for this indication, tocilizumab could potentially be effective.

- Can consider hospital admission for pain management in severe cases.

Patients can resume ICI if symptoms improve to grade 1. Recurrence of symptoms has been reported upon resuming therapy in some patients.

OTHER RHEUMATOLOGIC AND MUSCULOSKELETAL AEs

Sicca symptoms (dry eyes and mouth) have been reported in patients with ICI, with or without accompanying arthritis (25). Positive anti-Ro/SSA or anti-La/SSB antibodies have occasionally been identified. Caution must be exercised as many patients may report symptoms of dryness that can be attributed to the use of other commonly used chemotherapeutic agents (61).

Other rheumatologic irAEs that have been occasionally reported include: vasculitis of single organs (retina and uterus), lupus nephritis, sarcoidosis, scleroderma, remitting seronegative symmetrical synovitis with pitting edema syndrome, and eosinophilic fasciitis (1,6,12,60,62–66).

If any of these rare irAEs are suspected, a rheumatology consult is highly recommended for further evaluation and management, even if the patient complains of only mild symptoms, in order to prevent potential permanent organ damage (3,48). Guidelines for management for these syndromes when presenting as irAE are not available, but the general principles for more common irAE discussed before can be applied.

PATIENTS WITH PREEXISTING AUTOIMMUNE DISEASES RECEIVING ICI THERAPY

The presence of preexisting autoimmune disease in a patient with cancer should not, per se, be an absolute contraindication for ICI therapy. Those patients may be at higher risk of toxicity, but the available evidence suggests that much of the risk relates to flares and worsening of the preexisting autoimmune disease status, not necessarily to an increased incidence of de novo irAEs (5). Half of the reported patients in the literature had an exacerbation of their underlying autoimmune disease when receiving ICIs, while more than one-third had de novo irAEs, with colitis and hypophysitis being the most common, similar to what has been reported in trials. More flares of underlying autoimmune disease were reported with anti–PD-1/PD-L1 agents. Although the frequency of de novo irAEs may be similar in patients with or without autoimmune disease, they might be more severe in those with autoimmune disease, resulting in death from a serious AE in 2.4% of patients. No difference in the frequency of AEs was observed in patients with active versus inactive preexisting autoimmune disease at initiation of ICI. No clear evidence is currently available as to whether maintenance immunosuppressive treatment in those patients at initiation of ICI might have a protective effect on exacerbations of the preexisting autoimmune disease.

The guidelines for management of those patients are mostly similar to the aforementioned ICI musculoskeletal and rheumatologic irAEs, but the decision to initiate ICI therapy requires a multidisciplinary approach to weigh carefully the benefits and risks taking into account the prognosis of cancer, alternative effective therapies beyond ICI, severity of the underlying autoimmune disease, and the patient's preferences and tolerance for different risks. Close monitoring is required as most patients will need concomitant immunosuppressive therapy once they develop an irAE or flare. They may be able to continue ICI therapy or may require holding ICI until their irAEs are successfully managed, or permanent discontinuation, depending on the severity of the clinical manifestations and life-threatening risks.

CONCLUSION

The authors have provided expert opinion on the management of a wide range of musculoskeletal and rheumatologic side effects associated with ICI treatments. They rightly point out that the incidence of these side effects is likely to be underreported as mild degrees of muscle aches and joint stiffness are quite frequent and often overlooked. At the other extreme, symptoms can be so severe and debilitating that they take over in importance in patient management. In these cases, consults with specialist physicians skilled in their management becomes critical to achieve the best symptomatic and anticancer outcomes. This is particularly important for treatment with the many new biologic agents that are under study in treatment of these side effects particularly as they may have their own spectrum of side effects.

REFERENCES

1. Cappelli LC, Gutierrez AK, Bingham CO 3rd, et al. Rheumatic and musculoskeletal immune-related adverse events due to immune checkpoint inhibitors: a systematic review of the literature. *Arthritis Care Res*. 2016;69(11):1751–1763. doi:10.1002/acr.23177

2. Cappelli LC, Brahmer JR, Forde PM, et al. Clinical presentation of immune checkpoint inhibitor-induced inflammatory arthritis differs by immunotherapy regimen. *Semin Arthritis Rheum*. 2018;48(3):553–557. doi:10.1016/j.semarthrit.2018.02.011

3. Puzanov I, Diab A, Abdallah K, et al. Managing toxicities associated with immune checkpoint inhibitors: consensus recommendations from the Society for Immunotherapy of Cancer (SITC) Toxicity Management Working Group. *J Immunother Cancer*. 2017;5(1):95. doi:10.1186/s40425-017-0300-z

4. Calzascia T, Pellegrini M, Hall H, et al. TNF-alpha is critical for antitumor but not antiviral T cell immunity in mice. *J Clin Invest*. 2007;117(12):3833–3845.

5. Abdel-Wahab N, Shah M, Lopez-Olivo MA, et al. Use of immune checkpoint inhibitors in the treatment of patients with cancer and preexisting autoimmune disease: a systematic review. *Ann Intern Med*. 2018;168(2):121. doi:10.7326/m17-2073

6. Abdel-Wahab N, Shah M, Suarez-Almazor ME. Adverse events associated with immune checkpoint blockade in patients with cancer: a systematic review of case reports. *PLoS ONE*. 2016;11(7):e0160221. doi:10.1371/journal.pone.0160221

7. Calabrese L, Velcheti V. Checkpoint immunotherapy: good for cancer therapy, bad for rheumatic diseases. *Ann Rheum Dis*. 2016;76(1):1–3. doi:10.1136/annrheumdis-2016-209782

8. Pundole X, Shah M, Abdel-Wahab N, et al. Immune checkpoint inhibitors and inflammatory myopathies: data from the US Food and Drug Administration Adverse Event Reporting System. *Arthritis Rheumatol*. 2017;69(10):1192–1193.

9. Shah M, Tayar J, Abdel-Wahab N, et al. Myositis as a complication of checkpoint blockade at a comprehensive cancer center. *Arthritis Rheumatol*. 2017;69(10):3030–3030.

10. Abdel-Wahab N, Tayar JH, Diab A, et al. Inflammatory arthritis induced by the use of checkpoint inhibitors for immunotherapy of cancer. *J Immunother Cancer*. 2017;5(2):215–215.

11. Suarez-Almazor ME, Kim ST, Abdel-Wahab N, et al. Review: immune-related adverse events with use of checkpoint inhibitors for immunotherapy of cancer. *Arthritis Rheumatol*. 2017;69(4):687–699. doi:10.1002/art.40043

12. Barbosa NS, Wetter DA, Wieland CN, et al. Scleroderma induced by pembrolizumab: a case series. *Mayo Clin Proc*. 2017;92(7):1158–1163. doi:10.1016/j.mayocp.2017.03.016

13. U.S. Department of Health and Human Services. Common Terminology Criteria for Adverse Events (CTCAE) Version 4.03. 2010. http://www.hrc.govt.nz/sites/default/files/CTCAE%20manual%20-%20DMCC.pdf

14. Woodworth T, Furst DE, Alten R, et al. Standardizing assessment and reporting of adverse effects in rheumatology clinical trials II: the Rheumatology Common Toxicity Criteria v.2.0. *J Rheumatol*. 2007;34(6):1401–1414.

15. Dulos J, Carven GJ, van Boxtel SJ, et al. PD-1 blockade augments Th1 and Th17 and suppresses Th2 responses in peripheral blood from patients with prostate and advanced melanoma cancer. *J Immunother*. 2012;35(2):169–178. doi:10.1097/cji.0b013e318247a4e7

16. von Euw E, Chodon T, Attar N, et al. CTLA4 blockade increases Th17 cells in patients with metastatic melanoma. *J Transl Med*. 2009;7:35. doi:10.1186/1479-5876-7-35

17. Bailey SR, Nelson MH, Himes RA, et al. Th17 cells in cancer: the ultimate identity crisis. *Front. Immunol*. 2014;5:276. doi:10.3389/fimmu.2014.00276

18. Gracey E, Qaiyum Z, Almaghlouth I, et al. IL-7 primes IL-17 in mucosal-associated invariant T (MAIT) cells, which contribute to the Th17-axis in ankylosing spondylitis. *Ann Rheum Dis*. 2016;75(12):2124–2132. doi:10.1136/annrheumdis-2015-208902

19. Karczewski J, Dobrowolska A, Rychlewska-Hanczewska A, et al. New insights into the role of T cells in pathogenesis of psoriasis and psoriatic arthritis. *Autoimmunity*. 2016;49(7):435–450. doi:10.3109/08916934.2016.1166214

20. Kimura A, Kishimoto T. IL-6: regulator of Treg/Th17 balance. *Eur J Immunol*. 2010;40(7):1830–1835. doi:10.1002/eji.201040391

21. Noack M, Miossec P. Th17 and regulatory T cell balance in autoimmune and inflammatory diseases. *Autoimmun Rev*. 2014;13(6):668–677. doi:10.1016/j.autrev.2013.12.004

22. Raychaudhuri SP, Raychaudhuri SK. IL-23/IL-17 axis in spondyloarthritis-bench to bedside. *Clin Rheumatol*. 2016;35(6):1437–1441. doi:10.1007/s10067-016-3263-4

23. Yang J, Sundrud MS, Skepner J, et al. Targeting Th17 cells in autoimmune diseases. *Trends Pharmacol Sci*. 2014;35(10):493–500. doi:10.1016/j.tips.2014.07.006

24. Callahan MK, Yang A, Tandon S, et al. Evaluation of serum IL-17 levels during ipilimumab therapy: correlation with colitis. *J Clin Oncol*. 2011;29(15). doi:10.1200/jco.2011.29.15_suppl.2505

25. Cappelli LC, Gutierrez AK, Baer AN, et al. Inflammatory arthritis and sicca syndrome induced by nivolumab and ipilimumab. *Ann Rheum Dis*. 2016;76(1):43–50. doi:10.1136/annrheumdis-2016-209595

26. Diehl S, Rincon M. The two faces of IL-6 on Th1/Th2 differentiation. *Mol Immunol*. 2002;39(9):531–536. doi:10.1016/s0161-5890(02)00210-9

27. Kim ST, Tayar J, Trinh VA, et al. Successful treatment of arthritis induced by checkpoint inhibitors with tocilizumab: a case series. *Ann Rheum Dis*. 2017;76(12):2061–2064. doi:10.1136/annrheumdis-2017-211560

28. Weber JS, Kudchadkar RR, Yu B, et al. Safety, efficacy, and biomarkers of nivolumab with vaccine in ipilimumab-refractory or -naive melanoma. *J Clin Oncol*. 2013;31(34):4311–4318. doi:10.1200/jco.2013.51.4802

29. Wing K, Onishi Y, Prieto-Martin P, et al. CTLA-4 control over Foxp3+ regulatory T cell function. *Science*. 2008;322(5899):271–275. doi:10.1126/science.1160062

30. Okazaki T, Honjo T. The PD-1-PD-L pathway in immunological tolerance. *Trends Immunol*. 2006;27(4):195–201. doi:10.1016/j.it.2006.02.001

31. Barreto M, Santos E, Ferreira R, et al. Evidence for CTLA4 as a susceptibility gene for systemic lupus erythematosus. *Eur J Hum Genet*. 2004;12(8):620–626. doi:10.1038/sj.ejhg.5201214

32. Lee YH, Bae SC, Kim JH, et al. Meta-analysis of genetic polymorphisms in programmed cell death 1. Associations with rheumatoid arthritis, ankylosing spondylitis, and type 1 diabetes susceptibility. *Z Rheumatol*. 2015;74(3):230–239. doi:10.1007/s00393-014-1415-y

33. Lee YH, Kim JH, Seo YH, et al. CTLA-4 polymorphisms and susceptibility to inflammatory bowel disease: a meta-analysis. *Hum Immunol*. 2014;75(5):414–421. doi:10.1016/j.humimm.2014.02.020

34. Lee YH, Woo JH, Choi SJ, et al. Association of programmed cell death 1 polymorphisms and systemic lupus erythematosus: a meta-analysis. *Lupus*. 2009;18(1):9–15. doi:10.1177/0961203308093923

35. Li G, Shi F, Liu J, et al. The effect of CTLA-4 A49G polymorphism on rheumatoid arthritis risk: a meta-analysis. *Diagn Pathol*. 2014;9:157. doi:10.1186/s13000-014-0157-0

36. Liu JL, Zhang FY, Liang YH, et al. Association between the PD1.3A/G polymorphism of the PDCD1 gene and systemic lupus erythematosus in European populations: a meta-analysis. *J Eur Acad Dermatol Venereol*. 2009;23(4):425–432. doi:10.1111/j.1468-3083.2009.03087.x

37. Scalapino KJ, Daikh DI. CTLA-4: a key regulatory point in the control of autoimmune disease. *Immunol Rev*. 2008;223:143–155. doi:10.1111/j.1600-065x.2008.00639.x

38. Wu J, Zhang L, Zhou Y. The association between CTLA-4 (+49 A/G) polymorphism and susceptibility to ankylosing spondylitis: a meta-analysis. *Int J Rheum Dis*. 2015;19(12):1237–1243. doi:10.1111/1756-185x.12705

39. Belkhir R, Burel SL, Dunogeant L, et al. Rheumatoid arthritis and polymyalgia rheumatica occurring after immune checkpoint inhibitor treatment. *Ann Rheum Dis*. 2017;76(10):1747–1750. doi:10.1136/annrheumdis-2017-211216

40. Kimura T, Fukushima S, Miyashita A, et al. Myasthenic crisis and polymyositis induced by one dose of nivolumab. *Cancer Sci*. 2016;107(7):1055–1058. doi:10.1111/cas.12961

41. Gerdes LA, Held K, Beltrán E, et al. CTLA4 as immunological checkpoint in the development of multiple sclerosis. *Ann Neurol*. 2016;80(2):294–300. doi:10.1002/ana.24715

42. Godwin JL, Jaggi S, Sirisena I, et al. Nivolumab-induced autoimmune diabetes mellitus presenting as diabetic ketoacidosis in a patient with metastatic lung cancer. *J Immunother Cancer*. 2017;5:40. doi:10.1186/s40425-017-0245-2

43. Le Burel S, Champiat S, Routier E, et al. Onset of connective tissue disease following anti-PD1/PD-L1 cancer immunotherapy. *Ann Rheum Dis*. 2017;77(3):468–470. doi:10.1136/annrheumdis-2016-210820

44. Narita T, Oiso N, Taketomo Y, et al. Serological aggravation of autoimmune thyroid disease in two cases receiving nivolumab. *J. Dermatol*. 2015;43(2):210–214. doi:10.1111/1346-8138.13028

45. Shirai T, Sano T, Kamijo F, et al. Acetylcholine receptor binding antibody-associated myasthenia gravis and rhabdomyolysis induced by nivolumab in a patient with melanoma. *Jpn J Clin Oncol*. 2016;46(1):86–88. doi:10.1093/jjco/hyv158

46. Cappelli LC, Naidoo J, Bingham CO 3rd, et al. Inflammatory arthritis due to immune checkpoint inhibitors: challenges in diagnosis and treatment. *Immunotherapy*. 2017;9(1):5–8. doi:10.2217/imt-2016-0117

47. Albayda J, Bingham CO 3rd, Shah AA, et al. Metastatic joint involvement or inflammatory arthritis? A conundrum with immune checkpoint inhibitor-related adverse events. *Rheumatology*. 2018;57(4):760–762. doi:10.1093/rheumatology/kex470

48. Brahmer JR, Lacchetti C, Schneider BJ, et al. Management of immune-related adverse events in patients treated with immune checkpoint inhibitor therapy: American Society of Clinical Oncology Clinical Practice Guideline. *J Clin Oncol*. 2018;36(17):1714–1768. doi:10.1200/jco.2017.77.6385

49. Uemura M, Trinh VA, Haymaker C, et al. Selective inhibition of autoimmune exacerbation while preserving the anti-tumor clinical benefit using IL-6 blockade in a patient with advanced melanoma and Crohn's disease: a case report. *J Hematol Oncol*. 2016;9(1):81. doi:10.1186/s13045-016-0309-7

50. Behling J, Kaes J, Munzel T, et al. New-onset third-degree atrioventricular block because of autoimmune-induced myositis under treatment with anti-programmed cell death-1 (nivolumab) for metastatic melanoma. *Melanoma Res*. 2017;27(2):155–158. doi:10.1097/cmr.0000000000000314

51. Hunter G, Voll C, Robinson CA. Autoimmune inflammatory myopathy after treatment with ipilimumab. *Can J Neurol Sci*. 2009;36(4):518–520. doi:10.1017/s0317167100007939

52. Johnson DB, Balko JM, Compton ML, et al. Fulminant myocarditis with combination immune checkpoint blockade. *N Engl J Med*. 2016;375(18):1749–1755. doi:10.1056/nejmoa1609214

53. Laubli H, Balmelli C, Bossard M, et al. Acute heart failure due to autoimmune myocarditis under pembrolizumab treatment for metastatic melanoma. *J Immunother Cancer*. 2015;3:11. doi:10.1186/s40425-015-0057-1

54. Matson DR, Accola MA, Rehrauer WM, et al. Fatal myocarditis following treatment with the PD-1 inhibitor nivolumab. *J Forensic Sci*. 2017;63(3):954–957. doi:10.1111/1556-4029.13633

55. Yoshioka M, Kambe N, Yamamoto Y, et al. Case of respiratory discomfort due to myositis after administration of nivolumab. *J Dermatol*. 2015;42(10):1008–1009. doi:10.1111/1346-8138.12991

56. Sheik Ali S, Goddard AL, Luke JJ, et al. Drug-associated dermatomyositis following ipilimumab therapy: a novel immune-mediated adverse event associated with cytotoxic T-lymphocyte antigen 4 blockade. *JAMA Dermatol*. 2015;151(2):195–199. doi:10.1001/jamadermatol.2014.2233

57. Bernier M, Guillaume C, Leon N, et al. Nivolumab causing a polymyalgia rheumatica in a patient with a squamous non-small cell lung cancer. *J Immunother*. 2017;40(4):129–131. doi:10.1097/cji.0000000000000163

58. Garel B, Kramkimel N, Trouvin AP, et al. Pembrolizumab-induced polymyalgia rheumatica in two patients with metastatic melanoma. *Joint Bone Spine*. 2017;84(2):233–234. doi:10.1016/j.jbspin.2016.01.007

59. Nakamagoe K, Moriyama T, Maruyama H, et al. Polymyalgia rheumatica in a melanoma patient due to nivolumab treatment. *J Cancer Res Clin Oncol*. 2017;143(7):1357–1358. doi:10.1007/s00432-017-2410-x

60. Goldstein BL, Gedmintas L, Todd DJ. Drug-associated polymyalgia rheumatica/giant cell arteritis occurring in two patients after treatment with ipilimumab, an antagonist of ctla-4. *Arthritis Rheumatol*. 2014;66(3):768–769. doi:10.1002/art.38282

61. Naidu MU, Ramana GV, Rani PU, et al. Chemotherapy-induced and/or radiation therapy-induced oral mucositis—complicating the treatment of cancer. *Neoplasia*. 2004;6(5):423–431. doi:10.1593/neo.04169

62. Fadel F, El Karoui K, Knebelmann B. Anti-CTLA4 antibody-induced lupus nephritis. *N Engl J Med*. 2009;361(2):211–212. doi:10.1056/nejmc0904283

63. Gauci M-L, Baroudjian B, Laly P, et al. Remitting seronegative symmetrical synovitis with pitting edema (RS3PE) syndrome induced by nivolumab. *Semin Arthritis Rheum*. 2017;47(2):281–287. doi:10.1016/j.semarthrit.2017.03.003

64. Khoja L, Maurice C, Chappell M, et al. Eosinophilic fasciitis and acute encephalopathy toxicity from pembrolizumab treatment of a patient with metastatic melanoma. *Cancer Immunol Res*. 2016;4(3):175–178. doi:10.1158/2326-6066.cir-15-0186

65. Manusow JS, Khoja L, Pesin N, et al. Retinal vasculitis and ocular vitreous metastasis following complete response to PD-1 inhibition in a patient with metastatic cutaneous melanoma. *J Immunother Cancer*. 2014;2(1):41.doi:10.1186/s40425-014-0041-1

66. Minor DR, Bunker SR, Doyle J. Lymphocytic vasculitis of the uterus in a patient with melanoma receiving ipilimumab. *J Clin Oncol*. 2013;31(20):e356. doi:10.1200/jco.2012.47.5095

CHAPTER 7

IMMUNE-RELATED GASTROINTESTINAL TOXICITIES

Hamzah Abu-Sbeih, Daniel H. Johnson, and Yinghong Wang

INTRODUCTION

Gastrointestinal immune-related adverse events (irAEs) are among the most frequent adverse events (AEs) associated with checkpoint inhibition therapy and include the (a) gastrointestinal (GI) tract—although the colon is the most common involved segment, these toxicities can involve the entire GI tract including small intestine, stomach, esophagus, and the oral mucosa; (b) liver; and (c) pancreas. These toxicities can be severe and if left untreated, can be fatal. In this chapter, we summarize the epidemiological and clinical features, diagnostic evaluation, and management recommendations of these toxicities.

DIARRHEA AND COLITIS

Epidemiology and Clinical Presentation

- Immune-related diarrhea is among the most commonly reported irAEs, which occurs in up to 45% of patients receiving a monoclonal antibody against cytotoxic T-lymphocyte antigen 4 (CTLA-4) therapy. However, the incidence of immune-mediated diarrhea is lower in patients receiving a monoclonal antibody against programmed cell death 1 (PD-1) or its ligand (PD-L1), with only 5% to 20% of patients (1–8).
- Colitis is of less occurrence than diarrhea with immune checkpoint inhibitors (ICIs). Anti-CTLA-4 therapy can lead to immune-mediated colitis in 10% to 25% of patients. Conversely, anti-PD-1/PD-L1 might cause colitis in only 1% to 5% of patients (5–8).
- Of note, diarrhea and colitis associated with anti-CTLA-4 are dose dependent where they occur in up to 38% and 10%, respectively, of patients receiving 10 mg/kg versus 23% and 5%, respectively, in patients receiving 3 mg/kg ipilimumab (9).
- Transient diarrhea might occur following the first ICI infusion and is not immune-mediated, which should be distinguished from the immune-mediated diarrhea.
- Immune-mediated AEs of the GI tract might involve less frequently the small bowel, duodenum, or stomach (10).
- The onset of GI irAE is typically after the third ICI infusion on average; however, it might occur as early as after the first (11).
- The severity of GI irAE ranges from mild, transient diarrhea to severe, potentially life-threatening colitis that requires prolonged hospitalization and immunosuppressant treatment.

Published by Springer Publishing Company DOI: 10.1891/9780826172150.0007

- Alarming symptoms of severe colitis include abdominal pain, fever, abdominal distension, and blood or mucous in the stool.
- The recurrence of GI symptoms related to the initial irAE after several months of the discontinuation of ICI is not uncommon, and can occur in a similar fashion as chronic inflammatory bowel disease (12,13).

Diagnostic Approach (Table 7.1)

- Other causes of diarrhea, such as infectious and inflammatory diseases, should be excluded, first utilizing diagnostic serum and stool laboratory studies before confirming the diagnosis of ICI-related GI toxicity.
- Physicians may consider testing for HIV, tuberculosis, and hepatitis A and B prior to starting infliximab treatment.
- Radiological evaluation of ICI-related colitis by CT scan or fluorodeoxyglucose positron emission tomography (FDG-PET) study can be helpful for the characterization of the disease.

TABLE 7.1 Diagnostic Workup Recommendations for Patients With Immune-Mediated Diarrhea/Colitis

Grade of diarrhea/colitis	Recommendations
Grade 2	
	• Blood workup (CBC, CMP, TSH, ESR, CRP)
	• Stool workup (culture, CMV, *Clostridium difficile*, parasites and ova, viral etiology)
	• Fecal inflammatory markers (lactoferrin and calprotectin) are optional
	• Screening for HIV, TB, and hepatitis A and B before the initiation of infliximab in high-risk patients based on the recommendation of an infectious disease specialist
	• CT scan of the abdomen and pelvis should be considered in patients with alarming symptoms
	• Gastrointestinal endoscopic evaluation should be considered in selected patients
	• Repeat endoscopic evaluation if no response to immunosuppressant treatment, planning to resume ICI, or clinically indicated
Grade 3 and 4	
	• All workup studies listed in grade 2 should be completed immediately
	• Repeat endoscopy should be considered if no response to immunosuppressant treatment, planning to resume ICI, or clinically indicated

CBC, complete blood count; CMP, comprehensive metabolic panel; CMV, cytomegalovirus; CRP, C-reactive protein; ESR, erythrocyte sedimentation rate; ICI, immune checkpoint inhibitors; TB, tuberculosis; TSH, thyroid stimulating hormone.

- The findings of ICI-related colitis on CT scan might be normal or indicative of inflammation signs which include mesenteric vessel engorgement, bowel wall thickening, and colonic distension. The pattern of distribution on CT varies from segmental to diffuse involvement of the entire colon and small bowel (14).
- Colonoscopy is a useful diagnostic modality to assess for the distribution and gross endoscopic features of colitis in selected patients when deemed necessary. Certain gross endoscopic features, particularly colonic ulceration, can predict a steroid refractory disease (15,16,41).
- In some cases endoscopic evaluation shows normal appearance grossly, however, histological assessment reveals microscopic inflammatory features suggestive of ICI-related colitis (17).
- Microscopic histological features of ICI-related colitis are categorized as acute (cryptitis with neutrophilic infiltration, crypt micro-abscesses, and crypt epithelial cells apoptosis), chronic (lymphocyte infiltration of the lamina propria, crypt architectural distortion and atrophy, and Paneth cell metaplasia), or lymphocytic (expansion of the lamina propria with intraepithelial lymphocytosis) (16,17).

Management Recommendations (Table 7.2)

General Recommendations

- All patients receiving ICI should be educated about the symptoms of its related GI toxicity and the importance of informing their healthcare provider immediately in case they experienced any of the following signs:
  - Change in bowel habits
  - Abdominal pain
  - Nausea
  - Blood or mucous in the stool
  - Fever
  - Abdominal distension
  - Constipation or obstipation

TABLE 7.2 Management Recommendation for Patients With Diarrhea/Colitis

Grade of diarrhea/colitis (CTCAE V-4.03)	Recommendation
Grade 1: More than four stools per day over baseline; mild increase in ostomy output compared to baseline [Asymptomatic; clinical or diagnostic observations only; no intervention indicated]	• ICI can be continued if the grade of colitis does not exceed 1
	• Follow-up within 48 hours for disease progression
	• Routine blood and stool tests if symptoms persist longer than 48 hours
	• Bland diet recommendation and dehydration management
	• Anti-motility agents consideration after infection workup
	• Consider referral to gastroenterologist if diarrhea persists for more than 48 hours

(continued)

TABLE 7.2 Management Recommendation for Patients With Diarrhea/Colitis (*continued*)

Grade of diarrhea/colitis (*CTCAE V-4.03*)	Recommendation
Grade 2: Four to six stools per day over baseline; moderate increase in ostomy output compared to baseline [abdominal pain, mucus or blood in stool]	• Temporarily hold ICI
	• Outpatient blood and stool workup
	• Gastroenterologist consultation
	• Imaging and endoscopic evaluation when clinically needed
	• Prednisone 1 mg/kg/day immediately for colitis symptoms or if diarrhea persists after 48 to 72 hours
	○ If no improvement within 48 hours, increase the steroid dose to 2 mg/kg/day ○ If refractory to 2 mg/kg/day of steroid, start infliximab 5–10 mg/kg infusion
	○ If symptoms improve:
	■ Taper steroid over 4 to 6 weeks
	■ Resume ICI when toxicity grade returns to 1 and below and steroid tapered to less than 10 mg/day
	■ Continue anti-PD-1 or anti-PD-L1 and discontinue CTLA-4
	■ Dose reduction of ICI is not recommended
	• If colitis recurs on resuming:
	○ G ≤ 2: temporarily hold ICI
	○ G ≥ 3: permanently discontinue ICI
Grade 3: Seven or more stools per day over baseline; fecal incontinence; severe increase in ostomy output compared to baseline; diarrhea limiting self-care. **Grade 4:** Life-threatening consequences; need for urgent intervention [both grades: severe abdominal pain, change in bowel habits, medical intervention indicated, peritoneal signs]	• Withhold ICI for grade 3, and permanently discontinue ICI for grade 4
	• Hospitalization and consider ICU admission
	• Inflammatory markers, blood and stool infection workup
	• Imaging and endoscopy evaluation
	• Start IV prednisone 1–2 mg/kg/day immediately
	○ If improvement: follow instructions as in G2
	○ If no improvement: start prednisone 2 mg/kg/day for 72 hours, and infliximab infusion
	• Immunosuppressant agents (a) infliximab 5 mg/kg, can be repeated after 2 weeks if needed; or (b) vedolizumab 300 mg IV infusion if failing infliximab

CTCAE, common terminology criteria for adverse events; CTLA, cytotoxic T-lymphocyte antigen; ICI, immune checkpoint inhibitors; PD-1, programmed cell death 1; PD-L1, programmed cell death ligand 1.

• For ICI-related diarrhea/colitis grade 2 and above, clinicians should consider discontinuing the ICI permanently for patients receiving anti-CTLA-4 agents, whereas anti-PD-1/PD-L1 agents can be restarted when colitis improves to grade 1 or lower (18,19).

- For grade 2 or higher toxicity that improves to grade 1 or lower, reinitiation of anti-CTLA-4 with dose reduction is not recommended.
- Careful observation and management for signs of dehydration and electrolyte imbalance is a critical component of colitis treatment.
- Prophylactic use of steroids has not been proven effective in preventing immune-mediated AEs (20,21).
- Physicians should consult a gastroenterologist for grade 2 or above diarrhea and colitis.
- Endoscopic evaluation should be offered in colitis grade 2 or above to assess the severity of colitis, which may guide the need for infliximab treatment (16,41).
- Methylprednisone can be used with a dose equivalent to the recommended dose of prednisone (18,19).
- Studies reporting successful treatment of ICI-related GI toxicity with infliximab showed that the response to infliximab occurs usually within 24 to 72 hours, but in some instances a repeat dose is required. The counter effect of infliximab on ICI efficacy is not well established yet (22–26).
- Vedolizumab might be considered in patients with diarrhea/colitis of grade 3 and above that is refractory to steroid and infliximab (27,42).

HEPATITIS

Epidemiology and Clinical Presentation

- Anti-PD-1/PD-L1-related hepatotoxicity is reported in 0.5% to 3% of patients, however, the incidence of hepatotoxicity increases up to 20% in patients receiving anti-CTLA-4 therapy (5–8,28,29).
- The onset of hepatic injury is typically 6 to 12 weeks after the initiation of ICI treatment (5,30,31).
- The clinical presentation of hepatotoxicity ranges widely. The majority of patients are diagnosed incidentally on routine liver function tests. Only minority of patients present with symptoms that include right upper quadrant abdominal pain, fever, and other systemic symptoms.
- The pattern of hepatotoxicity is characteristically hepatocellular injury, while, cholestatic injury is of less frequent occurrence (32,33).

Diagnostic and Management Recommendations (Table 7.3)

- Obtaining liver function panel prior to the initiation of ICI treatment and before each infusion helps to detect and characterize liver injury.
- Exclusion of other causes of abnormal liver function laboratory panel should be sought first, that is, viral infection, alcohol, fatty liver diseases, concomitant medications, cancer metastasis, thromboembolic disease, and portal vein occlusion.
- Radiological examination of immune-mediated hepatitis should be considered when clinically indicated to evaluate the extent and confirm the diagnosis of the disease.

TABLE 7.3 Management Recommendations for Patients With Hepatitis

Grade of liver injury (*CTCAE V-4.3*)	Recommendation
Grade 1: AST and/or ALT: (> 3) times the ULN Total bilirubin: (1–1.5) times the ULN	• Continue ICI
	• Obtain hepatic function panel weekly
	• Reduce the frequency of blood tests when liver panel return to normal and remain stable
Grade 2: AST and/or ALT: (3–5) times the ULN Total bilirubin: (1.5–3) times the ULN	• Hold ICI
	• Rule out other causes of abnormal liver function panel
	• Give prednisone 0.5 to 1 mg/kg/day then 4 weeks taper
	• Monitor liver function panel twice weekly
	• Resume ICI: ○ prednisone taper to less than 10 mg/day ○ grade 1 or less liver injury
Grade 3 and 4: AST and/or ALT: (> 5) times the ULN Total bilirubin: (> 3) times the ULN	• Discontinue ICI
	• Monitor liver function panel every 24 to 48 hours
	• Give prednisone 1–2 mg/kg/day
	• Consider mycophenolate mofetil if no response after 72 hours
	• Taper off steroid over 4 weeks when liver function returns to grade 1 or less
	• Consider liver biopsy

ALT, alanine aminotransferase; AST, alanine aminotransferase; ICI, immune checkpoint inhibitors; ULN, upper limit of normal.

• Abnormal CT and MRI findings indicative of immune-mediated hepatitis include hepatomegaly, peri-portal edema, lymphadenopathy, and parenchymal enhancement (34,35).
• The radiological presentation of ipilimumab induced hepatitis correlates with the severity of the disease; however, the radiological findings are unspecific (34).
• Histological evaluation for immune-mediated hepatitis is indicated for grade 2 and above hepatitis in patients with severe complicated disease.
• The features of immune-mediated hepatitis on liver biopsy are similar to those of auto-immune hepatitis with hepatocyte injury pattern primarily, which includes features of sinusoidal histiocytic infiltrates, central hepatic vein damage, and endothelial inflammation. Biliary pattern of hepatic injury has also been reported, which includes portal inflammation and, very rarely, fibrin ring granulomas (34,36,37).
• Methylprednisone can be used with a dose equivalent to the recommended dose of prednisone.
• Infliximab is not recommended for immune-mediated hepatitis because of concerns for associated liver toxicity (18,38).

- In patients with baseline liver profile abnormalities secondary to metastases, a higher threshold should be used to prompt a liver toxicity work up and adjust ICI treatment regimen.

PANCREATITIS

- Elevated lipase and amylase have been reported in 1% to 15% of patients receiving ICI treatment (6,9).
- Immune-mediated acute pancreatitis is rare, occurring in less than 1% of patients receiving ICI (12,39,40).
- Pancreatic injury associated with ICI treatment is usually asymptomatic and is diagnosed incidentally.
- There is a paucity of data in the literature describing the clinical characteristics or treatment of ICI-related pancreatitis.
- The management of immune-mediated pancreatitis consists of steroids in addition to the traditional acute pancreatitis treatment of intravenous fluid, bowel rest, and hospital admission.
- For grade 2 pancreatitis that has resolved to grade 1 or lower, we recommend to consider restarting ICI therapy with close observation of lipase and amylase levels. For grade 3 pancreatitis or pancreatic necrosis, permanent discontinuation of ICI is recommended.

CONCLUSION

irAEs, specifically immune-related GI toxicities, are considered among the major limitations of ICI therapy. Not only do they limit the application of these drugs in the existing indication, but they also affect how new immunotherapeutic regimens are designed. With expansion of the therapeutic applications of ICIs in cancer treatment, proper diagnosis and management of these immune-related toxicities are vital both to the success of current regimens and to the development of more efficient immunotherapy strategies.

While following management algorithms mentioned in this chapter can reverse pathological damage caused by these toxicities and improve symptoms, patient education remains the most important tool for early recognition that can minimize morbidity and mortality. For example, diarrhea is one of the earliest clinical symptoms of immune-related colitis, thus strict and clear instruction to the patient to report these symptoms promptly will allow for earlier initiation of treatment. Rapid reversal of inflammation from these toxicities may decrease the risk of toxicity-related mortality, hasten symptom resolution, minimize the duration of immune suppression, and allow for faster reinitiation of ICI if not contraindicated.

REFERENCES

1. Michot JM, Bigenwald C, Champiat S, et al. Immune-related adverse events with immune checkpoint blockade: a comprehensive review. *Eur J Cancer*. 2016;54:139–148. doi:10.1016/j.ejca.2015.11.016
2. Dadu R, Zobniw C, Diab A. Managing adverse events with immune checkpoint agents. *Cancer J*. 2016;22(2):121–129. doi:10.1097/ppo.0000000000000186

3. Shepard B, Trower C, Hendrickson S. Toxic injury to the gastrointestinal tract after ipilimumab therapy for advanced melanoma. *J Am Osteopath Assoc*. 2018;118(1):40–44. doi:10.7556/jaoa.2018.007

4. Gupta A, Hodi FS, Wolchok JD, et al. Systematic review: colitis associated with anti-CTLA-4 therapy. *Aliment Pharmacol Ther*. 2015;42(4):406–417. doi:10.1111/apt.13281

5. Weber JS, Hodi FS, Wolchok JD, et al. Safety profile of nivolumab monotherapy: a pooled analysis of patients with advanced melanoma. *J Clin Oncol*. 2017;35(7):785–792. doi:10.1200/jco.2015.66.1389

6. Sznol M, Ferrucci PF, Hogg D, et al. Pooled analysis safety profile of nivolumab and ipilimumab combination therapy in patients with advanced melanoma. *J Clin Oncol*. 2017;35(34):3815–3822. doi:10.1200/jco.2016.72.1167

7. Larkin J, Hodi FS, Wolchok JD. Combined nivolumab and ipilimumab or monotherapy in untreated melanoma. *N Engl J Med*. 2015;373(13):1270–1271. doi:10.1056/NEJMc1509660

8. Weber J, Mandala M, Del Vecchio M, et al. Adjuvant nivolumab versus ipilimumab in resected stage iii or iv melanoma. *N Engl J Med*. 2017;377(19):1824–1835. doi:10.1056/nejmoa1709030

9. Ascierto PA, Del Vecchio M, Robert C, et al. Ipilimumab 10 mg/kg versus ipilimumab 3 mg/kg in patients with unresectable or metastatic melanoma: a randomised, double-blind, multicentre, phase 3 trial. *Lancet Oncol*. 2017;18(5):611–622. doi:10.1016/s1470-2045(17)30231-0

10. Gonzalez RS, Salaria SN, Bohannon CD, et al. PD-1 inhibitor gastroenterocolitis: case series and appraisal of 'immunomodulatory gastroenterocolitis'. *Histopathology*. 2017;70(4):558–567. doi:10.1111/his.13118

11. Bertrand A, Kostine M, Barnetche T, et al. Immune related adverse events associated with anti-CTLA-4 antibodies: systematic review and meta-analysis. *BMC Med*. 2015;13:211. doi:10.1186/s12916-015-0455-8

12. Cramer P, Bresalier RS. Gastrointestinal and Hepatic Complications of Immune Checkpoint Inhibitors. *Curr Gastroenterol Rep*. 2017;19(1):3. doi:10.1007/s11894-017-0540-6

13. Wang Y, Abu-Sbeih H, Mao E, et al. Immune-checkpoint inhibitor-induced diarrhea and colitis in patients with advanced malignancies: retrospective review at MD Anderson. *J Immunother Cancer*. 2018;6(1):37. doi:10.1186/s40425-018-0346-6

14. Kim KW, Ramaiya NH, Krajewski KM, et al. Ipilimumab-associated colitis: CT findings. *AJR Am J Roentgenol*. 2013;200(5):W468–W474. doi:10.2214/ajr.12.9751

15. Jain A, Lipson EJ, Sharfman WH, et al. Colonic ulcerations may predict steroid-refractory course in patients with ipilimumab-mediated enterocolitis. *World J Gastroenterol*. 2017;23(11):2023–2028. doi:10.3748/wjg.v23.i11.2023

16. Wang Y, Abu-Sbeih H, Mao E, et al. Endoscopic and histologic features of immune checkpoint inhibitor-related colitis. *Inflamm Bowel Dis*. 2018;24(8):1695–1705. doi:10.1093/ibd/izy104

17. Choi K, Abu-Sbeih H, Samdani R, et al. Can immune checkpoint inhibitors induce microscopic colitis or a brand new entity? *Inflamm Bowel Dis*. 2018. doi:10.1093/ibd/izy240

18. Puzanov I, Diab A, Abdallah K, et al. Managing toxicities associated with immune checkpoint inhibitors: consensus recommendations from the Society for Immunotherapy of Cancer (SITC) Toxicity Management Working Group. *J Immunother Cancer*. 2017;5(1):95. doi:10.1186/s40425-017-0300-z

19. Brahmer JR, Lacchetti C, Schneider BJ, et al. Management of immune-related adverse events in patients treated with immune checkpoint inhibitor therapy: American Society of Clinical Oncology Clinical Practice Guideline. *J Clin Oncol*. 2018;36(17):1714–1768. doi:10.1200/JCO.2017.77.6385

20. Weber J, Thompson JA, Hamid O, et al. A randomized, double-blind, placebo-controlled, phase II study comparing the tolerability and efficacy of ipilimumab administered with or without prophylactic budesonide in patients with unresectable stage III or IV melanoma. *Clin Cancer Res*. 2009;15(17):5591–5598. doi:10.1158/1078-0432.ccr-09-1024

21. Berman D, Parker SM, Siegel J, et al. Blockade of cytotoxic T-lymphocyte antigen-4 by ipilimumab results in dysregulation of gastrointestinal immunity in patients with advanced melanoma. *Cancer Immun*. 2010;10:11.

22. Pages C, Gornet JM, Monsel G, et al. Ipilimumab-induced acute severe colitis treated by infliximab. *Melanoma Res*. 2013;23(3):227–230. doi:10.1097/cmr.0b013e32835fb524

23. Tarhini A. Immune-mediated adverse events associated with ipilimumab CTLA-4 blockade therapy: the underlying mechanisms and clinical management. *Scientifica (Cairo).* 2013;2013:857519. doi:10.1155/2013/857519

24. Johnston RL, Lutzky J, Chodhry A, et al. Cytotoxic T-lymphocyte-associated antigen 4 antibody-induced colitis and its management with infliximab. *Dig Dis Sci.* 2009 ;54(11):2538–2540. doi:10.1007/s10620-008-0641-z

25. O'Connor A, Marples M, Mulatero C, et al. Ipilimumab-induced colitis: experience from a tertiary referral center. *Therap Adv Gastroenterol.* 2016;9(4):457–462. doi:10.1177 /1756283x16646709

26. Johnson DH, Zobniw CM, Trinh VA, et al. Infliximab associated with faster symptom resolution compared to corticosteroids alone for management of immune mediated enterocolitis. *J Immunother Cancer.*2018;6:103. doi:10.1186/s40425-018-0412-0.

27. Bergqvist V, Hertervig E, Gedeon P, et al. Vedolizumab treatment for immune checkpoint inhibitor-induced enterocolitis. *Cancer Immunol Immunother.* 2017;66(5):581–592. doi:10.1007/s00262-017-1962-6

28. Ali AK, Watson DE. Pharmacovigilance Assessment of Immune-Mediated Reactions Reported for Checkpoint Inhibitor Cancer Immunotherapies. *Pharmacotherapy.* 2017; 37(11):1383–1390. doi:10.1002/phar.2035

29. Foller S, Oppel-Heuchel H, Fetter I, et al. Adverse events of immune checkpoint inhibitors. *Urologe A.* 2017;56(4):486–491. doi:10.1007/s00120-017-0342-3

30. Ziemer M, Koukoulioti E, Beyer S, et al. Managing immune checkpoint-inhibitor-induced severe autoimmune-like hepatitis by liver-directed topical steroids. *J Hepatol.* 2017;66(3):657–659. doi:10.1016/j.jhep.2016.11.015

31. Spain L, Diem S, Larkin J. Management of toxicities of immune checkpoint inhibitors. *Cancer Treat Rev.* 2016;44:51–60. doi:10.1016/j.ctrv.2016.02.001

32. Boutros C, Tarhini A, Routier E, et al. Safety profiles of anti-CTLA-4 and anti-PD-1 antibodies alone and in combination. *Nat Rev Clin Oncol.* 2016;13(8):473–486. doi:10.1038/ nrclinonc.2016.58

33. Kwak JJ, Tirumani SH, Van den Abbeele AD, et al. Cancer immunotherapy: imaging assessment of novel treatment response patterns and immune-related adverse events. *Radiographics.* 2015;35(2):424–437. doi:10.1148/rg.352140121

34. Kim KW, Ramaiya NH, Krajewski KM, et al. Ipilimumab associated hepatitis: imaging and clinicopathologic findings. *Invest New Drugs.* 2013;31(4):1071–1077. doi:10.1007/s10637-013-9939-6

35. Alessandrino F, Tirumani SH, Krajewski KM, et al. Imaging of hepatic toxicity of systemic therapy in a tertiary cancer centre: chemotherapy, haematopoietic stem cell transplantation, molecular targeted therapies, and immune checkpoint inhibitors. *Clin Radiol.* 2017;72(7):521–533. doi:10.1016/j.crad.2017.04.003

36. Johncilla M, Misdraji J, Pratt DS, et al. Ipilimumab-associated hepatitis: clinicopathologic characterization in a series of 11 cases. *Am J Surg Pathol.* 2015;39(8):1075–1084. doi:10.1097/ pas.0000000000000453

37. Everett J, Srivastava A, Misdraji J. Fibrin ring granulomas in checkpoint inhibitor-induced hepatitis. *Am J Surg Pathol.* 2017;41(1):134–137. doi:10.1097/pas.00000 00000000759

38. Haanen JBAG, Carbonnel F, Robert C, et al. Management of toxicities from immunotherapy: ESMO Clinical Practice Guidelines for diagnosis, treatment and follow-up. *Ann Oncol.* 2017;28(suppl_4):iv119–iv142. doi:10.1093/annonc/mdx225

39. Hofmann L, Forschner A, Loquai C, et al. Cutaneous, gastrointestinal, hepatic, endocrine, and renal side-effects of anti-PD-1 therapy. *Eur J Cancer.* 2016;60:190–209. doi:10.1016/j. ejca.2016.02.025

40. Wolchok JD, Kluger H, Callahan MK, et al. Nivolumab plus ipilimumab in advanced melanoma. *N Engl J Med.* 2013;369(2):122–133. doi:10.1056/NEJMoa1302369

41. Abu-Sbeih H, Ali FS, Luo W, et al. Importance of endoscopic and histological evaluation in the management of immune checkpoint inhibitor-induced colitis. *J Immunother Cancer.* 2018;6(1):95. doi:10.1186/s40425-018-0411-1

42. Abu-Sbeih H, Ali FS, Alsaadi D, et al. Outcomes of vedolizumab therapy in patients with immune checkpoint inhibitor-induced colitis: a multi-center study. *J Immunother Cancer.* 2018;6(1):142. doi:10.1186/s40425-018-0461-4

CHAPTER 8

PNEUMOTOXICITY ASSOCIATED WITH IMMUNE CHECKPOINT BLOCKADES

Vickie R. Shannon

CLINICAL PEARLS

- Although pneumonitis is less common than many of the other immune-related adverse events (irAEs) associated with immune checkpoint inhibition, this adverse event (AE) accounts for some of the most severe and potentially lethal irAEs, and is one of the most frequent reasons for discontinuation of therapy.
- Both cytotoxic T-lymphocyte antigen 4 (CTLA-4) and programmed cell death 1 (PD-1) axis inhibitors may precipitate symptomatic pneumonitis. However, this adverse reaction is much more common among PD-1-treated patients.
- Nonspecific interstitial pneumonitis (NSIP) and cryptogenic organizing pneumonia (COP) are the two most common imaging and histopathological findings of patients with pneumonitis, although considerable heterogeneity exists.
- The images of iatrogenic pneumonitis can be difficult to differentiate from cancer progression in the lungs and often require a pathological verification.
- Early diagnosis and the use of high dose corticosteroids are the mainstay of therapy. Other immunosuppressive therapies should be considered if corticosteroids are unsuccessful. Treatment algorithms in the management of lung-related irAEs, including the timing of additional immunosuppressive therapies have not been validated in any evidence-based trials.
- Drug rechallenge may be feasible for some patients, depending on the grade of pneumonitis and response to therapy. The risks and benefits of restarting therapy should be carefully weighed in consultation with the patient, oncologist, and subspecialty team.

INTRODUCTION

A key responsibility of the immune system is to protect the host from exogenous pathogens by distinguishing self from nonself antigens. This process in orchestrated by complex co-stimulatory and co-inhibitory immunomodulatory signals that result in a dynamic state of equilibrium between immune attack and immune tolerance. Strategies that harness the immune system to fight cancer have involved blocking immune inhibitory signals, thereby tilting the equilibrium in favor of enhanced immune attack and tumor killing.

Published by Springer Publishing Company DOI: 10.1891/9780826172150.0008

Currently, three major classes of blocking agents have been developed which target inhibitory signaling via the CTLA-4, PD-1, or programmed cell death ligand 1 (PD-L1) pathways. These agents, referred to as immune checkpoint inhibitors (ICIs), have rapidly emerged as standard of care with positive outcomes for patients with a variety of advanced and metastatic malignancies and have joined the ranks of cytotoxic drugs, hormonal agents, and molecular targeted therapies in the medical management of cancer.

Unbalancing the immune system in favor of tumor killing has resulted in a unique spectrum of autoimmune and inflammatory toxicities, referred to as irAEs, that may affect virtually every major organ system. Although lung involvement is less common than other forms of irAEs, its consequences are potentially lethal. The expanding applications of ICIs in both solid and hematological malignancies and strategies that include complex combinations with standard cancer therapies that carry their own toxicity risk have resulted in a steady rise in the incidence, complexity, and lethality of lung-related irAEs.

This chapter provides an overview of the current knowledge of irAEs affecting the respiratory system and offers insights into the differential epidemiology and common clinical presentations associated with the three major classes of ICI therapies. Optimal treatment strategies, based on existing clinical experience, and clinical clues that facilitate prompt recognition of signs and symptoms will also be explored.

CLINICAL PRESENTATION

Epidemiology and Risk Factors

The earliest reports of lung-related irAEs varied widely across clinical trials. Pneumonitis is the most frequently reported adverse lung event in these trials, occurring in 1% to 11% of patients (1–5). Although rare, this AE is not trivial, as pneumonitis accounts for some of the most severe and potentially lethal irAEs observed in ICI clinical trials, and is one of the most frequent reasons for discontinuation of therapy (6–8).

Monotherapy

In a meta-analysis of 11 clinical trials of cancer patients receiving ICIs as monotherapy, all grade pneumonitis occurred in up to 11% of patients, with severe pneumonitis occurring in 2% of treated patients (1). Epidemiologic data derived from studies both within and outside of the clinical trial experience suggest that respiratory events (which includes shortness of breath, cough, and pneumonitis) are more common following anti-PD-1 (3%–14%) versus anti-CTLA-4 (1%–5%) therapies (5,9,10).

Combination Therapy

Combination strategies using concurrent or sequential anti-CTLA-4/PD-1 regimens confer higher rates and earlier onset of lung irAEs than either approach as monotherapy (4,11,12). The differential cellular and tissue distribution of CTLA-4 ligands versus PD-1 ligands may influence the susceptibility of organ-specific toxicity, however, the reason for toxicity disparities with CTLA-4 versus PD-1 blockade is not well understood.

Pneumonitis Risk and Cancer Type

Rates of ICI-related pneumonitis also vary with cancer type, with significantly higher rates observed among patients treated for lung and renal carcinomas versus melanoma (4). Non-small cell lung cancer (NSCLC) has been associated with both increased rates and severity of pneumonitis (4). The toxicity risk following CTLA-4 targeted therapies appears to be dose-dependent, however, no such relationship has not been associated with anti-PD-1/PD-L1 therapies (12–15).

Other Influencing Factors

While the influence of factors such as advanced age, preexisting fibrotic lung disease, hyperoxia, tobacco use history, and thoracic irradiation have been associated with drug-induced lung injury in general, the impact of these clinical factors on the risk of lung irAEs has not been established. In contrast to these data, in another investigation, more than one-half of patients who developed pneumonitis following PD-1 axis inhibition were current or former smokers (16). The influence of tobacco in augmenting the risk of lung-irAEs is unclear.

- In a recent study of patients with NSCLC treated with concurrent chemoradiation followed by anti-PD-L1 therapy versus placebo, rates of pneumonitis were predominantly low-grade in both groups, with only an incremental increase in grade 3/4 pneumonitis observed among the anti-PD-L1-treated patients (3.4% with anti-PD-L1 versus 2.6% with placebo) (17).
- The relevance of age in the development of irAEs is incomplete, as elderly patients were underrepresented in clinical trials. Several small studies suggest that tolerance in elderly patients ($\geq$ 65 years of age) to anti-CTLA-4 and anti-PD-1 axis therapies is similar to that of younger patients (<65 years of age), however results have been mixed. Reduced efficacy of these agents due to the effects of immunosenescence in elderly populations is a theoretical concern, although this concept has not been supported in several small studies (18–22).

Clinical Characteristics

Although considerable variability in pneumonitis onset has been reported, with toxicities emerging within 9 days to 19 months after the first cycle of ICI therapy, most events occur within the first 6 months of initiation of ICI therapies (5,16,23).

- Recipients of CTLA-4 inhibitors and patients with NSCLC may present earlier, within the first 3 months of therapy.
  - The earlier presentation among patients with lung cancer has been attributed to more vigilant lung imaging, limited pretreatment

pulmonary reserve, and/or increased lung parenchymal tumor burden in this group of patients (4).

- New or worsening cough and dyspnea are the most common presenting symptoms among ICI-treated patients with pneumonitis.
  ○ Rare reports of fever and chest pain have also been described.
- Tachycardia and hypoxia, when present, typically signal more advanced disease.
- Dyspnea and dry cough may occur without associated radiographic abnormalities in some cases.
- Radiographic abnormalities may precede symptoms of pneumonitis by days to weeks in up to 1/3 of patients (24).
- These nonspecific symptoms are challenging to distinguish from competing comorbid conditions, such as lymphangitic carcinomatosis, pneumonia, pulmonary edema, chronic obstructive pulmonary disease (COPD) exacerbation, alveolar hemorrhage, or preexisting lung disease.
- A high level of suspicion for ICI-treated patients who present with pulmonary symptoms is warranted.
- Extrapulmonary irAEs involving the skin, gastrointestinal, endocrine, and musculoskeletal organs occur in more than 50% of patients and should raise the index of suspicion (4,16).

The severity of pneumonitis is based on Common Terminology Criteria for Adverse Events (CTCAE) scores. This scoring system stratifies the severity of therapy-related organ toxicities by clinical symptoms with specific parameters based on the organ system involved:

Grade 1 pneumonitis: Compatible radiographic changes occurring in the absence of symptoms.

Grade 2 pneumonitis: Pneumonitis with associated symptoms that limit activities of daily living.

Grade 3 pneumonitis: Severe symptoms that limit self-care.

Grade 4 pneumonitis: Life-threatening respiratory compromise.

Grade 5 pneumonitis: Death related to pneumonitis.

The CTCAE scoring system has been widely used to establish guidelines for optimal management of irAEs. Signs and symptoms of early grade (1/2) pneumonitis may be subtle initially, but may rapidly progress to respiratory failure and death in 1% to 2% of patients. Thus, close monitoring of patients with all grades of pneumonitis is warranted (see section on management).

Pathophysiological and Radiographic Phenotypes of Pneumonitis

Considerable heterogeneity exists in imaging findings associated with ICI-related lung injury.

- Nonspecific interstitial pneumonitis (NSIP), suggested by interlobular septal thickening, often with subpleural reticulation, and organizing pneumonia, suggested by patchy consolidations, usually in peripheral distribution, are the most common CT findings (Figures 8.1 and 8.2).

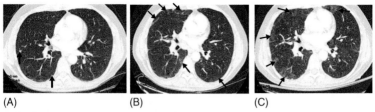

(A)   (B)   (C)

FIGURE 8.1 A 56-year-old man with bladder carcinoma, treated with a combination of Ipilimumab and Nivolumab after failing conventional therapy. Baseline CT of the chest (A) demonstrated emphysematous changes and predominantly right-sided subcentimeter pulmonary nodules (arrow). The patient presented on C2D1 of Nivolumab with severe shortness of breath and hypoxemia. An admitting chest CT demonstrated subtle bilateral, lower lobe predominant reticulonodular changes along with patchy airspace disease (B, arrows). The patient was started on antibiotics for presumed pneumonia and high-dose steroids with infliximab for suspicion of drug toxicity. Progression of airspace disease and reticular infiltrates were noted on repeat CT imaging on hospital day 7 (C). Despite aggressive therapy, the patient succumbed to respiratory failure on day 9 post hospitalization. Autopsy confirmed **NSIP with areas of early fibrotic change**.

NSIP, nonspecific interstitial pneumonitis.

- Additional observations include centrilobular nodules suggestive of hypersensitivity pneumonitis, bronchiectasis, nonspecific ground glass opacities, and mixed patterns.
- Honeycomb changes may be seen with more advanced disease.
- Chest CT is the preferred imaging modality, as plain films may fail to detect subtle findings in up to 25% of patients (25).
- Although no histopathological findings are pathognomonic for lung irAEs, bronchoscopy and lung biopsy remain valuable tools in discerning competing diagnoses.
- A lymphocyte-predominant inflammatory infiltrate on bronchoalveolar lavage (BAL) fluid is typical.
  ○ Peripheral and BAL eosinophilia may also been seen.

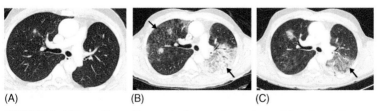

(A)   (B)   (C)

FIGURE 8.2 A 67-year-old man with progressive dyspnea and severe dyspnea 2 days after cycle 2 of Nivolumab therapy for primary lung adenocarcinoma. Admitting chest CT imaging (B) showed extensive bilateral ground glass opacities, subcentimeter nodules and bilateral patchy areas of consolidation with air bronchograms (B) which were new when compared to baseline studies (A). Bronchoscopically obtained microbiological evaluations were negative. Biopsies of the left lower lobe demonstrated inflammatory debris with plugging of the small airways and alveolar ducts, surrounded by a lymphocyte-rich infiltrate admixed with eosinophils, and consistent with **cryptogenic organizing pneumonia**. Significant symptomatic and radiographic improvement was seen on imaging studies following 4 weeks of high-dose steroids (C).

- The CD4:CD8 ratio is typically reduced in most drug-induced interstitial pneumonitides (26).
  - Elevated CD4:CD8 ratios are seen in the setting of sarcoidosis and may be used as an adjunct to this diagnosis.
- A cellular interstitial pneumonitis, organizing pneumonia, and diffuse alveolar damage are the most frequent findings on lung tissue samples (16,27).
- Pulmonary fibrosis has also been reported (28).

Other Adverse Lung Reactions Associated With Immune Checkpoint Therapies

Sarcoid-Like Granulomatous Reactions

Sarcoid-like granulomatous reactions have been described in up to 7% of patients following anti-CTLA-4 or PD-1 therapies and may occur as an isolated finding in the lungs or as a multi-organ system reaction (29–32). Both de novo sarcoid-like reactions as well as exacerbations of preexisting sarcoidosis have been described following CTLA-4 and PD-1 axis inhibition (33–36).

- Associated parenchymal nodules, subpleural micronodular opacities, and enlarged lymph nodes above and below the diaphragm are typically 18F-fluorodeoxyglucose-avid (FDG-avid) on PET-CT imaging (Figure 8.3).
  - These findings may mimic disease progression and pose particular diagnostic challenges.
- Biopsy evidence of noncaseating granulomas, elevated CD4:CD8 ratios, and the exclusion of competing diagnoses are supportive of the diagnosis.

The natural history of irAE-related sarcoidosis, associated risk factors, and treatment strategies for sarcoidosis in this setting have not been established.

- In one small restrospective study, sarcoid-like lymphadenopathy developed after a median interval of 3.2 months following initiation of ipilimumab with resolution of lymphadenopathy following drug withdrawal within 3.1 months of drug discontinuation (24).
- A short course of systemic steroids may be warranted in patients with critical end organ (ocular, myocardial, neurological, and renal), involvement, persistent fevers, associated erythema nodosum or sarcoid-related hypercalcemia.

Tumor Pseudoprogression

Immunotherapies may trigger an increase in tumor size or the development of new lesions as an early response to treatment. This is in stark contrast to conventional cytotoxic and molecular targeted therapies in which response to treatment is usually indicated by tumor shrinkage.

- The apparent increase in tumor burden following immunotherapy, known as tumor pseudoprogression, results from recruitment and

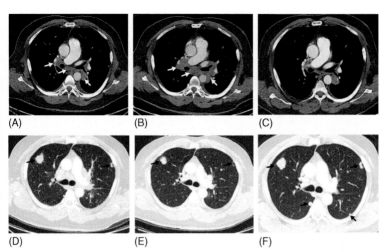

FIGURE 8.3 A 52-year-old man with extensively treated bladder cancer who presented with mild dry cough and dyspnea on exertion 3.5 months after initiating combination therapy with Nivolumab and Ipilimumab. Metastatic nodules of varying sizes and mildly enlarged mediastinal and hilar lymphadenopathy were noted at baseline (arrows, A, D). A small left-sided pleural effusion is also seen. Chest CT imaging upon admission (B, E) demonstrated marked increase in bihilar and mediastinal lymphadenopathy despite regression of the known pulmonary metastases (arrows). Endobronchial ultrasound-guided biopsies of the lymph nodes revealed noncaseating granulomas. Bronchoalveolar lavage fluid was culture- and AFB-smear negative. Findings were consistent with **ICI-induced sarcoidosis**. Discontinuation of both agents and initiation of steroids resulted in resolution of symptoms and significant reduction in lymph nodes 2 months later (C). Progression of parenchymal disease is noted despite regression of lymphadenopathy (F).

ICI, immune checkpoint inhibitors.

infiltration of cytotoxic T-lymphocytes and other immune cells into the tumor bed (Figure 8.4).

- Pseudoprogression is defined as a 25% increase in tumor burden following immunotherapy followed by spontaneous regression, typically within 4 weeks or more after the initial imaging study (37).

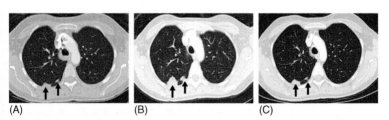

FIGURE 8.4 A 38-year-old woman with known lung metastases associated with renal cell carcinoma. Chest CT imaging at baseline (A) demonstrated pleural-based right upper lobe metastatic disease (arrows). Repeat CT imaging 22 days after cycle 1 of single agent pembrolizumab showed marked enlargement of the lung nodules (B). Despite apparent tumor progression, nivolumab therapy was continued without change. Repeat imaging one month later (C) showed significant improvement in the lung nodules. Findings are suggestive of tumor **pseudoprogression**.

- This rare immune phenomenon has been described following PD-1 and CTLA-4 blockade and is almost universally accompanied by symptomatic improvement.
- Suspicion of pseudoprogression should prompt repeat imaging at least 4 weeks after the initial study.
  - Symptom progression and/or tumor burden that remains increased on subsequent imaging studies suggests true tumor progression (38–41).

Airway Disease

T-lymphocyte activation and proliferation play a key role in the pathogenesis of inflammatory airway diseases, such as COPD and chronic bronchitis. The influence of immune checkpoints in the development of the bronchitic phenotype is complex.

- Emerging data suggest that CTLA-4 and PD-1 axis inhibitors may contribute to the pattern of exacerbation and lung damage characteristic of COPD and other chronic inflammatory airway disorders (42).
  - These observations have raised concerns regarding the use of ICIs in patients with preexisting inflammatory airway diseases.
- The development of bronchiolitis and COPD exacerbations following ICI-based therapies have been reported, but appear to be rare complications of these agents.

Pleural Effusions

Pleural and pericardial effusions have been reported during anti-PD-1 therapy. The fluid is typically lymphocyte-predominant and occurs early, within the first 6 to 8 weeks following initiation of therapy. Fluid regression tends to parallel response to therapy at other sites (41,43).

A partial list of FDA-approved checkpoint-directed agents and their associated pneumonitides are listed in Table 8.1.

Opportunistic Infections

Although ICI therapies have not been convincingly linked to the development of opportunistic infections, prolonged immunosuppressive therapies used in the treatment of irAEs may lead to the emergence of a variety of unusual and opportunistic fungal, mycobacterial, viral, and parasitic pathogens.

- In a recent retrospective study of melanoma patients with checkpoint-inhibitor-related irAEs treated with prolonged immunosuppression, opportunistic infections occurred in 13.5% of patients, with pneumonia being the most common form of infection and the most frequent cause of death.
- Anti-PD-1/CTLA-4 combination therapies were associated with the highest rates of serious infections, which is likely explained by the higher rates of irAEs among patients undergoing dual checkpoint inhibitor regimens and the associated need for prolonged immunosuppression (44,45).

TABLE 8.1 Radiographic and Histopathological Findings Following ICI Therapies

Agent	Target	Pneumonitis incidence (%)		Common pneumonitis-associated imaging and histologic findings			Median time to symptom onset (range)	Median time to symptom resolution (range)	Sarcoid-like hilar/mediastinal lymphadenopathy	Pleural effusions	Tumor pseudo-progression
		All grade	Grade 3-4	NSIP	Cryptogenic organizing pneumonia	Pulmonary fibrosis/ARDS					
Ipilimumab	CTLA-4	1.6–5	1	✓	✓	✓	First 3 to 4 months of therapy (0.9–9.1 months)	2.3 months (0.3–7.7 months)	✓		✓
Nivolumab	PD-1	5–12	1–3	✓	✓	✓	First 2.5 months of therapy (1.5–24.3 months)	1–3 months	✓	✓	✓
Pembrolizumab	PD-1	1.1%–2.6%	<1%	✓	✓	✓	First 5 months of therapy (0.3–84 weeks)	1–4 months	✓		✓
Atezolizumab Durvalumab Avelumab	PD-L1	0.5%–3%	1	✓	✓	✓	First 2.6 months of therapy (15 days–4.2 months)	0.5 months–3 months			

ARDS, acute respiratory distress syndrome; CTLA, cytotoxic T-lymphocyte antigen; ICI, immune checkpoint inhibitors; NSIP, nonspecific interstitial pneumonitis; PD-1, programmed cell death 1; PD-L1, programmed cell death ligand 1.

Infusion Reactions

Approximately 2% to 4% of ipilimumab-treated patients and less than 1% of patients treated with PD-1- and anti-PD-L1-targeted agents develop infusion reactions (IRs) (14,46). IRs occur most often during the first or second cycles of therapy. Postulated etiologic mechanisms of IRs include cytokine release and immunoglobulin E-mediated hypersensitivity reactions.

- Symptoms of flushing, pruritis, rash, chills, fever, dyspnea, dry cough, wheezing, nausea, hypotension, tachycardia, diaphoresis, and chest pain may occur during infusion or several hours after drug administration.
- Mild symptoms may be managed with antipyretics and by slowing the rate of infusion.
- Hospitalization and supportive care along with antihistamines, systemic corticosteroids, vasopressors, supplemental oxygen and bronchodilators are recommended for patients with more severe reactions.
- Considerations for drug rechallenge should be made on a case-by-case basis and all patients with a history of IRs to immunotherapy infusions should undergo antihistamine and antipyretic prophylaxis (10,14,47).

DIAGNOSTIC EVALUATION

Pneumonitis should be included in the differential of all ICI-exposed patients with unexplained pulmonary infiltrates and/or new onset respiratory symptoms. Our algorithm in the diagnostic evaluation of patients with suspected immune-related lung injury is depicted in Table 8.2.

- CT imaging of the chest is the key diagnostic tool in the radiologic investigation of patients with suspected ICI-related pneumonitis.
  - Plain chest films are not sufficiently sensitive, failing to detect radiographic abnormalities in nearly 25% of patients with pneumonitis, and are inadequate in distinguishing pneumonitis from competing diagnoses, such as infection, lymphangitic spread of disease and tumor progression.
- Consolidative and ground glass opacities, consistent with COP and nonspecific interstitial pneumonitis (NSIP), are the most frequent imaging findings on CT.
  - NSIP typically appears as peripheral ground glass and reticulonodular infiltrates with basilar predominance. Multifocal consolidations, hypersensitivity pneumonitis (HP), and pulmonary fibrosis have also been described (17,48).
- These radiographic findings may be confirmed upon histopathological analysis of lung tissue obtained bronchoscopically or by surgical lung biopsy.
  - However, there are no histopathological changes that are pathognomonic of immune-related pneumonitis versus pneumonitis arising from other causes.
- Immune-related pneumonitis remains a diagnosis of exclusion. Bronchoscopic examination is recommended to exclude competing

TABLE 8.2 Suggested Diagnostic Work-up and Management for Checkpoint Inhibitor-Associated Pneumonitis

Pneumonitis grade	Definition	Diagnostic evaluation	Management	Follow-up care	Rechallenge considerations
1	Asymptomatic radiographic abnormalities only	Chest CT imaging PFTs with 6MWT Consider Pulmonary and Infectious Disease consultations	• Withhold immunotherapy • Self-monitor symptoms and oxygen saturation (using personal pulse oximeter) daily Outpatient clinic follow up evaluations • Reimage prior to subsequent cycle of therapy (minimum 3-4 weeks following the initial chest CT)	If evidence of disease progression, treat as higher grade pneumonitis	Cautious resumption of therapy with close follow up may be considered once imaging abnormalities have resolved

2	New mild to moderate symptoms of cough, dyspnea, tachypnea causing limitations to normal activities of daily living	Chest CT imaging PFTs with 6MWT Pulmonary and Infectious Disease consult Bronchoscopy Consider lung biopsy for suspicious lesions or adenopathy	• Withhold immunotherapy
			• Monitor symptoms daily
			• Consider hospitalization
			• If not hospitalized, self-monitor symptoms and oxygen saturation (using personal pulse oximeter) daily
			• Initiate methylprednisolone 1 mg/kg/day (IV or oral equivalent)
			• Start prophylactic antibiotics for PCP and other opportunistic infections
			Day 2 of steroids/supportive care:
			  ○ *Symptoms improved* to grade 1, continue steroids at same dose over the ensuing week, then start slow steroid taper over 1 month, minimum
			  ○ *Symptoms worsening*—treat as grade 3-4
			Week 1-2 of steroids/supportive care:
			  ○ *Symptoms stable but not improved*—treat as grade 3-4
			• Start prophylactic antibiotics for PCP and other opportunistic infections
				Once stable and discharged from the hospital, close monitoring and slow steroid taper is recommended. Steroids should be tapered over an additional 4-6 weeks minimum to avoid pneumonitis flare-ups.	Cautious resumption of therapy with close follow up may be considered once imaging abnormalities have resolved on a case by case basis

(continued)

TABLE 8.2 Suggested Diagnostic Work-up and Management for Checkpoint Inhibitor-Associated Pneumonitis (continued)

Pneumonitis grade	Definition	Diagnostic evaluation	Management	Follow-up care	Rechallenge considerations

3	New, severe symptoms that self limit care Worsening hypoxia Respiratory compromise	Chest CT imaging Pulmonary and Infectious Disease consultation Bronchoscopy Consider lung biopsy for suspicious lesions, adenopathy	• Discontinue immunotherapy
			• Hospitalize
			• Consider ICU care
			• Initiate methylprednisolone 2 mg/kg/day IV
			• **Day 2 post steroids/supportive care:**
			  ○ *Worsening symptoms*—add additional immunosuppressive therapies (infliximab, cyclophosphamide, mycophenolate mofetil, azathioprine)
			  ○ *Symptoms improve back to baseline*—continue steroids at same dose over the ensuing week, then start slow steroid taper over 6–8 weeks, minimum
			• Start prophylactic antibiotics for PCP and other opportunistic infections
				Once stable and discharged from the hospital, close monitoring and slow steroid taper is recommended. Steroids should be tapered over an additional 6–8 weeks minimum to avoid pneumonitis flare-ups. Pulmonary outpatient clinic follow up with PFTs with 6MWT when stable	Permanent discontinuation of the drug is recommended

4	Life-threatening symptoms with impending respiratory failure	Chest CT imaging PFTs with 6MWT when stable Pulmonary and Infectious Disease consultation Bronchoscopy Consider lung biopsy for suspicious lesions, adenopathy	• Discontinue immunotherapy
			• Hospitalize
			• Transfer to higher level (ICU) care
			• Urgent intervention (intubation, BiPAP) is usually indicated
			• Initiate methylprednisolone 2 mg/kg/day IV
			• **Day 2 post steroids/supportive care:**
			  ○ *Worsening symptoms*—add additional immunosuppressive therapies (infliximab, cyclophosphamide, mycophenolate mofetil, azathioprine)
			  ○ *Symptoms improve back to baseline*—continue steroids at same dose over the ensuing 1–2 weeks, then start slow steroid taper over 8 weeks, minimum
			• Start prophylactic antibiotics for PCP and other opportunistic infections
				Once stable and discharged from the hospital, close monitoring and slow steroid taper is recommended. Steroids should be tapered over an additional 8 weeks minimum to avoid pneumonitis flare-ups. Pulmonary outpatient follow up with PFTs with 6MWT when stable	Permanent discontinuation of the drug is recommended

6MWT, 6 minute walk test; PCP, pneumocystis jirovecii pneumonia; PFT, pulmonary function testing.

diagnoses, such as infection. Biopsies of suspicious lymph nodes may be performed by endobronchial ultrasound (EBUS) or mediastinal lymph node sampling.

- Although a role for pulmonary function testing (PFT) and the 6 minute walk test (6 MWT) in the diagnosis of pneumonitis is unclear, these studies offer added information regarding functional performance, which may help to guide therapy. We, therefore, include PFTs and a 6 MWT as part of the pulmonary assessment and follow up of patients with suspected ICI-related pneumonitis.

MANAGEMENT AND OUTCOMES

Management of ICI-related pneumonitis is largely guided by the grade of clinical symptoms.

- Management recommendations for asymptomatic cases (grade 1), typically include cessation of the drug with close outpatient monitoring and repeat imaging in 2 to 4 weeks.
- In patients with grade 3/4 pneumonitis and patients with grade 2 pneumonitis who demonstrate progression of toxicity despite drug cessation, current consensus favors inpatient management with initiation of systemic corticosteroid therapy (17,49,50).
- A fibroscopy +/- a brochoalveolar lavage efficiently complete the functional pulmonary testing and help ruling out lung infection as well as tumor progression.
- Concerns regarding the potential for systemic corticosteroids in diminishing the efficacy of antitumor immunotherapies have not been substantiated in any clinical data.
  - In two separate studies of patients with melanoma, antitumor control was spared despite high doses of systemic corticosteroids and/or infliximab for management of anti-CTLA-4 induced irAEs.
  - Overall cancer treatment outcomes among patients receiving prolonged immunosuppression were not statistically different compared to patients not requiring immunosuppressive therapies (51,52).

Guidelines for steroid dosing and schedules are largely based on observational reports and clinical experience and have not been validated in any randomized clinical trials.

- As a general guide, we recommend initiation of a course of systemic steroids, dosed at 1 mg/kg, followed by a slow taper.
  - The initial steroid dose is continued over the ensuing 1 to 2 weeks or until symptoms have returned to grade 1 (asymptomatic CT abnormalities), at which time they may be slowly tapered.
  - The tapering schedule must be tailored to the severity of the pneumonitis event and response to initial therapy, and in general should occur over an additional 4 to 6 weeks.
  - Although most irAEs are steroid responsive, it is important to remember that the mechanism of action of the ICIs result in antitumor responses that persist long after these agents have been withdrawn.

Therefore, too rapid steroid taper may result in rebound symptoms of worse severity and duration.

- Higher dose steroids (2 mg/kg of prednisone or its equivalent) are recommended for more severe pulmonary toxicity (grade 3/4) and continued until clinical improvement is observed, then tapered over the ensuing 6 to 8 weeks (53).
  - Potential toxicities associated with prolonged high dose steroid therapy should be carefully considered in steroid dosing schedules and patients should be monitored closely while on steroid therapy.
- The addition of other immunosuppressive therapies, such as infliximab, azathioprine, mycophenolate mofetil, and cyclophosphamide should be considered in severe, steroid refractory cases in which no clinical improvement is noted after the first 48 to 96 hours of steroid therapy.
  - The clinical impact of additional immunosuppressive therapies remains unclear.
  - Pooled data, however, has not been favorable, with most patients succumbing to either acute respiratory failure from pneumonitis or secondary opportunistic infections that develop as a consequence of immunosuppression (16).
  - For all patients treated for 4 weeks or more with daily doses of 20 mg or higher of prednisone or its equivalent, it is recommended to do a pneumocystis prophylaxis with trimethoprim-sulfamethoxazole, pentamidine, or atovaquone, unless contraindicated. This practice follows guidelines issued by the National Comprehensive Cancer Network (NCCN) for the prevention of cancer-related infections.

In most patients, ICI-related pneumonitis improves or resolves with simple drug withdrawal or with drug cessation plus steroid therapy. Recurrent pneumonitis following completion of steroid therapy and in the absence of drug rechallenge (pneumonitis flare) may occur well after discontinuation of the offending ICI agent.

- Pneumonitis flares have been primarily reported following PD-1/PD-L1 therapies.
- Subsequent flare ups may present with a radiographic phenotype that is distinct from the initial presentation and clinical symptoms that are more severe than the initial symptoms.
- Longer courses of immunosuppressive therapy to achieve durable clinical improvement have been proposed, however the optimal choice, dose, and duration of immunosuppressive therapies in this setting have not been defined (16,54).
- Resumption of ICI therapy following resolution of grade 1/2 pneumonitis may be well tolerated in some patients. Recurrent pneumonitis in this setting, either with the same drug or an alternative ICI agent, has been reported in up to 25% of patients (55).
- Currently, there are no recognized clinical risk factors or serologic biomarkers that reliably identify rechallenge-tolerant versus rechallenge-intolerant patients.

- Considerations for drug rechallenge should be approached on a case-by-case basis, with permanent discontinuation of the agent if symptoms and/or radiographic abnormalities recur.

CONCLUSION

Over the past decade, unprecedented advances in the understanding of immune biology and its role in cancer development has led to a new era in pharmacotherapeutics in which immune-targeted therapies are frequently used in cancer management. The ICIs represent one new class of agents in cancer immunotherapy. ICI agents have become increasingly ubiquitous components of cancer treatment regimens and have precipitated a paradigm shift in the management of a rapidly expanding list of malignancies.

Cancer treatment strategies that contain CTLA-4 and PD-1/PD-L1-targeted therapies have gained the most clinical experience. Although ICIs avoid the indiscriminate cytotoxicity associated with conventional chemotherapy, these agents have been linked to the emergence of a unique spectrum of irAEs that may affect virtually every organ system. Lung-related irAEs are reportedly infrequent, but with variable clinical and histopathological presentations, and unpredictable evolution and sometimes fatal outcomes, clinical vigilance coupled with a high index of suspicion is warranted. Moreover, current published experience likely underestimates the incidence of clinically significant lung toxicity. These numbers are expected to grow as ICI-related toxicities are better recognized and as the clinical application of these agents in various tumor types continue to expand.

Despite the clinical success of ICIs in the management of a growing list of malignancies, critical questions with regard to identification, diagnostic evaluation, and optimal treatment strategies of irAEs remain. In addition, clinical and laboratory biomarkers that identify the patient at risk for immunotoxicity are largely unknown. Ongoing clinical trials may provide important answers to these concerns and inform critical decisions regarding the risk of drug rechallenge among patients with prior irAEs.

Current investigations include the development of other novel immune-based strategies, including modulation of additional immune checkpoint pathways and the use of complex approaches that target different immune mechanisms. Drug combinations using immunotherapy/conventional cytotoxic therapies, immunotherapy/targeted therapies and immunotherapy/radiation therapy are currently undergoing clinical trials. These novel immunotherapeutic approaches may not only increase in incidence of immunotoxicity, but change the landscape, timing, and intensity of toxicity profiles associated with these agents. Shared insights from a multidisciplinary team of experts in oncology, pulmonary medicine, radiology, pathology, and infectious diseases are needed to better understand and anticipate irAEs associated with this class of agents.

ACKNOWLEDGMENT

The author would like to thank Dr. Matthew Hellmann for his critique of the manuscript.

REFERENCES

1. Abdel-Rahman O, Fouad M. Risk of pneumonitis in cancer patients treated with immune checkpoint inhibitors: a meta-analysis. *Ther Adv Respir Dis.* 2016;10:183–193. doi:10.1177/1753465816636557

2. Delaunay M, Cadranel J, Lusque A, et al. Immune-checkpoint inhibitors associated with interstitial lung disease in cancer patients. *Eur Respir J.* 2017;50:1700050. doi:10.1183/13993003.00050-2017

3. Zimmer L, Goldinger SM, Hofmann L, et al. Neurological, respiratory, musculoskeletal, cardiac and ocular side-effects of anti-PD-1 therapy. *Eur J Cancer.* 2016;60:210–225. doi:10.1016/j.ejca.2016.02.024

4. Nishino M, Giobbie-Hurder A, Hatabu H, et al. Incidence of programmed cell death 1 inhibitor-related pneumonitis in patients with advanced cancer: a systematic review and meta-analysis. *JAMA Oncol.* 2016;2:1607–1616. doi:10.1001/jamaoncol.2016.2453

5. Eigentler TK, Hassel JC, Berking C, et al. Diagnosis, monitoring and management of immune-related adverse drug reactions of anti-PD-1 antibody therapy. *Cancer Treat Rev.* 2016;45:7–18. doi:10.1016/j.ctrv.2016.02.003

6. Weber JS, D'Angelo SP, Minor D, et al. Nivolumab versus chemotherapy in patients with advanced melanoma who progressed after anti-CTLA-4 treatment (CheckMate 037): a randomised, controlled, open-label, phase 3 trial. *Lancet Oncol.* 2015;16:375–384. doi:10.1016/s1470-2045(15)70076-8

7. Horvat TZ, Adel NG, Dang TO, et al. Immune-Related adverse events, need for systemic immunosuppression, and effects on survival and time to treatment failure in patients with melanoma treated with ipilimumab at memorial sloan kettering cancer center. *J Clin Oncol.* 2015;33:3193–3198. doi:10.1200/jco.2015.60.8448

8. Boutros C, Tarhini A, Routier E, et al. Safety profiles of anti-CTLA-4 and anti-PD-1 antibodies alone and in combination. *Nat Rev Clin Oncol.* 2016;13:473–486. doi:10.1038/nrclinonc.2016.58

9. Topalian SL, Hodi FS, Brahmer JR, et al. Safety, activity, and immune correlates of anti-PD-1 antibody in cancer. *N Engl J Med.* 2012;366:2443–2454. doi:10.1056/nejmoa1200690

10. Robert C, Schachter J, Long GV, et al. Pembrolizumab versus ipilimumab in advanced melanoma. *N Engl J Med.* 2015;372:2521–2532. doi:10.1056/nejmoa1503093

11. Hassel JC, Heinzerling L, Aberle J, et al. Combined immune checkpoint blockade (anti-PD-1/anti-CTLA-4): Evaluation and management of adverse drug reactions. *Cancer Treat Rev.* 2017;57:36–49. doi:10.1016/j.ctrv.2017.05.003

12. Callahan MK, Kluger H, Postow MA, et al. Nivolumab plus ipilimumab in patients with advanced melanoma: updated survival, response, and safety data in a phase i dose-escalation study. *J Clin Oncol.* 2017;36(4):391–398. doi:10.1200/jco.2017.72.2850

13. Wolchok JD, Kluger H, Callahan MK, et al. Nivolumab plus ipilimumab in advanced melanoma. *N Engl J Med.* 2013;369:122–133. doi:10.1056/nejmoa1302369

14. Larkin J, Hodi FS, Wolchok JD. Combined nivolumab and ipilimumab or monotherapy in untreated melanoma. *N Engl J Med.* 2015;373:1270–1271. doi:10.1056/nejmc1509660

15. Topalian SL, Sznol M, McDermott DF, et al. Survival, durable tumor remission, and long-term safety in patients with advanced melanoma receiving nivolumab. *J Clin Oncol.* 2014;32:1020–1030. doi:10.1200/jco.2013.53.0105

16. Naidoo J, Wang X, Woo KM, et al. Pneumonitis in patients treated with anti-programmed death-1/programmed death ligand 1 therapy. *J Clin Oncol.* 2017;35:709–717. doi:10.1200/jco.2016.68.2005

17. Antonia SJ, Villegas A, Daniel D, et al. Durvalumab after chemoradiotherapy in stage iii non-small-cell lung cancer. *N Engl J Med.* 2017;377:1919–1929. doi:10.1056/nejmoa1709937

18. Chiarion Sileni V, Pigozzo J, Ascierto PA, et al. Efficacy and safety of ipilimumab in elderly patients with pretreated advanced melanoma treated at Italian centres through the expanded access programme. *J Exp Clin Cancer Res.* 2014;33:30. doi:10.1186/1756-9966-33-30

19. Friedman CF, Wolchok JD. Checkpoint inhibition and melanoma: considerations in treating the older adult. *J Geriatr Oncol*. 2017;8:237–241. doi:10.1016/j.jgo.2017.04.003

20. Daste A, Domblides C, Gross-Goupil M, et al. Immune checkpoint inhibitors and elderly people: A review. *Eur J Cancer*. 2017;82:155–166. doi:10.1016/j.ejca.2017.05.044

21. Betof AS, Nipp RD, Giobbie-Hurder A, et al. Impact of age on outcomes with immunotherapy for patients with melanoma. *Oncologist*. 2017;22:963–971. doi:10.1634/theoncologist.2016-0450

22. Singh H, Kim G, Maher VE, et al. FDA subset analysis of the safety of nivolumab in elderly patients with advanced cancers. *J Clin Oncol*. 2016;34(15_suppl):10010. doi:10.1200/jco.2016.34.15_suppl.10010

23. Weber JS, Yang JC, Atkins MB, et al. Toxicities of immunotherapy for the practitioner. *J Clin Oncol*. 2015;33:2092–2099. doi:10.1200/jco.2014.60.0379

24. Tirumani SH, Ramaiya NH, Keraliya A, et al. Radiographic profiling of immune-related adverse events in advanced melanoma patients treated with ipilimumab. *Cancer Immunol Res*. 2015;3:1185–1192. doi:10.1158/2326-6066.cir-15-0102

25. Naidoo J, Page DB, Li BT, et al. Toxicities of the anti-PD-1 and anti-PD-L1 immune checkpoint antibodies. *Ann Oncol*. 2015;26:2375–2391. doi:10.1093/annonc/mdv383

26. Costabel U, Uzaslan E, Guzman J. Bronchoalveolar lavage in drug-induced lung disease. *Clin Chest Med*. 2004;25:25–35. doi:10.1016/s0272-5231(03)00143-6

27. Barjaktarevic IZ, Qadir N, Suri A, et al. Organizing pneumonia as a side effect of ipilimumab treatment of melanoma. *Chest*. 2013;143:858–861. doi:10.1378/chest.12-1467

28. Koelzer VH, Rothschild SI, Zihler D, et al. Systemic inflammation in a melanoma patient treated with immune checkpoint inhibitors-an autopsy study. *J Immunother Cancer*. 2016;4:13. doi:10.1186/s40425-016-0117-1

29. Montaudie H, Pradelli J, Passeron T, et al. Pulmonary sarcoid-like granulomatosis induced by nivolumab. *Br J Dermatol*. 2017;176:1060–1063. doi:10.1111/bjd.14808

30. Berthod G, Lazor R, Letovanec I, et al. Pulmonary sarcoid-like granulomatosis induced by ipilimumab. *J Clin Oncol*. 2012;30:e156–e159. doi:10.1200/jco.2011.39.3298

31. Kim C, Gao J, Shannon VR, et al. Systemic sarcoidosis first manifesting in a tattoo in the setting of immune checkpoint inhibition. *BMJ Case Rep*. 2016;2016:bcr2016216217. doi:10.1136/bcr-2016-21621

32. Cousin S, Toulmonde M, Kind M, et al. Pulmonary sarcoidosis induced by the anti-PD1 monoclonal antibody pembrolizumab. *Ann Oncol*. 2016;27:1178–1179. doi:10.1093/annonc/mdw125

33. Reddy SB, Possick JD, Kluger HM, et al. Sarcoidosis Following Anti-PD-1 and Anti-CTLA-4 Therapy for Metastatic Melanoma. *J Immunother*. 2017;40:307–311. doi:10.1097/cji.0000000000000181

34. Lomax AJ, McGuire HM, McNeil C, et al. Immunotherapy-induced sarcoidosis in patients with melanoma treated with PD-1 checkpoint inhibitors: case series and immunophenotypic analysis. *Int J Rheum Dis*. 2017;20:1277–1285. doi:10.1111/1756-185x.13076

35. Firwana B, Ravilla R, Raval M, et al. Sarcoidosis-like syndrome and lymphadenopathy due to checkpoint inhibitors. *J Oncol Pharm Pract*. 2017;23:620–624. doi:10.1177/1078155216667635

36. Kyi C, Carvajal RD, Wolchok JD, et al. Ipilimumab in patients with melanoma and autoimmune disease. *J Immunother Cancer*. 2014;2:35. doi:10.1186/s40425-014-0035-z

37. Brandsma D, Stalpers L, Taal W, et al. Clinical features, mechanisms, and management of pseudoprogression in malignant gliomas. *Lancet Oncol*. 2008;9:453–461. doi:10.1016/s1470-2045(08)70125-6

38. Therasse P, Arbuck SG, Eisenhauer EA, et al. New guidelines to evaluate the response to treatment in solid tumors. European Organization for Research and Treatment of Cancer, National Cancer Institute of the United States, National Cancer Institute of Canada. *J Natl Cancer Inst*. 2000;92:205–216. doi:10.1093/jnci/92.3.205

39. Eisenhauer EA, Therasse P, Bogaerts J, et al. New response evaluation criteria in solid tumours: revised RECIST guideline (version 1.1). *Eur J Cancer*. 2009;45:228–247. doi:10.1016/j.ejca.2008.10.026

40. Di Giacomo AM, Danielli R, Guidoboni M, et al. Therapeutic efficacy of ipilimumab, an anti-CTLA-4 monoclonal antibody, in patients with metastatic melanoma unresponsive to prior systemic treatments: clinical and immunological evidence from three patient cases. *Cancer Immunol Immunother*. 2009;58:1297–1306. doi:10.1007/s00262-008-0642-y

41. Wolchok JD, Hoos A, O'Day S, et al. Guidelines for the evaluation of immune therapy activity in solid tumors: immune-related response criteria. *Clin Cancer Res.* 2009;15:7412–7420. doi:10.1158/1078-0432.ccr-09-1624

42. Wilkinson TMA. Immune checkpoints in chronic obstructive pulmonary disease. *Eur Respir Rev.* 2017;26:170045. doi:10.1183/16000617.0045-2017

43. Kolla BC, Patel MR. Recurrent pleural effusions and cardiac tamponade as possible manifestations of pseudoprogression associated with nivolumab therapy- a report of two cases. *J Immunother Cancer.* 2016;4:80. doi:10.1186/s40425-016-0185-2

44. Kyi C, Hellmann MD, Wolchok JD, et al. Opportunistic infections in patients treated with immunotherapy for cancer. *J Immunother Cancer.* 2014;2:19. doi:10.1186/2051-1426-2-19

45. Del Castillo M, Romero FA, Arguello E, et al. The Spectrum of Serious Infections Among Patients Receiving Immune Checkpoint Blockade for the Treatment of Melanoma. *Clin Infect Dis.* 2016;63:1490–1493. doi:10.1093/cid/ciw539

46. Chung CH, O'Neil BH. Infusion reactions to monoclonal antibodies for solid tumors: immunologic mechanisms and risk factors. *Oncology (Williston Park).* 2009;23:14–17.

47. Ali AK, Watson DE. Pharmacovigilance Assessment of immune-mediated reactions reported for checkpoint inhibitor cancer immunotherapies. *Pharmacotherapy.* 2017;37:1383–1390. doi:10.1002/phar.2035

48. Nishino M. Immune-related response evaluations during immune-checkpoint inhibitor therapy: establishing a "common language" for the new arena of cancer treatment. *J Immunother Cancer.* 2016;4:30. doi:10.1186/s40425-016-0134-0

49. Balaji A, Verde F, Suresh K, et al. Pneumonitis From Anti-PD-1/ PD-L1 Therapy. *Oncology (Williston Park).* 2017;31:739–746:754.

50. Champiat S, Lambotte O, Barreau E, et al. Management of immune checkpoint blockade dysimmune toxicities: a collaborative position paper. *Ann Oncol.* 2016;27:559–574. doi:10.1093/annonc/mdv623

51. Downey SG, Klapper JA, Smith FO, et al. Prognostic factors related to clinical response in patients with metastatic melanoma treated by CTL-associated antigen-4 blockade. *Clin Cancer Res.* 2007;13:6681–6688. doi:10.1158/1078-0432.ccr-07-0187

52. Arriola E, Wheater M, Krishnan R, et al. Immunosuppression for ipilimumab-related toxicity can cause pneumocystis pneumonia but spare antitumor immune control. *Oncoimmunology.* 2015;4:e1040218. doi:10.1080/2162402x.2015.1040218

53. Michot JM, Bigenwald C, Champiat S, et al. Immune-related adverse events with immune checkpoint blockade: a comprehensive review. *Eur J Cancer.* 2016;54:139–148. doi:10.1016/j.ejca.2015.11.016

54. Nishino M, Ramaiya NH, Hatabu H, et al. PD-1 inhibitor-related pneumonitis in lymphoma patients treated with single-agent pembrolizumab therapy. *Br J Haematol.* 2016;180(5):752–755. doi:10.1111/bjh.14441.

55. Spain L, Diem S, Larkin J. Management of toxicities of immune checkpoint inhibitors. *Cancer Treat Rev.* 2016;44:51–60. doi:10.1016/j.ctrv.2016.02.001

CHAPTER 9

IMMUNE-RELATED ENDOCRINOPATHIES ASSOCIATED WITH IMMUNE CHECKPOINT INHIBITORS

Rajeev Sharma, Ha Nguyen, and Ramona Dadu

INTRODUCTION

Endocrine immune-related adverse events (irAEs) are commonly seen with cytotoxic T-lymphocyte antigen 4 (CTLA-4), programmed cell death 1 (PD-1), programmed cell death ligand 1 (PD-L1), and combination immune checkpoint inhibitor (ICI) therapy. The two most common endocrine irAEs include acute hypophysitis resulting in pituitary hormonal deficiencies (central hypothyroidism, central adrenal insufficiency, and hypogonadotropic hypogonadism), especially with anti-CTLA-4 drugs or combinations and thyroid disease or abnormalities in thyroid function tests, especially with anti-PD-1/PD-L1 drugs or combinations.

Other endocrinopathies, such as type 1 diabetes mellitus, primary adrenal insufficiency, hypogonadism, hypercalcemia, and primary hypoparathyroidism, have been reported as well, but are rare. The diagnostic dilemma in these patients is complicated by the fact that endocrine disease symptoms may overlap with underlying malignancy or masked by the empirical use of steroids. A low threshold for clinical suspicion and continuous patient education is therefore warranted in patients receiving ICIs.

THYROID ABNORMALITIES

Thyroid dysfunction is one of the common endocrine adverse effects of checkpoint inhibitor therapy. As thyroid function tests (TFTs) are routinely monitored before each ICI cycle, various thyroid abnormalities are identified in the absence of any symptoms most of the times.

- The spectrum of thyroid abnormality seen commonly is primary hypothyroidism, immune-related thyroiditis causing transient thyrotoxicosis followed by likely long-term hypothyroidism.
- Secondary hypothyroidism as sequela of hypophysitis is also seen.

An algorithm for diagnosis and treatment is summarized in Figure 9.1

Thyrotoxicosis (Also Known as Hyperthyroidism)

Thyrotoxicosis in setting of use of checkpoint inhibitor therapy is seen in about 0.4% to 14% patients across the various clinical trials (1,2). The most common cause of thyrotoxicosis is immune-mediated thyroiditis with Graves disease being very rare.

Published by Springer Publishing Company DOI: 10.1891/9780826172150.0009

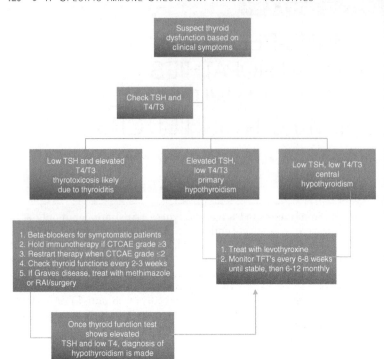

FIGURE 9.1 Diagnosis and management of checkpoint inhibitor thyroid dysfunction.

CTCAE, Common terminology criteria for adverse events; TFTs, thyroid function tests; TSH, thyroid-stimulating hormone.

Thyroiditis

Prevalence

Thyroiditis is very infrequently reported as a sole irAE. In most studies examining ICI-mediated thyroiditis, a distinction is made between hypothyroidism, hyperthyroidism, or thyroiditis cases, when in reality these are likely part of the same disease process.

- Thyroiditis is the most common cause of thyrotoxicosis, commonly seen with anti-PD-1/PD-L1 drugs or combinations (2–7).
  - The incidence of thyroiditis/hyperthyroidism varies from 4% with ipilimumab, 2.7% with nivolumab, and 3 to 7.8% with pembrolizumab.
  - The number of incidence is increased with combination therapies: 4.3% to 14% with nivolumab plus ipilimumab and 4.5% to 6% with pembrolizumab plus ipilimumab.

In a recent meta-analysis, within different classes of checkpoint inhibitors, combination therapy of anti-CTLA-4 and PD-1 had the highest incidence compared to single agent PD-1 or CTLA-4 inhibitor therapy.

- Among PD-1 inhibitors, pembrolizumab has an increased incidence of hyperthyroidism compared to nivolumab (3.8% versus 2.5%).
- Hyperthyroidism incidence was not significantly different in higher versus low-dose anti-PD-1 pembrolizumab (8).

Pathophysiology

The mechanism of thyroiditis is thought to be immune-mediated destruction of normal thyroid cells and release of preformed thyroid hormones, thyroxine (T4) and triiodothyronine (T3), into the circulation.

- One study from Mayo Clinic has shown more circulating CD56+CD16+ natural killer (NK) cells and an elevated human leukocyte antigen-DR isotype (HLA-DR) surface expression in the inflammatory CD14+ CD16+ monocytes in anti-PD-1-treated patients. The study proposes that the mechanism of thyroid destruction may include T cell, NK cell, and/or monocyte-mediated pathways and appears independent of thyroid autoantibodies (9).

Clinical Presentation

- Median time to develop hyperthyroidism is about 3 to 6 weeks after starting therapy.
- Many patients present with painless thyroiditis (10,11).
  - Most of the patients are asymptomatic or present with mild symptoms.
- Classic symptoms of more severe thyrotoxicosis include palpitation, tremors, increased sweating, thinning of hair, weight loss, insomnia, agitation, and mood changes.
- The symptoms are more pronounced in younger patients while elderly patients may present with no symptoms (apathetic hyperthyroidism) or with atrial fibrillation.
- As thyroiditis improves, it evolves into a hypothyroid phase in many patients.
  - In one study, the median time for transition from thyrotoxicosis to hypothyroidism was about 6 weeks (12).

Diagnosis

The laboratory diagnosis of thyrotoxicosis due to thyroiditis is dependent on the measurement of thyroid-stimulating hormone (TSH) and free T4 and total T3 levels.

- Classically, during the initial phase of thyroiditis (hyperthyroid phase, blood tests show low/suppressed TSH and elevated free T4 followed by either hypothyroidism (elevated TSH and low T4) or recovery (normal TSH/T4).
  - Therefore, a baseline TSH and T4 followed by serial values over time (usually 2 to 3 weeks) should be performed and thyroid hormone replacement initiated once hypothyroidism is diagnosed (13).
- Some researchers have shown that patients with baseline positive thyroid antibodies (anti-thyroglobulin [TgAb] or anti-thyroid peroxidase antibodies [TPOAb]) were more likely to have destructive thyroiditis,

and checking antibodies at baseline may help identify patients at high risk of thyroid disorders with use of checkpoint inhibitors (14)

Treatment

The checkpoint inhibitor-induced hyperthyroidism is usually managed symptomatically.

- Thyrotoxicosis symptoms due to thyroiditis are treated with beta-blockers.
  - The commonly used beta-blockers are nonspecific propranolol or more specific beta-1 blockers atenolol or metoprolol. The usual starting dose of atenolol is 25 to 50 mg daily with a goal heart rate of less than 90 per minute.
  - Repeat thyroid hormone panel should be performed every 2 to 3 weeks until hypothyroidism is diagnosed.
  - Once therapy with thyroid hormone is initiated, recheck thyroid tests in 6 to 8 weeks followed by every 6 to 12 months if stable clinically and biochemically (13) (Figure 9.1).
  - Antithyroid drugs like methimazole are almost never used, as the underlying pathology is destructive thyroiditis and not excess thyroid hormones production.
- Checkpoint inhibitors are recommended to be held for ≥ grade 3 thyroid irAEs (15).
  - The therapy with checkpoint inhibitors can be resumed after the patient has been adequately controlled for symptoms and is safe.

Recovery

A majority of the patients develop long-term hypothyroidism requiring thyroid hormone replacement.

Hyperthyroidism Due to Graves Disease

Hyperthyroidism due to Graves disease is uncommon in these patients and is reported with use of anti-CTLA-4 agents and not PD-1 inhibitors (10,16). However, this entity needs to be in differential diagnosis of thyrotoxicosis.

- The symptoms of thyroiditis and Graves disease may be similar with some notable differences.
  - Exophthalmos and pretibial myxedema are characteristic of Graves disease but are absent in thyroiditis.
  - Thyroid antibodies like thyroid-stimulating immunoglobulin (TSI) or TSH receptor antibodies (TRAbs) are commonly found in Graves disease.
  - If possible, in acute phase of thyrotoxicosis, a radioiodine uptake scan can differentiate between thyroiditis (low uptake) versus Graves disease (increased uptake).
- It is important to differentiate between the two, as management is different (symptomatic with thyroiditis versus thionamides, radioactive iodine therapy, or surgery in Graves).

Primary Hypothyroidism

Prevalence

The incidence of hypothyroidism ranges from 3.8% with ipilimumab to about 13.2% with combination therapy of ipilimumab and nivolumab (1,8).

- The odds of having hypothyroidism with PD-L1 inhibitor (e.g., atezolimumab) compared to anti-CTLA-4 agent ipilimumab are not significantly different.
- No significant differences in incidence of hypothyroidism were observed between PD-1 inhibitors nivolumab and pemrolizumab.
- There was no significant difference in hypothyroid incidence with use of higher or lower dose of anti-PD-1 agent pembrolizumab (8.2% versus 7.6%) (8).

Pathophysiology

Most of the cases of primary hypothyroidism are a sequel of previous thyroiditis episodes as result of destructive process in thyroid gland.

- Isolated primary hypothyroidism with use of checkpoint inhibitors is probably rare.

Clinical Presentation

The clinical manifestation of primary hypothyroidism is nonspecific and variable. Most patients are asymptomatic and the hypothyroidism is identified on routine laboratory testing.

- Hypothyroidism symptoms include weight gain, dry skin, fatigue, cold intolerance, constipation, somnolence, and menstrual abnormalities in women.
- On physical examination, bradycardia, hypertension (specifically diastolic), dry skin, nonpitting edema of the lower limbs, and delayed relaxation of deep tendon reflexes might be encountered.

Diagnosis

Laboratory examination characteristic of primary hypothyroidism shows elevated TSH and low T4. T3 may also be low on blood tests.

- Because the majority of these patients have hypothyroidism as a sequel of previous thyroiditis, one should be careful interpreting the tests during recovery phase.
  - In this situation, thyroid testing may show transient low TSH and T4 as TSH lags behind during the recovery, and this could be construed as central hypothyroidism.

Treatment

- Typically, patients are treated with synthetic T4 hormone (levothyroxine).
  - The starting dose is usually 1.6 to 1.7 µ/kg body weight.

- ○ In elderly and those with cardiac issues, a step-up dose regimen with lower starting dose is advised to prevent any side effects.
- ○ The drug is preferably taken on an empty stomach with water in the morning; if that's not possible, then at night about 3 to 4 hours after dinner as food might cause problems with absorption.
- ○ It is advisable to avoid taking levothyroxine with calcium, iron, bile acid resins, and caffeine.
- ○ A repeat thyroid test after 6 to 8 weeks is recommended to adjust the dose.
- Once a stable dose is achieved with normalization of TSH and patient feels asymptomatic, a longer follow-up visit can be advised.
- Over-replacement should be discouraged as it can lead to bone loss and adverse cardiac effects (15).
- Checkpoint inhibitors are recommended to be held for ≥ grade 3 irAEs (17).
- ○ The therapy with checkpoint inhibitors can be resumed after patient has resolution of symptoms to grade 2 or lower (13).

Recovery

There is sparse and conflicting data about the resolution of primary hypothyroidism after stopping ICI therapy. One study with pembrolizumab showed recovery in four out of seven patients while other did not (18,19).

IMMUNE-RELATED HYPOPHYSITIS

Incidence

- Immune-related hypophysitis (IH) occurs mainly in patients treated with anti-CTLA-4 antibodies (ipilimumab and tremelimumab) alone or in combination with other checkpoint inhibitors.
- ○ IH occurrence remains very rare in patients treated with single agent anti-PD-1 or PD-L1 antibodies.
- Due to lack of strict definitions, much difficulty in obtaining accurate data on incidence and prevalence of this disorder based on clinical trials is noted.
- ○ The prevalence varies greatly from 1% to 17%.
- ○ Several reports focused on endocrine irAEs (each case evaluated by an endocrinologist) report IH prevalence as 8% to 11% (18–21). A strict criterion for the definition of IH was not used in any of these studies.

Pathophysiology

The exact mechanism of IH is not clearly established. However, a study has demonstrated the roles of autoantibodies recognizing TSH, follicle-stimulating hormone (FSH), and adrenocorticotropic hormone (ACTH)-secreting cells and the activation of complement pathway through binding activity of Ipilimumab IgG1 or autoantibodies to CTLA-4, which is expressed in normal pituitary tissue, as possible mechanisms of IH (22).

Clinical Picture

The median time from starting ipilimumab to diagnosis of IH is 8 to 9 weeks, or after the third dose of ipilimumab.

- Headache and fatigue are most commonly seen, and can occur in 85% and 65% of patients, respectively.
  - Visual changes are uncommon. However, some patients remain asymptomatic.
- Clinical suspicion is frequently raised when routine TFT monitoring (as recommended in the package insert) shows evidence of central hypothyroidism, leading to further testing.
- The most common hormone deficiency appears to be central hypothyroidism (>90%), followed by central adrenal insufficiency (75%–86%), and hypogonadism (79%–84%) (19,23).
  - In our experience, involvement of all three pituitary axes occurs in half of the patients (23).
  - Prolactin level could be low in more than 50% of patients, but high levels were also reported.
  - Hyponatremia occurs in 55% of patients.
- Low levels of insulin growth factor-1 (IGF-1) could be present in 28% to 46% patients (19,23).
  - There is only one case of central diabetes insipidus associated with anti-PD-L1 (Avelumab) reported to date (24).
- MRI findings can be seen in 80% to 90% of patients; however, sometimes these findings may be subtle and may not be readily apparent without comparison with a baseline scan.
  - In our experience, 90% of patients had increased height of the gland when compared with baseline scans.
  - Other MRI abnormalities include stalk thickening (70%), suprasellar convexity (48%), and heterogeneous enhancement of the pituitary gland (37%) (25). Resolution of pituitary enlargement is common with all cases resolved on follow-up scans at 2 months (2,19,26,27).

There are no good predictors to help identify patients at risk.

- A progressive decline in TSH level was noted prior to the onset of symptom or IH diagnosis.
- On MRI of the sella, pituitary enlargement can precede the development of clinical and biochemical evidence of IH (19).

Diagnosis

Strict criteria for diagnostic confirmation of IH are not currently available. Based on previous retrospective data and clinical experience proposed confirmation criteria of IH include:

- ≥1 pituitary hormone deficiency (TSH or ACTH deficiency required) combined with an MRI abnormality.
- ≥2 pituitary hormone deficiencies (TSH or ACTH deficiency required) in the presence of headache and other symptoms.

- Central hypogonadism was commonly reported in many case series of IH.
  - However, because the gonadal hormones are sensitive to changes in acute illness, central hypogonadism was not required in the criteria.
  - Recently, the criteria have been validated in large cohort with excellent performance (23).

Management

- Management of confirmed IH includes replacement of deficient hormones (physiologic doses of steroids and thyroid hormone).
  - Gonadal hormone replacement might not be indicated in all cases.
- High doses of steroids may be necessary in the setting of severe headaches, vision changes, or adrenal crisis.
  - Recently, in a large cohort study performed at the University of Texas MD Anderson Cancer Center, high-dose steroids werenot proven to have more benefits in pituitary hormone recovery compared with physiologic doses of steroids (23). Similar findings have also been reported in other retrospective studies (28,29).
  - We recommend that high dose of steroids may not always be necessary.
- Physiologic dose of steroids can be used in the majority of IH patients with no life-threatening symptoms (19–21,23).

Both adrenal insufficiency and hypothyroidism appear to represent long-term sequelae of hypophysitis and lifelong hormonal replacement is needed in most cases.

- If patients have both adrenal insufficiency and hypothyroidism, it is important that glucocorticoid therapy should be initiated prior to thyroid hormone replacement.
- The administration of thyroid hormones in patient with untreated adrenal insufficiency can precipitate adrenal crisis.
  - It is difficult to report the incidence of recovery because of unclear criteria and inconsistency among studies. Recovery of thyroid was reported in 21% to 60% of patients.
  - Adrenal recovery is rarer and its incidence ranged from 0% to as high as 17%. Of note, follow up and reassessment of adrenal function were not clear in many studies.
- From 60% to 71% patients with central hypogonadism can achieve recovery (20,23,28).
  - In our experience, treatment with gonadal hormones may not have significant impact on gonadal hormone recovery as some patients were able to achieve recovery without gonadal hormonal replacement (23).
- Continuous monitoring with clinical assessment and repeat biochemical evaluation aimed to test for recovery is needed in order to appropriately treat these patients.

○ We recommend periodic assessment, such as every 3 months in the first year and every 6 months thereafter.

Recommendations for Diagnosis and Follow-Up (Figure 9.2)

Hold ICI if ≥ grade 2 irAE until work up is completed and appropriate hormone replacement is started.

• If central adrenal insufficiency: start physiologic steroid replacement: Hydrocortisone ~ 10 mg/m^2 (hydrocortisone 15 mg at 8 a.m., 5 mg at 3 p.m.)

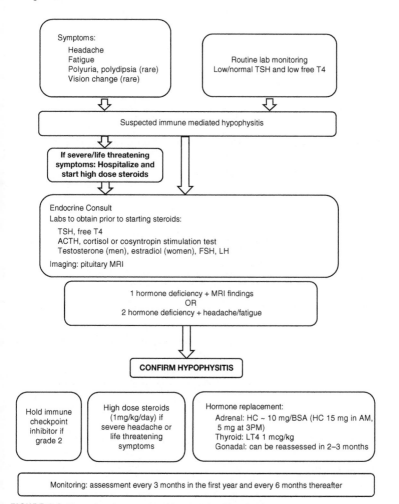

FIGURE 9.2 Diagnosis and management of immune-related hypophysitis.

ACTH, adrenocorticotropic hormone; FSH, follicle-stimulating hormone; LH, luteinizing hormone; TSH, thyroid-stimulating hormone.

- ○ Periodic assessment (e.g., every 3 months in the first year and every 6 months thereafter): clinical monitoring and repeat hormone levels (a.m. cortisol and ACTH and/or low-dose cosyntropin stimulation test) to assess recovery.
- If central hypothyroidism: start thyroid hormone (levothyroxine 1.6 mcg/kg).
  - ○ Repeat thyroid function testing 6 to 8 weeks after initiation of thyroid hormone and then periodically (e.g., every 3 months in the first year and every 6 months thereafter) to assess recovery.
- If central hypogonadism, repeat hormone levels in 2 to 3 months and consider testosterone in men or hormone replacement therapy in women if appropriate for cancer type.

For severe/life-threatening symptoms such as adrenal crisis, severe headache, and visual field deficiency:

- Hospitalize as appropriate.
- High-dose corticosteroid (prednisone 1 mg/kg/day) (or equivalent dose of methylprednisolone) in the acute phase, followed by taper over 1 month.
- Adrenal crisis should be managed per standard guidelines.
- If central hypothyroidism, replace thyroid hormone (see above) after corticosteroids have been initiated.

IMMUNE-MEDIATED DIABETES

Incidence

Immune-mediated diabetes related to ICI is a very rare but important AE. Its incidence was reported to be approximately 0.2% in a recent systematic review and meta-analysis (8).

- Checkpoint inhibitor immune-mediated diabetes has been reported in patients on anti-PD-1 or PD-L1 antibodies with or without anti-CTLA4 antibodies (30,31).
  - ○ To date, only one patient who developed immune-mediated diabetes from anti-CTLA4 antibody (Ipilimumab) use as a single agent has been described in the English literature (32).
- With regards to the pathophysiology, the PD-1 and PD-L1 pathway has been shown to play a critical role in regulating autoimmune diabetes.
  - ○ Blockade of PD-1 or PD-L1 can lead to rapid development of diabetes in animal models (33).
- In human studies, both humoral and cellular immunity have been proposed to be involved in the mechanism of the disease (34).

Clinical Picture

Clinically, immune-mediated diabetes can affect individuals with or without pre-existing diabetes.

- Patients can present with acute and new onset diabetes ketoacidosis, new hyperglycemia, or worsening glucose control in pre-existing diabetes.

- Time from drug administration to diabetes onset varied from 1 week to 5 months (31).

Diagnosis

- Most patients have evidence of decreased beta cell function with inappropriately low or undetectable C peptide levels.
- The presence of anti-GAD65 and/or insulin antibodies are common findings in these patients.
- Anti-islet cell and anti-zinc transporter antibodies can also be found. Majority of patients required long-term insulin therapy and follow-up (35).

Management

Although immune-mediated diabetes associated with checkpoint inhibitors is rare, patients can be acutely ill with diabetes ketoacidosis requiring hospitalization and need long-term therapy.

- An HbA1c or blood glucose should be obtained at baseline before the starting of ICIs.
- We recommend blood glucose be monitored before each cycle of drug administration and appropriate treatment be started promptly if needed.

PRIMARY ADRENAL INSUFFICIENCY

Immune-mediated primary adrenal insufficiency is a very rare endocrine AE related to ICIs.

- The majority of affected patients were using PD-1 antibodies or PD-L1 antibodies with only a few cases on CTLA-4 antibodies as a single agent.
  - In a recent systematic study and meta-analysis across 62 study cohorts, the incidence was 0.7%.
  - However, among the patients who received combination therapy (PD-L1/PD-1 antibodies and CTLA-4 antibodies), the reported incidence was higher (4.2%) (8).
- Hormonal studies can help differentiate primary adrenal insufficiency (high ACTH, low cortisol) from secondary adrenal insufficiency (low or normal ACTH, low cortisol).
- Replacement with glucocorticoid is per standard of care for primary adrenal insufficiency.
  - Long-term follow-up is recommended.

CONCLUSIONS FOR ENDOCRINE irAEs

There is significant variance in definitions of irAEs, their severity, as well as variation in how symptoms and signs may be attributable to other irAEs. Currently, there are no good predictors for either response or toxicity to immunotherapy.

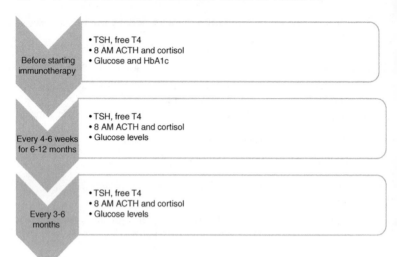

FIGURE 9.3 Proposed algorithm for routine monitoring in all patients treated with immunotherapy.

ACTH, adrenocorticotropic hormone; TSH, thyroid stimulating hormone.

- Therefore, identification of patients at risk, consistent communication between patients and medical teams, frequent monitoring, early recognition, and treatment of irAEs are critical in optimizing treatment outcomes.
- Additionally, in all patients receiving ICIs, routine monitoring for clinical signs and symptoms of endocrinopathies, and patient education are recommended.
- All patients should be tested before starting immunotherapy for thyroid (TSH and free T4), adrenal (early morning ACTH and cortisol), and glycemic control (glucose and HbA1c).
- Before each cycle, thyroid testing (TSH and free T4) should be repeated, along with a baseline metabolic panel to allow monitoring of glycemic trends.
  ○ Routine monitoring with early morning ACTH and cortisol levels should be considered (every month for 6 months, then every 3 months for 6 months, and then every 6 months for 1 year) (Figure 9.3).
- Once an immune-mediated endocrinopathy is diagnosed, appropriate treatment should be started promptly.
  ○ Long-term follow-up and reassessment of hormone function for possible recovery is recommended in all patients.

REFERENCES

1. Abdel-Rahman O, ElHalawani H, Fouad M. Risk of endocrine complications in cancer patients treated with immune check point inhibitors: a meta-analysis. *Future Oncol.* 2016;12(3):413–25. doi:10.2217/fon.15.222

2. Cukier P, Santini FC, Scaranti M, et al. Endocrine side effects of cancer immunotherapy. *Endocr Relat Cancer.* 2017;24(12):T331–T347. doi:10.1530/erc-17-0358

3. Weber J, Mandala M, Del Vecchio M, et al. Adjuvant nivolumab versus ipilimumab in resected stage III or IV melanoma. *N Engl J Med.* 2017;377:1824–1835. doi:10.1056/nejmoa1709030

4. Reck M, Rodriquez-Abreau D, Robinson AG, et al. Pembrolizumab versus chemotherapy for PD-L1-positive non-small-cell lung cancer. *N Engl J Med.* 2016;375:1823–1833. doi:10.1056/nejmoa1606774

5. Petrylak DP, Powles T, Bellmunt J, et al. A phase Ia study of MPDL3280A (anti-PDL1): updated response and survival data in urothelial bladder cancer (UBC). *J Clin Oncol.* 2015;33(15 suppl):4501.

6. Postow MA, Chesney J, Pavlick AC, et al. Nivolumab and ipilimumab versus ipilimumab in untreated melanoma. *N Engl J Med.* 2015;372:2006–2017. doi:10.1056/NEJMoa1414428

7. Atkins MB, Choueiri TK, Hodi FS, et al. Pembrolizumab plus low-dose ipilimumab in patients with advanced melanoma or renal cell carcinoma: data from the KEYNOTE-029 phase 1 study. *J Clin Oncol.* 2015;33(15 suppl):3009.

8. Barroso-Sousa R, Barry WT, Garrido-Castro AC, et al. Incidence of endocrine dysfunction following the use of different immune checkpoint inhibitor regimens: a systematic review and meta-analysis. *JAMA Oncol.* 2018;4(2):173–182. doi:10.1001/jamaoncol.2017.3064

9. Delivanis DA, Gustafson MP, Bornschlegl S, et al. Permbrolizumab-induced thyroiditis: comprehensive clinical review and insights into underlying involved mechanisms. *J Clin Endocrinol Metab.* 2017;102(8):2770–2780. doi:10.1210/jc.2017-00448

10. Yamauchi I, Sakane Y, Fukuda Y, et al. Clinical features of nivolumab-induced thyroiditis: a case series study. *Thyroid.* 2017;27(7):894–901. doi:10.1089/thy.2016.0562

11. Orlov S, Salari F, Kashat L, et al. Induction of painless thyroiditis in patients receiving programmed death 1 receptor immunotherapy for metastatic malignancies. *J Clin Endocrinol Metab.* 2015;100(5):1738–1741. doi:10.1210/jc.2014-4560

12. Lee H, Hodi FS, Giobbie-Hurder A, et al. Characterization of thyroid disorders in patients receiving immune checkpoint inhibition therapy. *Cancer Immunol Res.* 2017;5(12):1133–1140. doi:10.1158/2326-6066.cir-17-0208

13. Puzanov I, Diab A, Abdallah K, et al. Managing toxicities associated with immune checkpoint inhibitors: consensus recommendations from the Society for Immunotherapy of Cancer (SITC) Toxicity Management Working Group. *J Immunother Cancer.* 2017;5(1):95. doi:10.1186/s40425-017-0300-z

14. Kobayashi T, Iwama S, Yasuda Y, et al. Patients with antithyroid antibodies are prone to develop destructive thyroiditis by Nivolumab: a prospective study. *J Endocr Soc.* 2018;2(3):241–251. doi:10.1210/js.2017-00432

15. Garber JR, Cobin RH, Gharib H, et al. Clinical practice guidelines for hypothyroidism in adults: cosponsored by the American Association of Clinical Endocrinologists and the American Thyroid Association. *Thyroid.* 2012;22(12):1200–1235. doi:10.1089/thy.2012.0205

16. Borodic G, Hinkle DM, Cia Y. Drug-induced Graves disease from CTLA-4 receptor suppression. *Ophthal Plast Reconstr Surg.* 2011;27(4): e87–e88. doi:10.1097/iop.0b013e3181ef72a1

17. U.S. Department of Health and Human Services. *Common terminology criteria for adverse events.* 2010.

18. Ryder M, Callahan M, Postow MA, et al. Endocrine-related adverse events following ipilimumab in patients with advanced melanoma: a comprehensive retrospective review from a single institution. *Endocr Relat Cancer.* 2014;21(2):371–381. doi:10.1530/erc-13-0499

19. Faje A. Immunotherapy and hypophysitis: clinical presentation, treatment, and biologic insights. *Pituitary.* 2016;19(1):82–92. doi:10.1007/s11102-015-0671-4

20. Faje AT, Sullivan R, Lawrence D, et al. Ipilimumab-induced hypophysitis: a detailed longitudinal analysis in a large cohort of patients with metastatic melanoma. *J Clin Endocrinol Metab.* 2014;99(11):4078–4085. doi:10.1210/jc.2014-2306

21. Corsello SM, Barnabei A, Marchetti P, et al. Endocrine side effects induced by immune checkpoint inhibitors. *J Clin Endocrinol Metab.* 2013;98(4):1361–1375. doi:10.1210/jc.2012-4075

22. Iwama S, De Remigis A, Callahan MK, et al. Pituitary expression of CTLA-4 mediates hypophysitis secondary to administration of CTLA-4 blocking antibody. *Sci Transl Med.* 2014;6(230):230ra45. doi:10.1126/scitranslmed.3008002

23. Nguyen KS, Waguespack SG, Habra MA, et al. Immune-related Hypophysitis (irh) associated with checkpoint inhibitor therapy: diagnosis, characteristics and long term follow up in the endocrine society meeting 2018. Chicago, USA; 2018.

24. Zhao C, Tella SH, Del Rivero J, et al. Anti-PD-L1 Treatment Induced Central Diabetes Insipidus. *J Clin Endocrinol Metab.* 2018;103(2):365–369. doi:10.1210/jc.2017-01905

25. Komal Shah SA, Cabanillas M, Dadu R, et al. *Imaging Findings of Cancer Immunotherapy Induced Hypophysitis.* ASNR. 2015.

26. Pitteloud M, Dadu R, Cabanillas ME, et al. *Hypophysitis in the Age of Cancer Immunotherapy: Experience in a Large Cancer Center.* ENDO. 2015.

27. Byun DJ, Wolchok JD, Rosenberg LM, et al. Cancer immunotherapy—immune checkpoint blockade and associated endocrinopathies. *Nat Rev Endocrinol.* 2017;13(4):195–207. doi:10.1038/nrendo.2016.205

28. Min L, Hodi FS, Giobbie-Hurder A, et al. Systemic high-dose corticosteroid treatment does not improve the outcome of ipilimumab-related hypophysitis: a retrospective cohort study. *Clin Cancer Res.* 2015;21(4):749–755. doi:10.1158/1078-0432.ccr-14-2353

29. Honegger J, Buchfelder M, Schlaffer S, et al. Treatment of primary hypophysitis in Germany. *J Clin Endocrinol Metab.* 2015;100(9):3460–3469. doi:10.1210/jc.2015-2146

30. Chae YK, Chiec L, Mohindra N, et al. A case of pembrolizumab-induced type-1 diabetes mellitus and discussion of immune checkpoint inhibitor-induced type 1 diabetes. *Cancer Immunol Immunother.* 2017;66(1):25–32. doi:10.1007/s00262-016-1913-7

31. Kapke J, Shaheen Z, Kilari D, et al. Immune checkpoint inhibitor-associated Type 1 diabetes mellitus: case series, review of the literature, and optimal management. *Case Rep Oncol.* 2017;10(3):897–909. doi:10.1159/000480634

32. Yamazaki N, Kiyohara Y, Uhara H, et al. Phase II study of ipilimumab monotherapy in Japanese patients with advanced melanoma. *Cancer Chemother Pharmacol.* 2015;76(5):997–1004. doi:10.1007/s00280-015-2873-x

33. Guleria I, Gubbels Bupp M, Dada S, et al. Mechanisms of PDL1-mediated regulation of autoimmune diabetes. *Clin Immunol.* 2007;125(1):16–25. doi:10.1016/j.clim.2007.05.013

34. Hughes J, Vudattu N, Sznol M, et al. Precipitation of autoimmune diabetes with anti-PD-1 immunotherapy. *Diabetes Care.* 2015;38(4):e55–e57. doi:10.2337/dc12-0321

35. Priyanka Iyer CB, Lavis VR, Varghese JM, et al. *Checkpoint inhibitor mediated insulin dependent diabetes: a cancer center experience.* In *The Endocrine Society meeting 2018.* 2018.

CHAPTER 10

NEUROLOGIC ADVERSE EVENTS AND NEUROLOGIC COMPLICATIONS

Haroon Ahmad, Jasmin Jo, Elizabeth Gaughan, and Camilo Fadul

INTRODUCTION

Neurologic adverse events (AEs) caused by a direct effect of the drug on the nervous system are frequently the dose-limiting toxicity in patients receiving chemotherapy for cancer. The approval and widespread use of new molecules and biologicals for the treatment of cancer has resulted in the description of unique and severe neurologic toxicities that, although associated with, are not directly caused by the therapy. For example, the association of posterior reversible encephalopathy syndrome (PRES) with bevacizumab was only recognized after more widespread use of the drug (1).

Immune-related adverse events (irAEs) are the most frequent and potentially life-threatening toxicities associated with immune checkpoint inhibitors (ICIs). About 10% of the patients treated with these medications may have mild-to-moderate neurologic symptoms, but severe immune-mediated neurologic complications occur in less than 1% of the patients (2). Though rare, awareness of their clinical presentation is necessary because early recognition and adequate management will dictate the outcome.

The incidence of neurologic complications associated with ICI is difficult to ascertain because, although there are meta-analysis and reports of large series, many are single or small case reports that are not well documented and causality cannot be definitely established (Table 10.1). Some patients may suffer nonspecific neurologic symptoms that may be constitutional and usually resolve spontaneously, while some of the severe neurologic toxicities ascribed to ICI may be caused by the cancer itself or other oncologic treatments. Furthermore, it is recognized that the incidence will vary according to the drug's mechanism of action (cytotoxic T-lymphocyte antigen 4 [CTLA-4], programmed cell death 1 [PD-1], and programmed cell death ligand 1 [PD-L1] blockade) and the combination of agents (2,3).

This chapter will describe the reported severe immune-related neurologic syndromes associated with ICI, while providing recommendations on diagnostic approach and management. The neurologic immune-mediated AEs range from involvement of the cortex (encephalitis) to the muscle (myositis) and the syndromes will be branded according to the area of the nervous system affected. Optic neuritis, hypophysitis, and myositis will be covered in other chapters.

Published by Springer Publishing Company DOI: 10.1891/9780826172150.0010

TABLE 10.1 Reported Incidences of Neurologic Adverse Events

Drug	Grade 3/4 (3) (%)	Any grade (3) (%)
Ipilimumab	0.8	3.0
All CTLA-4 ICI	0.7	3.8
Nivolumab	0.4	5.2
Pembrolizumab	0.2	6.3
All PD-1 ICI	0.4	6.1
Combination CTLA4+PD-1	0.7	12.0

CTLA-4, cytotoxic T-lymphocyte antigen 4; ICI, immune checkpoint inhibitors; PD-1, programmed cell death 1.

Source: Adapted from Cuzzubbo S, Javeri F, Tissier M, et al. Neurological adverse events associated with immune checkpoint inhibitors: Review of the literature. *Eur J Cancer*. 2017;73:1–8. doi:10.1016/j.ejca.2016.12.001

AEs BY NEUROLOGIC LOCALIZATION

Brain

Encephalitis

Encephalitis is a general term used for inflammation of the brain parenchyma caused by a number of etiologies including autoimmune, infectious, paraneoplastic, or idiopathic.

- Symptoms can include fever, nuchal rigidity, encephalopathy, or seizures.
- Diagnosis is usually made through central nervous system (CNS) imaging and cerebrospinal fluid (CSF) analysis; the latter would typically show an increase in the number of leukocytes, low glucose, and increased protein concentration.

According to clinical trials data, the frequency of ICI-induced autoimmune encephalitis is low. The incidence is estimated to be 0.1 to less than 1% with a higher probability during combined or sequential anti-CTLA-4/anti-PD-1 therapy than during anti-PD-1 or anti-PD-L1 monotherapy (4).

Our literature review identified 11 cases of encephalitis purportedly caused by anti-CTLA-4, anti-PD-1, anti-PD-L1, or combination therapy (Table 10.2).

- The onset of symptoms after ICI therapy varied widely, with two cases developing after the first course (5,11) and one not until the 36th course of anti-PD-1 therapy (8).
- The presentations generally fit the usual pattern of encephalitis: with acute to subacute onset confusion or cognitive changes.
  - One patient had seizures and MRI revealed findings suggestive of frontal lobe inflammation (9).
- The diagnosis in all cases was established by CNS imaging and/or CSF analysis.

TABLE 10.2 Encephalitis Cases

Cases	Age/sex	ICI	Primary cancer	Cycles to onset	Presentation	Diagnostic findings	Treatment	Outcome	Ref
1	71M	Ipi 3 mg/kg q3 weeks	MEL	1	Brainstem Encephalitis	Increased protein CSF, normal WBC, no malignant cells	Stopped Ipi, High dose steroids	Improvement in 24 hours	(5)
2	64M	Ipi 10 mg/kg q3 weeks	Prostate Carcinoma	NR	Encephalopathy, possibly secondary to thyroiditis	Normal CSF and normal MRI.	High dose steroids	Improvement in 3 days	(6)
3	NR	Ipi	MEL	NR	Autoimmune meningoencephalitis	NR	NR	NR	(7)
4	78M	No 3 mg/kg q3 weeks	NSCLC	14	Autoimmune Encephalitis	MRI normal, CSF increased protein and pleocytosis.	Steroids and AEDs	Improved fully in 24 hours	(4)
5	51F	Pem 10 mg/kg q2 weeks	MEL	36	Encephalopathy. Concurrent fasciitis	MRI with subcortical T2 enhancing lesions. CSF normal	Steroids	Partial response	(8)
6	66M	Pem 2 mg/kg q3 weeks	MEL	6	Encephalitis with seizures	MRI with T2 hyperintensities bilaterally. Biosy showed neuropil with diffuse microglial activation and focal perivascular inflammation with lymphocytic infiltrates	Supportive care and AEDs and stopped Pem	Complete response 2–4 months follow-up MRI	(9)

(continued)

TABLE 10.2 Encephalitis Cases (*continued*)

Cases	Age/sex	ICI	Primary cancer	Cycles to onset	Presentation	Diagnostic findings	Treatment	Outcome	Ref
7	NR	Pem	MEL	1 year	Limbic encephalitis	Antibody negative, MRI hyperintensity in limbic structures. CSF with pleocytosis	Steroids	No improvement, but no progression	(10)
8	59F	ATZ	Urothelial carcinoma	1	Encephalitis	MRI with enhancing lesion, CSF normal	Steroids	Partial improvement in 5 days	(11)
9	NR	Ipi + Pem	MEL	NR	Brainstem encephalitis	NR	NR	Patient died	(12)
10-11	NR	Ipi 3 mg/kg+ Nivo 1 mg/kg	NR	NR	Limbic encephalitis and anti-NMDA receptor encephalitis	NR	Prednisone for 1st, steroids and Ritux for 2nd	Improvement	(13)

AChR Ab, acetylcholine receptor antibody; ATZ, atezolizumab; AEDs, anti-epilepsy drugs; CSF, cerebrospinal fluid; EMG, electromyography study; ICI, immune checkpoint inhibitors; Ipi, ipilimumab; IVIG, Intravenous immunoglobulin; MEL, melanoma; MKD, mg/kg/dose; MP, methylprednisolone; Nivo, nivolumab; NR, not reported; NSCLC, non-small cell lung cancer; Pem, pembrolizumab; PLEX, plasma exchange; Pyrido, pyridostigmine; RCC, renal cell carcinoma; RNS, repetitive nerve stimulation; SCC, squamous cell carcinoma; SF-EMG, Single fiber EMG.

*Exacerbation of previous history of myasthenia gravis.

- ○ One patient was confirmed to have N-methyl-D-aspartate (NMDA) receptor antibodies, which causes autoimmune encephalitis (13). The link between ICI therapy and NMDA receptor antibodies may have been coincidental.
- Of the 10 cases with reported outcomes, 80% had partial to full recovery with steroid therapy or supportive care and the time interval for improvement varied from days to months.
  - ○ One patient, with brainstem encephalitis from combination therapy, died from the encephalitis (12), while another had no response to steroid treatment (10). It is worth mentioning that two of the cases listed, and some that were excluded, may have been encephalopathies secondary to other etiologies, still associated with ICI therapy, such as thyroid storm after thyroiditis or abnormal endocrine function from hypophysitis.

These scenarios highlight the difficulty in suspecting and confirming that the symptoms are the result of ICI-mediated encephalitis.

Meningitis

Meningitis is the inflammation of the leptomeninges caused by infectious, autoimmune, neoplastic, paraneoplastic, or idiopathic etiologies. In a review of 12 clinical trials including 3,763 patients with melanoma receiving nivolumab with or without ipilimumab, there were five (0.13%) cases of meningitis reported (14). In another review, aseptic meningitis was estimated to occur in 0.1% to 0.2% of patients treated with ipilimumab with onset of symptoms between 1 and 7 weeks following ICI initiation (2).

The diagnosis is usually clinical and aided by CSF analysis that shows lymphocytic pleocytosis. All cases were associated with ipilimumab, one in combination with nivolumab (15) (Table 10.3).

- Patients presented in typical fashion, with fever, nuchal rigidity, and some with somnolence.
- Most received empirical antibiotics upon presentation, but it was discontinued after CSF cultures were negative for infection.
  - ○ Except for one case, all had to complete a near complete resolution with steroid therapy or supportive care.
  - ○ One patient did not respond to high-dose steroids, but later recovered with intravenous immunoglobulin (IVIG) (17).

These cases are a diagnostic challenge, as patients on ICI therapy are certainly predisposed to infectious and carcinomatous meningitis. Recognition of possible ICI-induced aseptic meningitis with rapid diagnostics and intervention can lead to improved patient outcomes.

CNS Demyelinating Disease

The CNS demyelinating diseases include multiple sclerosis, demyelination caused by toxic or metabolic disease, or developmental disorders. They often present with focal neurologic impairment which can be relapsing-remitting or progressive.

TABLE 10.3 Meningitis Cases

Cases	Age/sex	ICI	Primary cancer	Cycles to onset	Presentation	Diagnostic findings	Treatment	Outcome	Ref
1	NR	Ipi	MEL	1	Aseptic meningitis	CSF Increased pressure, protein, and leukocytosis	Oral steroids	Improved over 1 to 2 days	(16)
2	NR	Ipi	MEL	4	Meningo-radiculo-neuritis	CSF showed elevated protein and lymphocytic pleocytosis	High-dose steroids, IVIG	Worsened with steroids. Improved with IVIG. Recovered over 2 years.	(17)
3	59M	Ipi	MEL	NR	Aseptic meningitis		NR	NR	(18)
4–5	NR, NR	Ipi	NR	2	Aseptic meningitis	CSF showed mild pleocytosis, second normal. Both brain MRIs normal.	Supportive care, oral steroids	Complete resolution, first in 10 days, second in 8 weeks	(15)
6	52F	Ipi	MEL	4 weeks after initiation	Aseptic meningitis	CSF showed lymphocytosis, MRI showed new metastatic lesions	Empiric antibiotic and steroids	Complete response	(19)
7	NR	Ipi+Nivo	NR	1	Aseptic Meningitis	CSF showed lymphocytosis, MRI normal	Supportive	Complete response in 7 weeks, able to resume ICI therapy	(15)

CSF, cerebrospinal fluid; ICI, immune checkpoint inhibitors; Ipi, ipilimumab; IVIG, intravenous immunoglobulin; MEL, melanoma; Nivo, nivolumab; NR, not reported.

- In the instance of ICI therapy, it is postulated that autoimmune attacks on the nerve sheaths cause demyelination and resemble the pseudo-tumoral demyelinating lesions (tumefactive multiple sclerosis,) as enhanced myelin specific T-cell response has been characterized after ipilimumab therapy (20).
  - One patient developed acute tumefactive demyelinating multifocal brain lesions two days after the fourth cycle of nivolumab, having previously received ipilimumab (21). Despite high-dose steroids, the patient died (Table 10.4).
  - One case was identified of primary demyelination from ipilimumab, followed by nivolumab. This presentation is similar to the disease course of tumefactive multiple sclerosis, which can be rapidly progressive and fatal despite prompt therapy.
  - Another case reported, although without detailed information, had an exacerbation of pre-existing multiple sclerosis after starting ipilimumab for the treatment of melanoma (22) (Table 10.4).

With more case series (including patients with pre-existing autoimmune neurologic disease) treated with ICI, a guideline could be developed to assist neurologists in these difficult situations.

Posterior Reversible Encephalopathy Syndrome

PRES is caused by interstitial edema in the posterior regions of the brain. It is postulated that only the posterior circulation is affected because of lack of autoregulation of the blood vessels.

- Patients present with encephalopathy, headaches, visual changes, and focal neurologic deficits.
- The mechanism for ICI to cause PRES is not well understood. It is typically treated with aggressive blood pressure control, anti-seizure drugs, and supportive care.
  - Three cases of PRES were identified, all of which reported relatively early onset of symptoms: within one to four cycles of ICI (Table 10.5) (23–25). Of the two with reported outcomes, one had partial recovery with supportive care only and one had full recovery with steroids, IVIG, and plasmapheresis.

Cerebellar

There is only one case reported of a patient with a cerebellar syndrome after treatment with pembrolizumab for non-small cell lung cancer (NSCLC) (26).

- The patient presented with isolated ataxia after the 11th cycle of therapy, and despite normal MRI findings, the clinical presentation was concerning enough for the ICI to be stopped and the patient recovered to baseline shortly afterwards.

Spinal Cord

Inflammatory spinal cord disease, or myelitis, is a potentially debilitating condition presenting with motor, sensory, and sphincter-related symptoms and caused by many etiologies, including demyelination.

TABLE 10.4 CNS Demyelinating Disease Cases

Cases	Age/sex	ICI	Primary cancer	Cycles to onset	Presentation	Diagnostic findings	Treatment	Outcome	Ref
1	NR	Ipi	MEL	NR	Multiple sclerosis exacerbation	MRI showing new enhancing lesions	NR	NR	(22)
2	60M	Ipi, followed by Nivo, 3 mg/kg q2 weeks	MEL	4 (Nivo)	Tumefactive demyelination	MRI showing tumefactive lesions, CSF showed oligoclonal bands, increased protein, and myelin basic protein	Steroids, IVIG	No improvement, patient died	(21)

CNS, central nervous system; CSF, cerebrospinal fluid; ICI, immune checkpoint inhibitors; Ipi, ipilimumab; MEL, melanoma; Nivo, nivolumab; NR, not reported.

TABLE 10.5 PRES Cases

Cases	Age/sex	ICI	Primary cancer	Cycles to onset	Presentation	Diagnostic findings	Treatment	Outcome	Ref
1	58F	Ipi	Vaginal Melanoma	1	PRES	MRI findings consistent with PRES	AEDs and supportive care	Improved	(23)
2	18M	Nivo, 3 mg/kg q3 weeks	Hodgkin's Lymhoma	4	PRES	MRI findings of PRES. CSF normal	Steroids, IVIG, PLEX	Fully Recovered	(24)
3	58M	Pem	Non-Hodgkin's Lyrmphoma	1	PRES	NR	NR	NR	(25)

AEDs, anti-epilepsy drugs; CSF, cerebrospinal fluid; Nivo, nivolumab; NR, not reported; Pem, pembrolizumab; PLEX, plasma exchange; PRES, posterior reversible encephalopathy syndrome.

- In the case of ICI therapy, an autoimmune attack on the spinal cord parenchyma is the likely etiology, similar to the enhanced myelin specific T-cell response mentioned earlier (20).
- The incidence of spinal cord disorders is unknown, but it is possible that it is underdiagnosed as there are a plethora of grade 1/2 neurologic AE cases reported, such as numbness, weakness, gait disturbances, which may be caused by not fully worked up spinal cord lesions.
  - Three cases of myelitis, all caused by ipilimumab, have been reported (Table 10.6). The patients presented with varying degrees of weakness, usually in a subacute timeframe and onset of symptoms after the second cycle (27,28).
  - One patient had no improvement with steroids (29), the other two had partial recoveries.

The initial evaluation of suspected myelitis requires spinal cord MRI with and without contrast. Without cessation of therapy and early immunosuppressive management, the neurologic impairment can be irreversible.

Peripheral Nervous System

Peripheral nervous system AEs are thought to occur in less than 3% of patients treated with ICI.

- According to their temporal profile they are divided in acute and chronic forms, and include cranial nerve palsies, meningoradiculoneuritis, diffuse or focal neuropathies, and enteric neuropathy.
- Most reported cases are mild-to-moderate in severity and did not require discontinuation of ICI or initiation of immunosuppressive therapy (2,3,30). Severe cases have been increasingly reported and are discussed below.

Cranial Neuropathies

Cranial nerves, nerve roots, or cranial nerve nuclei can be affected by inflammation, infection, or mass effect. In six out of seven cases of cranial nerve palsy reported after ICI therapy, the seventh cranial nerve was affected causing unilateral facial paralysis. The other case affected the sixth cranial nerve and presented with acute onset horizontal diplopia (31).

- All but one of the ICI-induced cranial neuropathies were secondary to ipilimumab, with one case from nivolumab, and one after combination therapy (Table 10.7).
  - All seven cases developed symptoms within 6 weeks of ICI initiation.
  - Each of them also had complete or near-complete resolution with steroids.
  - One case had resolution of a unilateral facial nerve palsy with steroids, but it recurred on the opposite side later in the course of ipilimumab (32). Both sides of the face returned to normal after about 6 months.

TABLE 10.6 Myelitis Cases

Cases	Age/ sex	ICI	Primary cancer	Cycles to onset	Presentation	Diagnostic findings	Treatment	Outcome	Ref
1	NR	Ipi	NR	NR	Progressive necrotic myelopathy	NR	Steroids and infliximab	No improvement	(29)
2	62M	Ipi	MEL	2	Transverse myelitis	MRI showed focal T2 hyperintensity at T9-T10 level. CSF showed pleocytosis	Steroids	Improvement over 2 weeks	(27)
3	58M	Ipi	MEL	2	Myelitis with paraplegia	NR	Steroids and IVIG	Partial response	(28)

CSF, cerebrospinal fluid; Ipi, ipilimumab; IVIG, intravenous immunoglobulin; MEL, melanoma; NR, not reported.

TABLE 10.7 Peripheral Neuropathy Cases

Cases	Age/sex	ICI	Primary cancer	Cycles to onset	Presentation	Diagnostic findings	Treatment	Outcome	Ref
1	NR	Ipi	SCLC	NR	Unilateral facial weakness	NR	NR	NR	(33)
2	NR	Ipi	NR	2	Unilateral facial weakness, occurring twice	NR	Steroids	Improved over 6 months	(32)
3	NR	Ipi	NR	2	Unilateral facial weakness	NR	Steroids	Rapid improvement	(34)
4	61F	Ipi, 3 mg/kg, q3 weeks	MEL	1	Unilateral facial weakness	MRI normal	Supportive care	Improved	(35)
5	NR	Ipi 3 mg/kg q3 weeks (after failed Nivo)	NR	1	Unilateral facial weakness	NR	Steroids	Improved over 2 weeks	(36)
6	45M	Ipi 3 mg/kg + Nivo 1 mg/kg, q3 weeks	MEL	1	Unilateral facial weakness	MRI and CSF normal	Steroids and antiviral	Resolution in 7 days	(37)
7	83M	Nivo	NR	1	Horizontal diplopia, lateral rectus palsy	NR	Steroids	Resolved with steroids	(31)

CSF, cerebrospinal fluid; ICI, immune checkpoint inhibitors; Ipi, ipilimumab; MEL, melanoma; Nivo, nivolumab; NR, not reported; SCLC, small cell lung cancer.

Prompt recognition of an isolated cranial neuropathy is critical in patients being treated with ICI, as they could be mistaken and mistreated for ischemic strokes or progression of neoplastic disease. As illustrated by the reported cases, cessation of the immunotherapy with steroid administration usually resolves the cranial neuropathy.

Meningoradiculoneuritis

Meningoradiculoneuritis denotes a clinical syndrome caused by inflammatory involvement of meninges with cranial and/or spinal nerve roots, characterized by headache, intense radicular pain, facial palsies, and polyneuropathy. This condition is a recognized complication of chronic Lyme's disease.

- Two cases of ICI-related meningoradiculoneuritis have been reported with a postulated mechanism related to T-cell-mediated inflammation and autoimmunity (17,32).
  - The first case was a man treated with nivolumab for melanoma, who complained of weakness of both arms with pain on elevation 9 weeks after initiation of treatment. Brain and cervical spine MRI studies were unrevealing for the cause of his symptoms. Anti-PD-1 treatment was discontinued and his symptoms improved with steroids (32).
  - The second case was a man with melanoma who presented with vertigo, dizziness, cervicalgia, and headache 10 weeks after initiation of ipilimumab. His symptoms progressed over the following week resulting in flaccid tetraplegia, sensory deficit, severe ataxia, facial diplegia, dysarthria, and dysphagia. Diagnostic work-up ruled out other potential causes for his symptoms. Thoracolumbar MRI revealed global nerve roots enhancement suggestive of arachnoiditis. He improved after ipilimumab was stopped and received treatment with high-dose steroids and IVIG, with almost complete recovery 24 months after symptom onset.

Acute Inflammatory Demyelinating Polyneuropathy

Acute inflammatory demyelinating polyneuropathy (AIDP) or Guillain–Barré syndrome (GBS) is an autoimmune polyneuropathy that presents with acute, rapidly progressive, ascending weakness, decreased or absent reflexes, sensory deficits, and autonomic dysfunction (38). The pathophysiology of GBS involves antibodies directed against the cell surface gangliosides expressed in peripheral nerve axolemma.

- An enhanced T-cell immunity is hypothesized to play a role in ICI-induced AIDP (16,39,40). AIDP is estimated to occur in 0.1% to 2% of patients treated with ICI (2).
  - A recent report from the FDA Adverse Event Reporting System (FAERS) database identified 121 (0.3%) cases of GBS out of 35,726 total reported AEs from ICI therapy (41).
- We identified nine reported cases with melanoma who developed ICI-induced AIDP (see Table 10.8).

TABLE 10.8 AIDP Cases

Cases	Age/sex	ICI	Onset	Primary cancer	Presentation	EMG	CSF	Treatment	Outcome	Ref
1	77/M	Ipi (3 mkd q3 wk) and Nivo (1 mkd q3wk)	1 wk after 3rd cycle	MEL	Rapidly progressive distal sensory and motor deficits and areflexia	Delayed motor conduction velocity with CB in median and ulnar with absent F waves	Elevated protein (86 mg/dl), normal cells	IVIG	Improved	(42)
2	77/M	Ipi (NR)	3 days after 3rd cycle	MEL	Hoarseness, distal weakness and numbness, areflexia	Consistent with AIDP with 2° axonal features	Elevated IgG	IVIG and MP	Improved	(39)
3	65/M	Ipi (NR)	2 wk after 2nd cycle	MEL	Quadriparesis, distal hypesthesia, areflexia	Generalized, symmetric, sensorimotor neuropathy	Elevated protein (1.6 g/L), normal cells	Tacrolimus, MP and PLEX	Died from multiorgan failure	(43)
4	45/F	Pem (2 mkd q3 wk)	Before 3rd cycle	MEL	Paresthesia and hypesthesia of all limbs, leg weakness, facial paralysis	Multifocal demyelination with conduction block	Elevated protein (0.56 g/L), mild pleocytosis (45/mm³)	Pred and IVIG	Improved	(44)
5	63/M	Ipi (NR)	3 wk after 4th cycle	MEL	Sensory loss B hands and feet, gait unsteadiness, mild tetraparesis, areflexia	Median/ulnar absent SNAP and low CMAP; prolonged H-reflexes	Elevated protein (0.89 g/L), normal cells	IVIG	Died of respiratory insufficiency	(16)

(continued)

Cases	Age/sex	ICI	Onset	Primary cancer	Presentation	EMG	CSF	Treatment	Outcome	Ref
TABLE 10.8 AIDP Cases *(continued)*										
6	57/F	Ipi (3 mkd q3wk)	1 wk after 3rd cycle	MEL	Ascending sensory and motor function of limbs, inability to walk, areflexia	Generalized motor and sensory demyelinating polyneuropathy	Elevated protein (1.67 g/L), normal cells	MP	Improved	(40)
7	NR/M	Pem (NR)	After 6th cycle	MEL	Length-dependent UE/LE weakness and numbness	Severe length dependent peripheral neuropathy with axonal and demyelinating features	NA	Prednisone	Improved	(26)
8	NR/M	Pem (NR)	After 20th cycle	MEL	Facial weakness, dyspnea and dysarthria	Demyelinating polyneuropathy	Elevated protein (1.92 g/L), mild pleocytosis (12/mm³)	IVIG	Improved	(26)

AIDP, acute inflammatory demyelinating polyneuropathy; CSF, cerebrospinal fluid; ICI, immune checkpoint inhibitors; EMG, electromyography study; Ipi, Ipilimumab; IVIG, intravenous immunoglobulin; MEL, melanoma; MP, methylprednisolone; NR, not reported; Pem, pembrolizumab; PLEX: plasma exchange; UE/LE..

- ○ Five cases were associated with ipilimumab with one of these patients treated in combination with nivolumab, and three cases associated with pembrolizumab.
- ○ Onset of symptoms occurred after an average of three to four cycles, with one outlier occurring after the 20th cycle. Six of the nine cases presented with rapidly progressive motor and sensory deficits as well as areflexia; one patient with hoarseness, dyspnea, and dysarthria; and two patients with facial palsy.
- ○ Abnormalities in electromyography (EMG) and nerve conduction studies (NCS) consistent with GBS including slowed nerve conduction velocities, conduction blocks, and absent or prolonged F and H waves.
- ○ The characteristic GBS findings of elevated CSF protein with normal cell count (cytoalbuminologic dissociation) were seen in four cases and two cases associated with high protein and mild pleocytosis (12 and 45 cells/mm^3).
- Immunosuppressive treatment and discontinuation of ICI resulted in clinical improvement in six out of nine cases.
  - ○ Five patients received IVIG, two of whom also received steroids; one patient received a combination of plasmapheresis, steroids, and tacrolimus. Interestingly, two cases improved with steroids alone, a treatment option typically not effective in classic non-ICI-induced GBS.
  - ○ One patient died due to respiratory insufficiency and one patient died of multi-organ failure.

GBS is a rare but potentially life-threatening AE and should be suspected in patients presenting with progressive weakness after treatment with ICI.

Chronic Inflammatory Demyelinating Polyradiculoneuropathy

Chronic inflammatory demyelinating polyradiculoneuropathy (CIDP) is a chronic (greater than 8 weeks) autoimmune neuropathy typically presenting with symmetric proximal and distal weakness with sensory deficits of extremities, associated with electrophysiological evidence of demyelinating neuropathy. The disease course can be monophasic, relapsing-remitting, or progressive in nature (45). CIDP is mediated by both humoral and cellular immune mechanisms, leading to the recurrence of demyelination, remyelination, interstitial edema, and endoneural inflammatory infiltrates (46).

- Four cases of ICI-induced CIDP have been reported, related to administration of ipilimumab, pembrolizumab, and nivolumab for melanoma (Table 10.9).
  - ○ All patients presented after first cycle, except for one patient who had symptom onset after the sixth cycle.
  - ○ All patients presented with length-dependent weakness and sensory deficits as well as areflexia, and one patient developed autonomic dysfunction.
  - ○ The peak of symptoms occurred 5 and 12 weeks from symptom onset in two patients, while the other two patients initially

TABLE 10.9 CIDP Cases

Cases	Age/sex	ICI	Primary cancer	Cycles to onset	Onset to max. severity	Presentation	EMG	CSF	Treatment	Outcome	Ref
1	44/M	Ipi (NR)	MEL	1 wk after 1st cycle	5 wk	Length-dependent numbness and weakness UE/LE and face; areflexia	Suggestive of CIDP	Normal protein and WBC	PLEX	Improved	(27)
2	85/F	Ipi (3 mkd q3 wk x 4 doses), then Pem (2 mkd q3 wk)	MEL	Between 6th and 7th cycle	12 wk	Painful paresthesia and weakness of arms then legs; areflexia	Multifocal demyelination with conduction block	Elev. Protein (0.74 g/L), normal cells	Pred, MP and PLEX	No improvement	(44)
3	85/F	Nivo (2 mkd q3 wk)	MEL	2 wk after 1st cycle	2 wk, but had exacerbation 8 wk after onset.	Length dependent numbness and weakness; areflexia; Fluctuating deficits	Prolonged F-wave latency, slight delay in motor CV with CB, normal range of distal latency and diminished SNAP	Elevated protein (3.58 g/L), slight pleocytosis (11/mm^3)	IVIG and pred	Improved	(46)
4	49/F	Ipi (3 mkd) and Nivo (1 mkd)	MEL	5 days after 1st cycle	1.5 week, but had exacerbation 4 weeks later	Paresthesia, symmetric sensorimotor and autonomic neuropathy; Areflexia; Postural hypotensionand constipation	Acute generalized motor predominant neuropathy with patchy slowing of CV	Elevated protein (1.15 g/L), slight pleocytosis (15/mm^3)	IVIG, MP followed by pred; PLEX, Ritux, MF	Improved	(47)

CB, conduction block; CIDP, chronic inflammatory demyelinating polyradiculoneuropathy; CSF, imaging and cerebrospinal fluid; CV, conduction velocity; EMG, electromyography study; ICI, immune checkpoint inhibitors; Ipi, ipilimumab; IVIG, intravenous immunoglobulin; MF, mycophenolate mofetil; MEL, melanoma; MP, methylprednisolone; NR, not reported; Pem, pembrolizumab; PLEX, plasma exchange; SNAP, sensory nerve action potential; UE/LE, upper extremity/lower extremity; WBC, white blood cell count.

presented with GBS-like rapid onset neuropathy, but experienced exacerbation of symptoms after 1 to 2 months, both in the setting of tapering steroids.
- ○ Electrophysiological studies revealed abnormalities typically seen in demyelinating neuropathies.
- ○ Expected cytoalbuminologic dissociation was only seen in one case, while two cases had elevated protein with mild pleocytosis (11 and 15 cells/mm^3).
- Improvement occurred in all patients, except for one, after discontinuation of ICI therapy and administration of immunosuppressive therapy including plasmapheresis, steroids, and IVIG.
  - ○ One of two patients who experienced symptom exacerbation was given higher steroid dose, while the other patient was treated with IVIG, rituximab, higher dose of prednisone, and mycophenolate mofetil.

Neuromuscular Junction

Myasthenia Gravis

Myasthenia gravis (MG) is an autoimmune disease affecting the neuromuscular junction (NMJ) resulting in fatigable weakness involving the ocular, bulbar, neck, limbs, and respiratory muscles. It is caused by antibodies against the acetylcholine receptor (AchR) or muscle-specific tyrosine kinase (MuSK).

- ICI-triggered autoimmunity is hypothesized to be related to dysregulation of pre-existing immune response to self-antigens (48).
  - ○ De-novo MG is estimated to develop in 0.1% to 0.2% of patients who received ICI. Exacerbation of underlying MG has also been reported (2,49).
  - ○ In the recent analysis of FAERS, a total of 142 (0.4%) of 35,726 total reported AEs were related to neuromuscular junction disease; 112 (0.3%) of patients developed MG, 22 (0.06%) myasthenic syndrome, and eight (0.02%) ocular myasthenia (41).
- Our literature review identified 27 reported cases of MG related to ICI (see Table 10.10).
  - ○ Four patients (15%) had exacerbation of previous diagnosis of MG. Patient's age in this population were older compared to those with idiopathic MG (49,50).
  - ○ The most common primary malignancy was melanoma in 14 (52%) patients, followed by NSCLC in eight (30%) and other cancer types in five (18%) patients including squamous cell carcinoma of the bladder, small cell lung cancer, renal cell cancer, uterine carcinoma, and colon cancer.
  - ○ Seventeen (63%) patients received nivolumab, seven (26%) received pembrolizumab, and four (15%) received ipilimumab. One patient received combination of ipilimumab and nivolumab. The onset of MG symptoms occurred after an average of 2 cycles.

TABLE 10.10 Myasthenia Gravis Cases

Cases	Age/sex	ICI	Onset	Primary cancer	AChR antibody	EMG	Treatment	Outcome	Ref
1	75/M	Nivo (NR)	After 2nd cycle	SCC of the bladder	+	+ Decrement on RNS	Pyrido and IVIG	MG improved, but patient enrolled to hospice and died	(50)
2	84/M	Pem (NR)	After 2 cycles	Melanoma	+	NA	Prednisone, pyrido, IVIG	MG improved. Pt died from respiratory failure and hypotensive shock	(51)
3	63/M	Pem (NR)	2 wk after 1st cycle	Melanoma	+	NA	Pyrido, prednisone, MP, IVIG, PLEX	MG worsened and patient died	(52)
4	69/M	Ipi (3 mkd q3 wk)	Several days after 3rd cycle	Melanoma	+	+ Decrement on RNS	Pyrido, MP, PLEX	MG improved	(53)
5	73/M	Ipi (10 mkd)	After 2nd cycle	Melanoma	+	NA	Steroids, pyrido	MG improved. Pt died due to disease progression	(53)
6	70/M	Ipi (NR)	After 2nd cycle	Melanoma	+	+ Decrement on RNS	PLEX, MP, IVIG, pyrido	MG improved	(27)
7	71/F	Pem (NR)	After 4th cycle	Uterine carcinoma	− (MuSKAb negative)	+ Jitter on SF-EMG	Pyrido, prednisone	MG improved	(54)
8	70/M	Ipi and Nivo (NR)	16 days after 1st cycle	SCLC	+	+ Decrement on RNS	Prednisone, PLEX, MP, IVIG	Initial improvement, but developed worsening and patient died	(55)

(continued)

TABLE 10.10 Myasthenia Gravis Cases (continued)

Cases	Age/sex	ICI	Onset	Primary cancer	AChR antibody	EMG	Treatment	Outcome	Ref
9*	59/F	Pem (q3 wk)	After 3rd cycle	Melanoma	+	+ Decrement on RNS	PLEX, IVIG, and prednisone	MG improved	(56)
10	65/M	Nivo (292 mg q2 wk)	10 days after 2nd cycles	NSCLC	– (MuSKAb negative)	NA prior to MG treatment; Normal RNS after MG treatment	Pyrido	MG improved	(57)
11	81/M	Nivo (3 mkd q2 wk)	After 3rd cycle	NSCLC (adenocarcinoma)	–	- RNS; +jitter on SF-EMG	Prednisone	MG improved	(58)
12*	75/M	Pem (2 mkd q3 wk)	After 2nd cycle	Melanoma	+	NA	Pyrido, prednisone, PLEX, IVIG, rituximab	MG improved	(48)
13	65/M	Nivo (3 mkd q2 wk)	1 day after 2nd cycle	RCC	+	Neuropathic changes seen on EMG. RNS not performed	High-dose steroids and IVIG	Patient died due to MG	(59)
14*	75/M	Pem	5 wk after initiation (after 2nd or 3rd cycle)	Melanoma	+	NA	MP and IVIG	MG improved	(60)

(continued)

TABLE 10.10 Myasthenia Gravis Cases (*continued*)

Cases	Age/sex	ICI	Onset	Primary cancer	AChR antibody	EMG	Treatment	Outcome	Ref
15	69/F	Pem (NR)	Shortly after 3rd cycle	Melanoma	–	NA	MP, pyrido, PLEX	MG worsened with new brain metastases. Patient died	(32)
16–27 (total 12 cases; *1 case)	Age:73.5 ±6.3 Sex: 6 M, 6 F	Nivo (2 mkd q3 wk in 5 pts; 3 mkd q2 wk in 6 pts; 0.3 mkd in 1 pt)	4 pts after 1st cycle; 5 pts after 2nd cycle; 2 pts after 3rd cycle; 1 pt after 4th cycle	5 melanoma 6 NSCLC 1 colon	10 + 2 − 1 + for anti-striated muscle Ab	2 of 7 pts had decrement seen in RNS; 1 pt had jitter in SF-EMG	5 Pyrido 10 prednisone 5 MP 6 IVIG 4 PLEX 1 other	2 pharmacologic remission 2 minimal symptoms 5 improved 1 unchanged 2 died	(49)

AChR, acetylcholine receptor; ICI, immune checkpoint inhibitors; Ipi, ipilimumab; IVIG, intravenous immunoglobulin; MP, methylprednisolone; NA, not applicable; Nivo, nivolumab; NR, not reported; NSCLC, non-small cell lung cancer; Pem, pembrolizumab; PLEX, plasma exchange; RNS, repetitive nerve stimulation; SCC, squamous cell carcinoma.

- Only one patient experienced purely ocular symptoms with ptosis and diplopia and the rest of the patients presented in combination with bulbar weakness such as dysphagia and dysarthria as well as limb weakness.
- About 13% of patients presented with limb and bulbar weakness without ocular symptoms.
- Compared to patients with idiopathic MG, ICI-related MG demonstrated a higher frequency of bulbar weakness and dyspnea on presentation.
- Three patients had associated myocarditis, which complicates the clinical picture in those who predominantly presented with dyspnea as a manifestation of bulbar involvement of MG.
- Over one-third of patients required respiratory support; seven patients were supported by noninvasive positive pressure ventilation, while three patients necessitated mechanical ventilation.

- Serologic tests demonstrated 21 (78%) patients were positive for AChR antibody, one patient was positive for anti-striated muscle antibody, and none were positive for anti-MuSK antibodies.
  - Elevated creatine kinase (CK) concentrations (ranging from 1,200 to 10,386 U/L) were seen in 16 (59%) patients, which may signify associated myositis.
  - In patients who underwent EMG testing, typical findings associated with MG were reported in 10 patients.

- ICI therapy was initially discontinued in all patients. Treatment options of ICI-related MG is in general similar to the management of idiopathic MG (51).
  - Immunosuppressive treatment alone or in combination including steroids in 19 (70%), IVIG in 11 (41%), and plasmapharesis in 11 (41%) were administered; one patient received rituximab. IVIG and plasmapheresis are known to work rapidly in patients with acute myasthenic crisis.
  - Steroids can increase the risk of acute MG worsening and should be used with caution when administered alone (50).
  - Pyridostigmine, an acetylcholinesterase inhibitor, was administered in 15 (55%) patients. Improvement of MG was reported in 16 (59%) patients, five (19%) had unchanged or minimal symptoms, while six (22%) patients developed worsening of MG and died.

- FAERS analysis of 263 patients with ICI-associated GBS (46%) and neuromuscular junction disorder (54%) reported 64% of patients required hospitalization, 17% were reported as life-threatening events, 7% resulted in disability, and 22% of patients died (41).

Early recognition and timely intervention could potentially avoid fatal cases of ICI-related MG. Initiation of therapy is recommended if there is a high clinical suspicion, even prior to availability of serologic and electrophysiologic test results. Discontinuation of ICI and initiation of immunosuppressive therapies are an appropriate treatment approach for patients with ICI-related MG.

Management

The cornerstones of managing ICI-induced neurologic AEs is early discontinuation of ICI therapy and initiation of immunosuppressive therapy including intravenous (IV)/per os (oral) (PO) steroids, IVIG, or plasmapheresis.

- We recommend that ICI therapy be stopped for severe AEs and a neurology consult be initiated.
- Holding of ICI and neurologic evaluation should also be considered for any new onset of unexplained neurologic symptoms.
- Steroids should be initiated first after cessation of ICI and often are sufficient in treating the symptoms. Further immunosuppressive therapy should follow for refractory cases, but generally under the guidance of a multidisciplinary team.

An additional note should be made for the four pre-existing MG and one pre-existing multiple sclerosis cases reported. It appears reasonable to consider ICI therapy in patients with preexisting neurologic autoimmune disease.

- Preexisting non-neurologic autoimmune disease is not considered a contraindication to starting ICI.
  - In a case series using ipilimumab, it was noted that exacerbations were readily manageable with standard therapies when started in a timely fashion (61).
- We recommend, however, a detailed discussion with the patient about possible exacerbation of their neurologic illness while on ICI therapy.

More data need to be collected in order to develop guidelines in such situations.

CONCLUSION

Severe neurologic AEs associated with ICI therapy are rare, being MG cases most frequently reported. With increased use of ICI, however, we expect the frequency of neurologic irAE to increase. As experience with these agents expands, we will better be able to understand the immune-mediated pathogenesis mechanisms and develop more rationale management recommendations.

REFERENCES

1. Gluske P, Recht L, Lane B. Reversible posterior leukoencephalopathy syndrome and bevacizumab. *N Engl J Med.* 2006;354(9):980–982; discussion 980–982. doi:10.1056/nejmc052954

2. Touat M, Talmasov D, Ricard D, et al. Neurological toxicities associated with immune-checkpoint inhibitors. *Curr Opin Neurol.* 2017;30(6):659–668. doi:10.1097/wco.0000000000000503

3. Cuzzubbo S, Javeri F, Tissier M, et al. Neurological adverse events associated with immune checkpoint inhibitors: review of the literature. *Eur J Cancer.* 2017;73:1–8. doi:10.1016/j.ejca.2016.12.001

4. Schneider S, Potthast S, Komminoth P, et al. PD-1 Checkpoint Inhibitor Associated autoimmune encephalitis. *Case Rep Oncol.* 2017;10(2):473–478. doi:10.1159/000477162

5. Dheeraj Kalladka KB. Ipilimumab induced encephalitis: a case report. *Immunome Res*. 2015;11(2):092. doi:10.4172/1745-7580.1000092

6. Carl D, Grüllich C, Hering S, et al. Steroid responsive encephalopathy associated with autoimmune thyroiditis following ipilimumab therapy: a case report. *BMC Res Notes*. 2015;8:316. doi:10.1186/s13104-015-1283-9

7. Stein MK, Summers BB, Wong CA, et al. Meningoencephalitis following Ipilimumab Administration in metastatic melanoma. *Am J Med Sci*. 2015;350(6):512–513. doi:10.1097/maj.0000000000000584

8. Khoja L, Maurice C, Chappell M, et al. Eosinophilic fasciitis and acute encephalopathy toxicity from pembrolizumab treatment of a patient with metastatic melanoma. *Cancer Immunol Res*. 2016;4(3):175–178. doi:10.1158/2326-6066.cir-15-0186

9. Mandel JJ, Olar A, Aldape KD, et al. Lambrolizumab induced central nervous system (CNS) toxicity. *J Neurol Sci*. 2014;344(1–2):229–231. doi:10.1016/j.jns.2014.06.023

10. Salam S, Lavin T, Turan A. Limbic encephalitis following immunotherapy against metastatic malignant melanoma. *BMJ Case Rep*. 2016;2016:bcr2016215012. doi:10.1136/bcr-2016-215012

11. Levine JJ, Somer RA, Hosoya H, et al. Atezolizumab-induced encephalitis in metastatic bladder cancer: a case report and review of the literature. *Clin Genitourin Cancer*. 2017;15(5):e847–e849. doi:10.1016/j.clgc.2017.03.001

12. Bossart S, Thurneysen S, Rushing E, et al. Case report: encephalitis, with brainstem involvement, following checkpoint inhibitor therapy in metastatic melanoma. *Oncologist*. 2017;22(6):749–753. doi:10.1634/theoncologist.2016-0366

13. Williams TJ, Benavides DR, Patrice K-A, et al. Association of Autoimmune Encephalitis with combined immune checkpoint inhibitor treatment for metastatic cancer. *JAMA Neurol*. 2016;73(8):928–933. doi:10.1001/jamaneurol.2016.19

14. Larkin J, Chmielowski B, Lao CD, et al. Neurologic Serious Adverse Events Associated with nivolumab plus ipilimumab or nivolumab alone in advanced melanoma, including a case series of encephalitis. *Oncologist*. 2017;22(6):709–718. doi:10.1634/theoncologist.2016-0487

15. Spain L, Walls G, Julve M, et al. Neurotoxicity from immune-checkpoint inhibition in the treatment of melanoma: a single centre experience and review of the literature. *Ann Oncol*. 2017;28(2):377–385. doi:10.1093/annonc/mdw558

16. Bot I, Blank CU, Boogerd W, et al. Neurological immune-related adverse events of ipilimumab. *Pract Neurol*. 2013;13(4):278–280. doi:10.1136/practneurol-2012-000447

17. Bompaire F, Mateus C, Taillia H, et al. Severe meningo-radiculo-neuritis associated with ipilimumab. *Invest New Drugs*. 2012;30(6):2407–2410. doi:10.1007/s10637-011-9787-1

18. Oishi K, Nakao M, Maeda S, et al. A case of aseptic meningitis without neck rigidity occurring in a metastatic melanoma patient treated with ipilimumab. *Eur J Dermatol*. 2017;27(2):193–194. doi:10.1684/ejd.2016.2943

19. Voskens CJ, Goldinger SM, Loquai C, et al. The price of tumor control: an analysis of rare side effects of anti-CTLA-4 therapy in metastatic melanoma from the ipilimumab network. *PLoS One*. 2013;8(1):e53745. doi:10.1371/journal.pone.0053745

20. Lucca LE, Hafler DA. Co-inhibitory blockade while preserving tolerance: checkpoint inhibitors for glioblastoma. *Immunol Rev*. 2017;276(1):9–25. doi:10.1111/imr.12529

21. Maurice C, Schneider R, Kiehl T-R, et al. Subacute CNS demyelination after treatment with nivolumab for melanoma. *Cancer Immunol Res*. 2015;3(12):1299–302. doi:10.1158/2326-6066.cir-15-0141

22. Gettings EJ, Hackett CT, Scott TF. Severe relapse in a multiple sclerosis patient associated with ipilimumab treatment of melanoma. *Mult Scler*. 2015;21(5):670. doi:10.1177/1352458514549403

23. Maur M, Tomasello C, Frassoldati A, et al. Posterior reversible encephalopathy syndrome during ipilimumab therapy for malignant melanoma. *J Clin Oncol*. 2012;30(6):e76–e78. doi:10.1200/jco.2011.38.7886

24. Tchapyjnikov D, Borst AJ. Immune-related neurological symptoms in an adolescent patient receiving the checkpoint inhibitor nivolumab. *J Immunother*. 2017;40(7):286–288. doi:10.1097/cji.0000000000000177

25. LaPorte J, Solh M, Ouanounou S. Posterior reversible encephalopathy syndrome following pembrolizumab therapy for relapsed Hodgkin's lymphoma. *J Oncol Pharm Pract.* 2017;23(1):71–74. doi:10.1177/1078155215620922

26. Kao JC, Liao B, Markovic SN, et al. Neurological Complications Associated with anti-programmed death 1 (PD-1) antibodies. *JAMA Neurol.* 2017;74(10):1216–1222. doi:10.1001/jamaneurol.2017.1912

27. Liao B, Shroff S, Kamiya-Matsuoka C, et al. Atypical neurological complications of ipilimumab therapy in patients with metastatic melanoma. *Neuro Oncol.* 2014;16(4):589–593. doi:10.1093/neuonc/nou001

28. O'Kane GM, Lyons TG, Colleran GC, et al. Late-onset paraplegia after complete response to two cycles of ipilimumab for metastatic melanoma. *Oncol Res Treat.* 2014;37(12):757–760. doi:10.1159/000368316

29. Abdallah AO, Herlopian A, Ravilla R, et al. Ipilimumab-induced necrotic myelopathy in a patient with metastatic melanoma: A case report and review of literature. *J Oncol Pharm Pract.* 2016;22(3):537–542. doi:10.1177/1078155215572932

30. Hottinger AF. Neurologic complications of immune checkpoint inhibitors. *Curr Opin Neurol.* 2016;29(6):806–812. doi:10.1097/wco.0000000000000391

31. Zimmer L, Goldinger SM, Hofmann L, et al. Neurological, respiratory, musculoskeletal, cardiac and ocular side-effects of anti-PD-1 therapy. *Eur J Cancer.* 2016;60:210–225. doi:10.1016/j.ejca.2016.02.024

32. Altman AL, Golub JS, Pensak ML, et al. Bilateral facial palsy following ipilimumab infusion for melanoma. *Otolaryngol Head Neck Surg.* 2015;153(5):894–895. doi:10.1177/0194599815606701

33. Arriola E, Wheater M, Galea I, et al. Outcome and biomarker analysis from a multicenter phase 2 study of ipilimumab in combination with carboplatin and etoposide as first-line therapy for extensive-stage SCLC. *J Thorac Oncol.* 2016;11(9):1511–1521. doi:10.1016/j.jtho.2016.05.028

34. Johnson DB, Friedman DL, Berry E, et al. Survivorship in immune therapy: assessing chronic immune toxicities, health outcomes, and functional status among long-term ipilimumab survivors at a single referral center. *Cancer Immunol Res.* 2015;3(5):464–469. doi:10.1158/2326-6066.cir-14-0217

35. Luke JJ, Lezcano C, Hodi FS, et al. Antitumor granuloma formation by CD4+ T cells in a patient with rapidly progressive melanoma experiencing spiking fevers, neuropathy, and other immune-related toxicity after treatment with ipilimumab. *J Clin Oncol.* 2015;33(6):e32–e35. doi:10.1200/jco.2013.49.7735

36. Numata S, Iwata Y, Okumura R, et al. Bilateral anterior uveitis and unilateral facial palsy due to ipilimumab for metastatic melanoma in an individual with human leukocyte antigen DR4: a case report. *J Dermatol.* 2018;45(1):113–114. doi:10.1111/1346-8138.13779

37. Zecchini JM, Kim S, Yum K, et al. Development of bell's palsy after treatment with ipilimumab and nivolumab for metastatic melanoma: a case report. *J Immunother.* 2018;41(1):39–41. doi:10.1097/cji.0000000000000184

38. Dash S, Pai AR, Kamath U, et al. Pathophysiology and diagnosis of Guillain-Barré syndrome - challenges and needs. *Int J Neurosci.* 2015;125(4):235–240. doi:10.3109/00207454.2014.913588

39. Rupareliya CS, Naqvi S, Jani VB. Acute Inflammatory demyelinating polyneuroradiculopathy with ipilimumab in metastatic melanoma: a case report and review of literature. *Cureus.* 2017;9(6):e1310. doi:10.7759/cureus.1310

40. Wilgenhof S, Neyns B. Anti-CTLA-4 antibody-induced Guillain-Barré syndrome in a melanoma patient. *Ann Oncol.* 2011;22(4):991–993. doi:10.1093/annonc/mdr028

41. Garcia CR, Cox JN, Villano JL. Myasthenia gravis and Guillain-Barré syndrome adverse events with immune checkpoint inhibitors, in 2018 ASCO-SITC Clinical Immuno-Oncology Symposium. *J Clin Oncol.* 2018;36(5_suppl):37–37. doi:10.1200/jco.2018.36.5_suppl.37

42. Supakornnumporn S, Katirji B. Guillain-Barré syndrome triggered by immune checkpoint inhibitors: a case report and literature review. *J Clin Neuromuscul Dis.* 2017;19(2):80–83. doi:10.1097/cnd.0000000000000193

43. Gaudy-Marqueste C, Monestier S, Franques J, et al. A severe case of ipilimumab-induced Guillain-Barré syndrome revealed by an occlusive enteric neuropathy: a differential diagnosis for ipilimumab-induced colitis. *J Immunother.* 2013;36(1):77–78. doi:10.1097/cji.0b013e31827807dd

44. De Maleissye M, Nicolas G, Saiag P. Pembrolizumab-induced demyelinating polyradiculopathy. *N Engl J Med.* 2016;375(3):296–297. doi:10.1056/nejmc1515584

45. Eftimov F, van Schaik I. Chronic inflammatory demyelinating polyradiculoneuropathy: update on clinical features, phenotypes and treatment options. *Curr Opin Neurol.* 2013;26(5):496–502. doi:10.1097/wco.0b013e328363bfa4

46. Tanaka R, Maruyama H, Tomidokoro Y, et al. Nivolumab-induced chronic inflammatory demyelinating polyradiculoneuropathy mimicking rapid-onset Guillain-Barré syndrome: a case report. *Jpn J Clin Oncol.* 2016;46(9):875–878. doi:10.1093/jjco/hyw090

47. Gu Y, Menzies AM, Long GV, et al. Immune mediated neuropathy following checkpoint immunotherapy. *J Clin Neurosci.* 2017;45:14–17. doi:10.1016/j.jocn.2017.07.014

48. Phadke SD, Ghabour R, Swick BL, et al. Pembrolizumab therapy triggering an exacerbation of preexisting autoimmune disease: a report of 2 patient cases. *J Investig Med High Impact Case Rep.* 2016;4(4):2324709616674316. doi:10.1177/2324709616674316

49. Suzuki S. Nivolumab-related myasthenia gravis with myositis and myocarditis in Japan. *Neurology.* 2017;89:1127–1134. doi:10.1212/wnl.0000000000004359

50. Chang E, Sabichi AL, Sada YH. Myasthenia gravis after nivolumab therapy for squamous cell cercinoma of the bladder. *J Immunother.* 2017;40:114–115. doi:10.1097/cji.0000000000000161

51. Alnahhas I, Wong J. A case of new-onset antibody-positive myasthenia gravis in a patient treated with pembrolizumab for melanoma. *Muscle Nerve.* 2017;55(6):E25–E26. doi:10.1002/mus.25496

52. March KL, Samarin MJ, Sodhi A, et al. Pembrolizumab-induced myasthenia gravis: a fatal case report. *J Oncol Pharm Pract.* 2017;24(2):146–149. doi:10.1177/1078155216687389

53. Johnson DB, Saranga-Perry V, Lavin PJM, et al. Myasthenia gravis induced by ipilimumab in patients with metastatic melanoma. *J Clin Oncol.* 2015;33(33):e122–e124. doi:10.1200/jco.2013.51.1683

54. Gonzalez NL, Puwanant A, Lu A, et al. Myasthenia triggered by immune checkpoint inhibitors: new case and literature review. *Neuromuscul Disord.* 2017;27(3):266–268. doi:10.1016/j.nmd.2017.01.002

55. Loochtan AI, Nickolich MS, Hobson-Webb LD. Myasthenia Gravis Associated with ipilimumab an dnivolumab in the treatment of small cell lung cancer. *Muscle Nerve.* 2015;52(2):307–308. doi:10.1002/mus.24648

56. Zhu J, Li Y. Myasthenia gravis exacerbation associated with pembrolizumab. *Muscle Nerve.* 2016;54(3):506–507. doi:10.1002/mus.25055

57. Polat P, Donofrio PD. Myasthenia gravis induced by nivolumab therapy in a patient with non-small-cell lung cancer. *Muscle Nerve.* 2016;54(3):507. doi:10.1002/mus.25163

58. Sciacca G, Nicoletti A, Rampello L, et al. Benign form of myasthenia gravis after nivolumab treatment. *Muscle Nerve.* 2016;54(3):507–509. doi:10.1002/mus.25212

59. Lopez D, Calvo A, Fershko A. Myasthenia gravis and rhabdomyolysis in a patient with advanced renal cell cancer treated with nivolumab: a case report and review of literature. *Br J Med Health Res.* 2015;2(12).

60. Lau KH, Kumar A, Yang IH, et al. Exacerbation of myasthenia gravis in a patient with melanoma treated with pembrolizumab. *Muscle Nerve.* 2016;54(1):157–161. doi:10.1002/mus.25141

61. Johnson DB, Sullivan RJ, Ott PA, et al. Ipilimumab therapy in patients with advanced melanoma and preexisting autoimmune disorders. *JAMA Oncol.* 2016;2(2):234–240. doi:10.1001/jamaoncol.2015.4368

CHAPTER 11

CARDIOVASCULAR TOXICITIES RELATED TO IMMUNE CHECKPOINT INHIBITORS

Pankit Vachhani, Igor Puzanov, and Javid J. Moslehi

INTRODUCTION

Chemotherapies, targeted therapies, and immunotherapies constitute major pillars of cancer therapeutics. Cardiovascular toxicity, resulting from both cytotoxic and targeted cancer therapies, has been well described (1,2). Cardiovascular toxicity has also been observed with "traditional" immunotherapies (such as IL-2) and cancer vaccines. Recently, cardiovascular complications, including a number of cases of fulminant myocarditis cases, have been reported secondary to immune checkpoint inhibitors (ICIs). The current U.S. Food and Drug Administration (FDA) approved ICI therapies are all monoclonal antibodies that target two distinct immune checkpoint pathways regulated by cytotoxic T-lymphocyte antigen 4 (CTLA4; ipilimumab) and programmed cell death 1 (PD-1; nivolumab and pembrolizumab) and programmed cell death ligand 1 (PD-L1) (atezolizumab, avelumab, and durvalumab).

The detailed mechanisms of action of ICI have been reviewed elsewhere in this book. In this chapter, we first briefly describe the epidemiology of cardiotoxicity from ICI therapies. Then, we review the pathology, potential presentations of ICI-induced cardiotoxicity, and suggest diagnostic and management pathways. And finally, we conclude with future directions of research in ICI-induced cardiotoxicity, one of the most exciting subfields of cardio-oncology.

EPIDEMIOLOGY

Cardiovascular toxicities, unlike many other organ toxicities from ICI therapies, are rare (3,4). Fulminant myocarditis has been the focus of much of the cardiology and oncology communities over the past year due to a series of case reports. The true incidence of ICI-associated myocarditis in the community is unknown.

- From the clinical trial population, a pooled analysis of four studies in 576 patients with advanced melanoma who received nivolumab monotherapy identified 10 patients with any grade treatment-related cardiac adverse events (AEs) (1.7%) but only 1 patient (0.2%) had a grade 3/4 AE (5).
- Pharmacovigilance data of patients treated with ipilimumab and nivolumab, or both, showed that among 20,594 patients, only 18

Published by Springer Publishing Company DOI: 10.1891/9780826172150.0011

drug-related severe myocarditis events had occurred—thus amounting to an incidence rate of 0.09% (6). The incidence was slightly higher in those patients who received combination therapy (0.27%) vs. nivolumab alone (0.06%) (6). However, about half of all these cases were fatal. The median time to diagnosis of myocarditis was 17 days after first administration of ICI therapy (6).

The rarity can be adjudged by the large number of major clinical trials that have not noted any cardiotoxicities (7). Furthermore, many comprehensive reviews on immune-related adverse events (irAEs) and their management from various groups have nil or minimal mention of cardiotoxicities (3,8–10).

- However, recent efforts suggest that cardiovascular toxicity is an ongoing concern given the number of ICI clinical trials. The FDA, for example, held a one day symposium to discuss pathophysiology, screening, diagnosis, and management of cardiovascular toxicities of immunotherapy (11).
- In addition, with the emergence of combination therapies, one would suspect a higher incidence of myocarditis.
- Finally, previous ICI trials did not screen for cardiac issues routinely, thus less severe cases would be missed.

Current literature on cardiotoxicities from ICI therapies is largely limited to case reports and small case series (Table 11.1) (12). Potential reasons for underestimation of ICI-related cardiotoxicity include the varying definitions of cardiotoxicity, obscurity of Common Terminology Criteria for Adverse Events (CTCAEs) entries for some cardiac adverse events, as well as lack of monitoring and exclusion of patients with moderate-to-severe heart disease on clinical trials (4,13). Nevertheless, the severity of cardiotoxicities, including the report of many fatal cases, and the probability of a far higher incidence than currently estimated, gives gravity to this topic.

PATHOPHYSIOLOGY

Preclinical studies have demonstrated the underpinnings of ICI-induced cardiotoxicity (7).

- PD-1 and PD-L1 are expressed in the human cardiomyocytes after injury (7).
  - PD-1-deficient mice develop dilated cardiomyopathy and myocarditis (27–29).
  - Further, genetic deletion of PD-L1/PD-L2 and treatment with anti-PD-L1 agent in an autoimmune mouse background may transform transient myocarditis into lethal disease (30).
  - PD-1 limits T-cell-mediated myocarditis in murine models (31).
  - Recently, ischemic-reperfused rat hearts were shown to have increased expression of PD-1 and PD-L1 on cardiomyocytes (32).
  - Myocarditis has also been noted in CTLA-4-deficient mice (33,34).

TABLE 11.1 Summary of Reported Cases of Cardiac Toxicities From ICI, ATG, irAE, IVIG, I, LVEF, N, P, RBBB, and RV

Case	ICI; number of doses prior to cardiac irAE	Cardiac and other irAEs	Immunosuppressive therapies besides corticosteroids	Outcome from cardiac irAE
Laubli et al., 2015 (14)	P; 5	Acute heart failure, myocarditis	-	Survived
Berg et al., 2017 (15)	I; 1	Acute heart failure with progressive conduction delay, colitis	-	Fatal
Behling et al., 2017 (16)	N; 2	Progressive conduction delay, myositis		Fatal
Arangalage et al., 2017 (17)	I+N; 1	Fulminant myocarditis hyperthyroidism, myositis	IVIG, plasma exchange, tacrolimus	Survived
Johnson et al., 2017 (18)	I+N; 1	Myocarditis with progressive conduction delay, myositis	-	Fatal
	I+N; 1	Myocarditis with progressive conduction delay, myositis	infliximab	Fatal
Heinzerling et al., 2016 (19)	I+N -> N; 3	Myocarditis, cardiomyopathy, thyroiditis, hypophysitis	-	Survived
	I; 4	Cardiomyopathy	(no steroids)	Survived
	I; 2	Myocardial fibrosis, hepatitis	-	Fatal
	I; 3	Heart failure, colitis, hypophysitis	(no steroids)	Survived
	I; 4	Myocarditis, heart failure, uveitis	-	Survived
	I; 2	Myocarditis	(no steroids)	Fatal
	P; 9	Cardiac arrest	-	Survived
	I; 2	Myocarditis, hepatitis	-	Fatal

(continued)

TABLE 11.1 Summary of Reported Cases of Cardiac Toxicities From ICI, ATG, irAE, IMG, I, LVEF, N, P, RBBB, and RV *(continued)*

Case	ICI; number of doses prior to cardiac irAE	Cardiac and other irAEs	Immunosuppressive therapies besides corticosteroids	Outcome from cardiac irAE
Giesler et al., 2015 (20)	I; 4	Takatsubo-like cardiomyopathy, colitis	(no steroids)	Survived
Tadokoro et al., 2016 (21)	N; 3	Myocarditis, heart failure	-	Survived
Yun et al., 2015 (22)	I; 4	Pericardial effusion, acute fibrinous pericarditis, hypothyroidism	-	Survived
Jain et al., 2017 (12)	I+N; 1	Heart failure, advanced heart block	ATG	Survived
Semper et al., 2017 (23)	N; 9	Incomplete RBBB, septal hypokinesia, myocarditis, impaired LVEF	-	Survived
Zimmer et al., 2016 (24)	P; 2	Atrial flutter, impaired LVEF, ventricular arrhythmia, myocarditis	-	Fatal
	N; 17	Takatsubo-like cardiomyopathy, cardiac arrest	-	Survived
Tay et al., 2017 (25)	N; 2	Ventricular arrhythmias, impaired LVEF, myocarditis, myositis	Infliximab, ATG, mycophenolate	Survived
Reddy et al., 2017 (26)	I+N; 1	Evolution to complete heart block, impaired LVEF, RV dilatation, reduced RV systolic function, apical akinesis, anteroseptal hypokinesis, possible myocarditis	Mycophenolate	Survived

ATG, antithymocyte globulin; ICI, immune checkpoint inhibitors; I, ipilimumab; irAE, immune-related adverse event; IVIG, intravenous immunoglobulin; LVEF, left ventricular ejection fraction; N, nivolumab; P, pembrolizumab; RBBB, right bundle branch block; RV, right ventricle.

Together, these preclinical findings underscore the important roles that PD-1 and CTLA-4 immune checkpoints play in controlling cardiac homeostasis and how abrogation of these checkpoints can cause cardiac disease.

- In an eight-patient series of ICI-related cardiotoxicity, six patients underwent endomyocardial biopsy (EMB) (19).
  ○ Findings including myocardial inflammation with lymphocytes, fibrosis, myocyte hypertrophy, myocyte vacuolization, as well as the presence of multinucleated giant cells and eosinophils were noted.
- In another series of two patients with fulminant myocarditis secondary to dual therapy with nivolumab and ipilimumab, EMB demonstrated lymphocytic infiltrates within the myocardium, cardiac sinus, and atrioventricular nodes (6).
  ○ Notably, T-cell infiltrates in the myocardium, skeletal muscle, and tumor demonstrated clonality, raising the possibility of the lymphocytes targeting a common antigen.
- Recent data suggest that ICI are associated with other cardiovascular toxicities besides myocarditis. These include vasculitis, pericarditis and arrhythmias (40). More data are needed to better delineate these ICI-associated cardiovascular toxicities.

PRESENTATION

ICI-related cardiotoxicities may have protean manifestations—from subclinical findings to severe congestive heart failure (4,12). Clinical cardiotoxicity may itself have a multitude of manifestations.

- Some patients may have nonspecific symptoms (like fatigue and malaise), while others may have syncope or palpitations (due to arrhythmias), dyspnea, cough, peripheral edema, and weight gain (suggestive of heart failure) (4,12).
- Cardiac arrest as a presenting finding has also been noted (34,35).
- Examination findings may be notable for hypotension, jugular venous distention, pitting edema, cardiac murmurs, irregular rhythm, and pulmonary crepitations (12).

Patients may also present with either history of or the concurrent presence of other organ toxicities secondary to ICI therapies (4).

- In particular, emerging experience suggests a possible overlap or association between myositis (myalgias, rhabdomyolysis), myocarditis, and pericarditis (fever, pleuritic chest pain, diffuse ST elevation on ECG) (4).
- Similarly, some experts have noted an overlap between myasthenia gravis (fluctuating degree and a variable combination of ocular, bulbar, facial, limb, and respiratory muscle weakness—presenting as ptosis, diplopia, dysphagia, dysarthria, hypophonia, and dyspnea amongst others) and myocarditis as well.

While the care providers must always remain alert toward the development of cardiotoxicity, there are few situations which demand heightened vigilance. As implied before, these include, based on current literature and experience:

- Development of cardiac symptoms in a patient who started ICI therapy less than 12 weeks prior.
- Development of other organ toxicities secondary to ICI.
- Any patient receiving dual anti-CTLA-4 and anti-PD-1 blockade therapy.

Limited experience has not shown any correlation of cardiotoxicity with preexisting auto-immune conditions.

EVALUATION

Baseline and Follow-Up Surveillance

Until recently, most clinical trials did not require monitoring for cardiotoxicity. Clinical practice, similarly, did not routinely survey for cardiotoxicity. However, guidelines are just starting to suggest routine cardiotoxicity evaluation. For example, the Toxicity Management Working Group of the Society for Immunotherapy of Cancer (SITC) recommended:

- A judicious combination of biomarkers including troponin I or T, and an ECG in all patients prior to administration of first ICI therapy (4).
  - These tests should be done at baseline and following the start of ICI.
- Additionally, the guideline suggested a two-dimensional echocardiography (2D-Echo) in high-risk patients with cardiac history, symptoms of dyspnea, or if the initial tests were abnormal.
- The guideline recommended consideration for routine ECGs and cardiac biomarkers in patients with symptomatology suspicious for cardiotoxicity or if the initial battery of investigations were abnormal, although the ideal intervals for repeat testing are currently unknown.

The American Society of Clinical Oncology (ASCO) recommends individualized follow-up in consultation with cardiology. It should be noted that there is currently a paucity of evidence supporting or refuting baseline evaluations. In Table 11.2, we have provided a time frame of the most basic of baseline investigations that providers can consider.

Diagnosis

Myocarditis—an inflammatory condition of the heart muscle (i.e., myocardium) is one of the most common manifestations of cardiotoxicity from immunotherapies, including ICI. However, it is important to note that myocarditis has many different etiologies and it is often a diagnosis of exclusion (35,36).

- Myocarditis has a long differential diagnosis including heart failure and acute coronary syndrome with which it has overlapping presentation signs, symptoms, and laboratory findings.

TABLE 11.2 Suggested Baseline and Follow-up Investigations for Surveillance of Cardiotoxicity From Immune Checkpoint Inhibitor Therapy. The Investigations Synchronize With Routine Clinic Visits for Toxicity Checks. More Frequent and Expanded Monitoring Consisting of BNP/NT pro-BNP and Total CK May Be Considered in Patients at Higher Risk of Developing Cardiotoxicity (History of Cardiac Disease, Dual Inhibitor Therapy, and History of Autoimmune Conditions)

Investigation	Baseline (week 1 or before)	During week											
		1	2	3	4	5	6	7	8	9	10	11	12
Troponin-I and ECG (q2-week drug schedule)	✓			✓		✓		✓		✓		✓	
Troponin-I and ECG (q3-week drug schedule)	✓				✓			✓			✓		
Echocardiogram (for high-risk patients)	✓												

Drug regimen:
Every 2-weeks:
Nivolumab (Opdivo), avelumab (Bavencio), durvalumab (Imfinzi)
Every 3-weeks:
Ipilimumab (Yervoy), pembrolizumab (Keytruda), atezolizumab (Tecentriq), ipilimumab plus nivolumab

- Myocarditis can itself result in conduction abnormalities, wall motion abnormalities, and heart failure.
  - Abnormal surveillance tests or symptoms/signs consistent with cardiotoxicity should prompt immediate and comprehensive work-up.
  - Troponin-I, B-type natriuretic peptide (BNP) or N-terminal (NT) pro-BNP, CK, ECG, and 2D-Echo should be performed urgently if not done already.
- Chest radiograph or computed tomography angiography should be considered to evaluate pulmonary embolism, pneumonitis, and pulmonary edema from any cause (4).
  - Troponin-I and troponin-T are both specific markers of cardiomyocyte damage (37). However, BNP and NT pro-BNP are markers of myocardial stretch which could be normal in milder cases of myocarditis (37).
  - Because myocarditis is often a diagnosis of exclusion, other cardiac etiology should be ruled out including acute coronary syndrome.
- ECG may show normal or nonspecific abnormalities.
  - Findings may include nonspecific ST changes, single atrial or ventricular ectopic beats, complex atrial or ventricular arrhythmias, as well as heart blocks (4,36).
  - Q waves and regional or diffuse ST elevations (reminiscent of acute myocardial infarction or pericarditis) may also be seen (36).
  - 2D-Echo might demonstrate impaired ventricular function, wall motion abnormalities, or left ventricular dilation; however, a subset of patients with ICI-associated myocarditis have preserved cardiac function (36).

- Extrapolating data from other forms of myocarditis, cardiovascular magnetic resonance (CMR) may serve as the cardiac imaging test of choice (37).
- It helps detect various features found in myocarditis including inflammatory hyperemia, edema, myocyte necrosis and scar (pathognomonic features), changes in ventricular size and geometry (structural changes), and wall motion abnormalities (function), besides accompanying pericardial effusion (36,38,39).
- Importantly, the specific pattern of late gadolinium enhancement in myocarditis can generally distinguish myocarditis from ischemic cardiomyopathy related findings (36).
- Other cardiac imaging, including cardiac positron emission tomography (PET) scans, may be useful in specific cases.
- While invasive, the importance of obtaining an endomyocardial biopsy (EMB) in uncertain or complicated cases cannot be overstated. EMB may be particularly important as the medical community begins to define what is essentially a new clinical syndrome. The key in EMB is in identifying immune infiltrates not typical of ischemic heart disease (37).

Early treatment might improve outcomes of patients with myocarditis. However, it is important to note that treatment with immunosuppressive agents prior to specific diagnostic modalities—CMR or EMB—may increase the chance of false negativity.

- Given that various etiologies can cause myocarditis, it is wise to rule out at least viral myocarditis, either through serologic tests or polymerase chain reaction (PCR) testing on blood or EMB samples, as it is the most commonly identified cause of lymphocytic myocarditis (35,36).

MANAGEMENT

Present management guidelines are based largely on anecdotal evidence and from extrapolation of management of other ICI-associated organ toxicities.

- One algorithm developed for two ongoing trials with patients at high risk of ICI-induced myocarditis, suggests screening patients with troponin and ECG.
- For asymptomatic abnormalities of cardiac biomarkers or EKG findings, ICI therapy should be held while the investigations are repeated and findings normalize (4,37).
  - ICI therapy could be restarted if the findings normalized, although heightened monitoring should be pursued (4,37).
- For patients with symptoms or severe abnormal cardiac biomarkers, ICI therapy should be discontinued permanently (4,37).
  - Additional investigations to identify the precise underlying cardiotoxicity (e.g., acute coronary syndrome or myocarditis) should be performed as outlined in the preceding section.

Beyond holding or discontinuing ICI therapy, the management of myocarditis involves two aspects—immunosuppression and adjunct measures.

- High-dose corticosteroids should be started immediately upon high suspicion of myocarditis.
  - Methylprednisolone 1 to 2 mg/kg to up to 1,000 mg daily for 3 to 5 days at least or until biomarkers/EKG findings normalize, followed by gradual tapering over 4 to 6 weeks, is recommended (4,37).
  - Cases refractory to steroid therapy have been noted in literature.
- Additional immunosuppressive measures should be added at the earliest signs of refractoriness or severe cardiotoxicity.
  - Infliximab may be used; however, it is contraindicated in patients with moderate or severe heart failure.
  - Rabbit or horse anti-thymocyte globulin (ATG), tacrolimus, or mycophenolate could be used instead based on their efficacy in patients with cardiac allograft rejection (37). Reports of successful outcomes using ATG, tacrolimus, and mycophenolate, amongst other therapies, in fulminant myocarditis exist in the literature, although all are case reports (12,17,25).
  - Adjunct therapies should be pursued concurrent to immunosuppressive therapies. Anti-arrhythmic management should be started early and cardiac pacing should be considered in patients with high-grade conduction abnormalities (4,12).
  - Medical management of heart failure and additional hemodynamic support, if required, should be provided simultaneously (4,12).
  - The importance of early consultation and joint management with cardiology specialists (including heart failure, transplant, and electrophysiology specialists) cannot be overstated.

CONCLUSION

The lack of cardiotoxicity surveillance and exclusion of patients with various cardiovascular toxicities from cancer clinical trials has probably led to an underestimation of the true incidence of ICI-related cardiotoxicity. Prospective studies of biomarkers, EKG, and imaging findings are needed to identify subclinical cardiotoxicities. Most reports of ICI-related cardiotoxicity are secondary to ipilimumab, nivolumab, or pembrolizumab. While cardiotoxicity has been noted with other ICI therapies in clinical trials, more data is needed to identify if such therapies have similar or different cardiotoxicity rates and types.

Additional preclinical data on the plausibility of cardiotoxicity using ICI therapies, including those currently in development that target other immune-checkpoints like TIM-3 and LAG-3, is needed to better understand the pathophysiology, predict, and treat outcomes. Similarly, identification of biomarkers that predict ICI-related cardiotoxicities or toxicities in general is much needed to personalize surveillance and management of patients. Given the rarity of cardiotoxicity from ICI, prospective studies on treatment are unlikely to occur. As such, development of large multicenter databases will be crucial to better define toxicity characteristics and identify management options to treat the toxicities. That, along with long-term data from clinical trials, will help identify late cardiotoxicities of ICI therapies, if any.

REFERENCES

1. Moslehi JJ. Cardiovascular toxic effects of targeted cancer therapies. *N Engl J Med.* 2016;375:1457–1467. doi:10.1056/nejmra1100265

2. Li W, Croce K, Steensma DP, et al. Vascular and metabolic implications of novel targeted cancer therapies:focus on kinase Inhibitors. *J Am Coll Cardiol.* 2015;66:1160–1178. doi:10.1016/j.jacc.2015.07.025

3. Michot JM, Bigenwald C, Champiat S, et al. Immune-related adverse events with immune checkpoint blockade: a comprehensive review. *Eur J Cancer.* 2016;54:139–148. doi:10.1016/j.ejca.2015.11.016

4. Puzanov I, Diab A, Abdallah K, et al. Managing toxicities associated with immune checkpoint inhibitors: consensus recommendations from the Society for Immunotherapy of Cancer (SITC) Toxicity Management Working Group. *J Immunother Cancer.* 2017;5:95. doi:10.1186/s40425-017-0300-z

5. Weber JS, Hodi FS, Wolchok JD, et al. Safety profile of nivolumab monotherapy: a pooled analysis of patients with advanced melanoma. *J Clin Oncol.* 2017;35:785–792. doi:10.1200/jco.2015.66.1389

6. Johnson DB, Balko JM, Compton ML, et al. Fulminant myocarditis with combination immune checkpoint blockade. *N Engl J Med.* 2016;375:1749–1755. doi:10.1056/nejmoa1609214

7. Varricchi G, Galdiero MR, Tocchetti CG. Cardiac Toxicity of immune checkpoint inhibitors: cardio-oncology meets immunology. *Circulation.* 2017;136:1989–1992. doi:10.1161/circulationaha.117.029626

8. Spain L, Diem S, Larkin J. Management of toxicities of immune checkpoint inhibitors. *Cancer Treat Rev.* 2016;44:51–60. doi:10.1016/j.ctrv.2016.02.001

9. Haanen JBAG, Carbonnel F, Robert C, et al. Management of toxicities from immunotherapy: ESMO clinical practice guidelines for diagnosis, treatment and follow-up. *Ann Oncol.* 2017;28:iv119–iv142. doi:10.1093/annonc/mdx225

10. Friedman CF, Proverbs-Singh TA, Postow MA. Treatment of the immune-related adverse effects of immune checkpoint inhibitors: a review. *JAMA Oncol.* 2016;2:1346–1353. doi:10.1001/jamaoncol.2016.1051

11. US Food and Drug Administration. FDA Public Workshop: Assessment of Cardiovascular Toxicities in Immuno-oncology Trials. 2018. https://www.fda.gov/Drugs/NewsEvents/ucm574741.htm

12. Jain V, Bahia J, Mohebtash M, et al. Cardiovascular complications associated with novel cancer immunotherapies. *Curr Treat Options Cardiovasc Med.* 2017;19:36. doi:10.1007/s11936-017-0532-8

13. Moslehi JJ, Johnson DB, Sosman JA. Myocarditis with immune checkpoint blockade. *N Engl J Med.* 2017;376:292. doi:10.1056/nejmc1615251

14. Laubli H, Balmelli C, Bossard M, et al. Acute heart failure due to autoimmune myocarditis under pembrolizumab treatment for metastatic melanoma. *J Immunother Cancer.* 2015;3:11. doi:10.1186/s40425-015-0057-1

15. Berg DD, Vaduganthan M, Nohria A, et al. Immune-related fulminant myocarditis in a patient receiving ipilimumab therapy for relapsed chronic myelomonocytic leukaemia. *Eur J Heart Fail.* 2017;19(5):682–685. doi:10.1002/ejhf.806

16. Behling J, Kaes J, Münzel T, et al. New-onset third-degree atrioventricular block because of autoimmune-induced myositis under treatment with anti-programmed cell death-1 (nivolumab) for metastatic melanoma. *Melanoma Res.* 2017;27(2):155–158. doi:10.1097/CMR.0000000000000314

17. Arangalage D, Delyon J, Lermuzeaux M, et al. Survival after fulminant myocarditis induced by immune-checkpoint inhibitors. *Ann Intern Med.* 2017;167:683–684. doi:10.7326/l17-0396

18. Johnson DB, Balko JM, Compton ML, et al. Fulminant myocarditis with combination immune checkpoint blockade. *N Engl J Med.* 2016;375(18):1749–1755.

19. Heinzerling L, Ott PA, Hodi FS, et al. Cardiotoxicity associated with CTLA4 and PD1 blocking immunotherapy. *J Immunother Cancer.* 2016;4:50. doi:10.1186/s40425-016-0152-y

20. Geisler BP, Raad RA, Esaian D, et al. Apical ballooning and cardiomyopathy in a melanoma patient treated with ipilimumab: a case of takotsubo-like syndrome. *J Immunother Cancer.* 2015;3:4. doi:10.1186/s40425-015-0048-2

21. Tadokoro T, Keshino E, Makiyama A, et al. Acute lymphocytic myocarditis with anti-PD-1 antibody nivolumab. *Circ Heart Fail.* 2016;9(10):e003514. doi:10.1161/CIRCHEARTFAILURE.116.003514

22. Yun S, Vincelette ND, Mansour I, et al. Late onset ipilimumab-induced pericarditis and pericardial effusion: a rare but life threatening complication. *Case Rep Oncol Med.* 2015;2015:794842. doi:10.1155/2015/794842

23. Semper H, Muehlberg F, Schulz-Menger J, et al. Drug-induced myocarditis after nivolumab treatment in a patient with PDL1- negative squamous cell carcinoma of the lung. *Lung Cancer.* 2016;99:117–119. doi:10.1016/j.lungcan.2016.06.025

24. Zimmer L, Goldinger SM, Hofmann L, et al. Neurological, respiratory, musculoskeletal, cardiac and ocular side-effects of anti-PD-1 therapy. *Eur J Cancer.* 2016;60:210–225. doi:10.1016/j.ejca.2016.02.024

25. Tay RY, Blackley E, McLean C, et al. Successful use of equine anti-thymocyte globulin (ATGAM) for fulminant myocarditis secondary to nivolumab therapy. *Br J Cancer.* 2017;117:921–924. doi:10.1038/bjc.2017.253

26. Reddy N, Moudgil R, Lopez-Mattei JC, et al. Progressive and reversible conduction disease with checkpoint inhibitors. *Can J Cardiol.* 2017;33:1335.e13–1335.e15. doi:10.1016/j.cjca.2017.05.026

27. Nishimura H, Okazaki T, Tanaka Y, et al. Autoimmune dilated cardiomyopathy in PD-1 receptor-deficient mice. *Science.* 2001;291:319–322. doi:10.1126/science.291.5502.319

28. Wang J, Okazaki IM, Yoshida T, et al. PD-1 deficiency results in the development of fatal myocarditis in MRL mice. *Int Immunol.* 2010;22:443–452. doi:10.1093/intimm/dxq026

29. Okazaki T, Tanaka Y, Nishio R, et al. Autoantibodies against cardiac troponin I are responsible for dilated cardiomyopathy in PD-1-deficient mice. *Nat Med.* 2003;9:1477–1483. doi:10.1038/nm955

30. Lucas JA, Menke J, Rabacal WA, et al. Programmed death ligand 1 regulates a critical checkpoint for autoimmune myocarditis and pneumonitis in MRL mice. *J Immunol.* 2008;181:2513–2521. doi:10.4049/jimmunol.181.4.2513

31. Tarrio ML, Grabie N, Bu DX, et al. PD-1 protects against inflammation and myocyte damage in T cell-mediated myocarditis. *J Immunol.* 2012;188:4876–4884. doi:10.4049/jimmunol.1200389

32. Baban B, Liu JY, Qin X, et al. Upregulation of programmed death-1 and its ligand in cardiac injury models: interaction with GADD153. *PLoS One.* 2015;10:e0124059. doi:10.1371/journal.pone.0124059

33. Waterhouse P, Penninger JM, Timms E, et al. Lymphoproliferative disorders with early lethality in mice deficient in Ctla-4. *Science.* 1995;270:985–988. doi:10.1126/science.270.5238.985

34. Boutros C, Tarhini A, Routier E, et al. Safety profiles of anti-CTLA-4 and anti-PD-1 antibodies alone and in combination. *Nat Rev Clin Oncol.* 2016;13:473–486. doi:10.1038/nrclinonc.2016.58

35. Cooper L. Etiology and pathogenesis of myocarditis. In: Yeon S, ed. *UpToDate.* Waltham, MA: UpToDate Inc; 2018.

36. Cooper L. Clinical manifestations and diagnosis of myocarditis in adults. In: Yeon S, ed. *UpToDate.* Waltham, MA: UpToDate Inc; 2018.

37. Wang DY, Okoye GD, Neilan TG, et al. Cardiovascular toxicities associated with cancer immunotherapies. *Curr Cardiol Rep.* 2017;19:21. doi:10.1007/s11886-017-0835-0

38. Friedrich MG, Marcotte F. Cardiac magnetic resonance assessment of myocarditis. *Circ Cardiovasc Imaging.* 2013;6:833–839. doi:10.1161/circimaging.113.000416

39. Friedrich MG, Sechtem U, Schulz-Menger J, et al. Cardiovascular magnetic resonance in myocarditis: a JACC white paper. *J Am Coll Cardiol.* 2009;53:1475–1487.

40. Salem JE, Manouchehri A, Moey M, et al. Cardiovascular toxicities associated with immune checkpoint inhibitors: an observational, retrospective, pharmacovigilance study. *Lancet Oncol.* 2018;19(12):1579–1589. doi:10.1016/S1470-2045(18)30608-9

CHAPTER 12

RENAL TOXICITIES ASSOCIATED WITH IMMUNE CHECKPOINT INHIBITORS

Ala Abudayyeh, Maen Abdelrahim, and Laurence Albiges

INTRODUCTION

Immune checkpoint inhibitor (ICI) had a major clinical success in clinical oncology and impacted the treatment paradigm in many cancers and has been expanded in the adjuvant setting (1–3). Immune-related adverse events (irAEs) are well-described toxicities that are closely associated with ICI therapies and can involve any organ in the human body (4). Skin, gut, endocrine, lung, and musculoskeletal irAEs are relatively common, whereas cardiovascular, hematologic, renal, neurologic, and ophthalmologic are less common (5). The adverse events (AEs) have been associated with improved survival outcomes (6,7). Unlike other common irAEs, renal toxicity associated with ICI is usually asymptomatic and present only with acute kidney injury (AKI) defined by elevated creatinine levels, which in cancer patients is very nonspecific findings and can be due to multiple etiologies. The lack of a definitive, noninvasive, diagnostic test may lead to under- or delayed diagnosis of true immune-related renal toxicity.

Therapy guidelines for the multidisciplinary management of irAEs have been published by the Society for Immunotherapy of Cancer (SITC) and the American Society of Clinical Oncology (ASCO), European Society of Medical Oncology (ESMO), and more recently the National Comprehensive Cancer Network (NCCN) (4,8–10); however, the data on renal management is limited.

In this chapter, we will discuss and summarize the published data on immune-related nephrotoxicity, including the epidemiology and clinicopathological features as well as a recommendation on the management of renal immune toxicity in the setting of ICI.

EPIDEMIOLOGY

- Incidence of immune-related renal toxicity has been reported as low as 2% when nivolumab alone to 4.9% with 1.7% of grade 3/4 toxicity when a combination of nivolumab and ipilimumab has been used (7,8,11).
- As reported with other irAEs, renal toxicities occurred more frequently with the combination or sequential anti-cytotoxic T-lymphocyte antigen 4 (CTLA-4)/anti-programmed cell death 1 (PD-1) (12,13).
- A study by Cortazar et al. looked at the incidence of AKI in 3,695 patients on clinical trials treated with ICI, where the overall incidence of AKI was 2.2%. The incidence of grade III or IV AKI or need for dialysis was 0.6%. Most of the AKIs related to the ipilimumab occurred in

Published by Springer Publishing Company DOI: 10.1891/9780826172150.0012

the first 3 months of therapy, whereas most of the AKIs related to the PD-1 inhibitors occurred after 3 to 12 months of therapy (14).

- Although the incidence of renal toxicity based on case reports and clinical trial is low, we believe that it is much higher and not reported. When defining AKI based on AKI network criteria in a population of 99 patients, incidence of AKI has been reported to be from 9.9% to as high as 29% (15).

CLINICAL PRESENTATION AND DIAGNOSIS

- Newly elevated (above base line) and persistent serum creatinine level.
- Rule out other etiologies such as (a) infection (urinary tract infection [UTI]), (b) nephrotoxic agents (drugs, IV contrast), (iii) postrenal or obstructive causes (progressive disease, etc.), (iv) pre-renal: fluid imbalance (azotemia), and (v) exacerbation of preexisting, subclinical, and autoimmune nephropathy.
- Close monitoring of serum creatinine and frequency depend on severity of the toxicity, we recommend testing not longer than 7 days if grade 1/2.
- Urine analysis often show pyuria (white blood cells [WBC]> 0), subnephrotic proteinuria with rare cases of eosinophilia, rash, or fevers as typical of acute intestinal nephritis (AIN) (16). Sometimes the urine analysis may not be revealing if the patient is already on immune suppression.
- For empirically treating immune renal toxicity or more often to treat pre/co-existing other organ irAE (such as colitis, hepatitis, etc.).
- Nephrology consult is recommended, kidney biopsy is often required especially for high-grade toxicity or patient with suspicious or known preexisting nephropathy.

PATHOLOGICAL FEATURES

Acute Tubulointerstitial Nephritis

- The most commonly associated renal toxicity with ICI has been acute tubulointerstitial nephritis (ATIN) with some reports of granulomatous interstitial nephritis (14,17–19)
  - Since CTLA-4 activity is in the lymphoid organs regulating peripheral tolerance, it has been demonstrated in CTLA-4-deficient mice a lymphoproliferative disease develops with multi-organ lymphocytic infiltration and tissue destruction just as present with ATIN induced by ICI (20,21).
  - PD-1 regulates tolerance primarily at the level of target organs. In mice models PD-1, programmed cell death ligand 1 (PD-L1) were important inhibitory regulators of CD8(+) T-cells in tubulointerstitial inflammation and provide protection from ischemic reperfusion injury (22,23).
  - The exact immune biology of ICI-induced renal toxicity is yet to be elucidated; however, what has become evident is the delayed response after exposure to ICI which is not typical of ATIN.

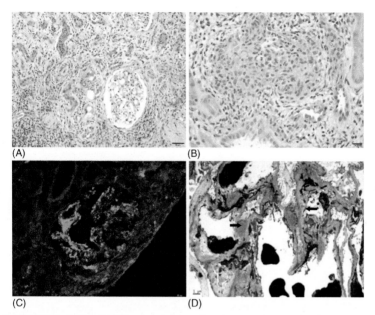

FIGURE 12.1 (A, H&E, 20×). There was a single case of granulomatous tubulointerstitial nephritis (B, H&E, 40×) which had C3-only granular deposits (C, C3 immunofluorescence, 40×) with corresponding rare, large subepithelial electron dense deposits (D, electron microscopy).

Source: Images provided courtesy of Amanda Tchakarov from McGovern Medical School, UTHealth, The University of Texas Health Science Center at Houston.

Renal Toxicity and Glomerulonephritis

- A recent abstract has reported on membranous nephropathy, antineutrophil cytoplasmic antibodies (ANCA) vasculitis, IgA nephropathy, C3 glomerulopathy, AA type amyloid, and the typical AIN after ICI (24) (Figures 12.1–12.4).

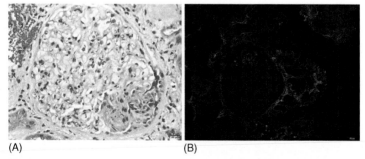

FIGURE 12.2 Pauci-immune glomerulonephritis characterized by focal, segmental glomerulonecrosis (A, H&E, 40×) without immune complex deposition (B, IgG immunofluorescence, 20×).

Source: Images provided courtesy of Amanda Tchakarov from McGovern Medical School, UTHealth, The University of Texas Health Science Center at Houston.

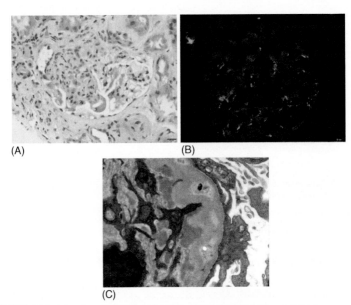

(A)   (B)

(C)

FIGURE 12.3 IgA nephropathy, one of which was characterized by segmental mesangial and endocapillary hypercellularity seen on H&E (A, 40×). There were IgA-dominant immune complex deposits (B, IgA immunofluorescence, 40×) with numerous mesangial electron dense deposits ultrastructurally (C, electron microscopy).

Source: Images provided courtesy of Amanda Tchakarov from McGovern Medical School, UTHealth, The University of Texas Health Science Center at Houston.

- One of the cases in the series with AIN had aggressive T-cell infiltration with CD4+ and CD8+ T-cell infiltration, and further demonstrated in another case in the literature (24,25).
- Other biopsy-proven kidney manifestations were published as case reports after ICI use included: lupus nephropathy, thrombotic microangiopathy (TMA), nephrotic syndrome (focal segmental glomerulosclerosis [FSGS]), two cases of minimal-change disease (MCD) (26), membranous nephropathy, pauci-immune glomerulonephritis (27), and two cases of IgA nephropathy (28–33). The etiology of the reported kidney toxicity is not yet clear. Suggested mechanisms include direct lymphocytic cellular infiltration of renal interstitium, immune complex-mediated kidney injury, lupus nephritis, IgA, microangiopathic hemolytic anemia TMA, or release of cytokines leading to podocyte foot process effacement (minimal-change disease and focal segmental glomerulosclerosis).
- Treatment of the glomerulonephritis (GN) induced by ICI includes steroids but also necessitates treatment of the GN with other immunosuppressive medications as indicated for the disease identified after renal biopsy. Case reports and our experience has GN treatment from steroids alone to a combination of steroids with rituximab, infliximab, mycophenolate mofetil, and cyclosporine (24,29,30,34).

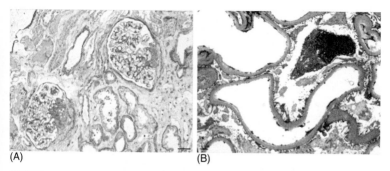

FIGURE 12.4 A case of AIN with eosinophils (A, H&E, 40×) and focal glomeruli with segmental sclerosis (A, PAS, 20×). Podocyte foot processes were preserved (B, electron microscopy), consistent with secondary FSGS.

Source: Images provided courtesy of Amanda Tchakarov from McGovern Medical School, UTHealth, The University of Texas Health Science Center at Houston.

Renal irAEs With Preexisting Renal Glomerulonephritis

- Another interesting notion is the higher likelihood of patients with preexisting autoimmune disorders to develop irAE on ICI. This would impact the kidney since primary renal diseases are attributed to de Novo autoimmune induction. There are limited data available about management of these patients. But clinicians should be cautious and check urine analysis at baseline and 2 to 4 weeks with initiation of ICI to detect any proteinuria or hematuria which could be early signs of re-induction of GN.

- In a recent meta-analysis by Abdel-Wahab et al., among 123 patients, 92 (75%) had irAEs of which 50 patients (41%) had exacerbation of their current autoimmune symptoms, 31 (25%) had new irAEs, and 11 (9%) had both.

- Interestingly, two cases had *preexisting autoimmune nephritis (IgA nephropathy and IgM nephropathy)* (35).

In a prospective study of 45 patients with cancer and preexisting autoimmune or inflammatory disease who were treated with anti-PD-1 antibodies, the study demonstrated that patients with preexisting autoimmune disease were more likely to have irAEs. Overall survival in the group with autoimmune disease versus the group without was no different (36).

- *Extrarenal* irAE in published case series have *preceded* renal irAEs, such as hypophysitis, colitis, hypothyroidism, dermatitis, pneumonitis, adrenal insufficiency, and myositis (14,17,24). Other irAEs have occurred between 2 and 14 weeks prior to renal irAE.

We have summarized in Table 12.1 all published renal irAEs reported and ICI-associated renal toxicity.

Immunotherapy and its impact on CKD: Chronic kidney disease (CKD) and cancer have a bidirectional relationship. This is evident in the observations that cancer and/or its treatments can lead to CKD and that CKD is a risk factor for cancer development. A number of observational

TABLE 12.1 Reported irAEs and ICI-Associated Renal Toxicity

Reference	Renal manifestation	Checkpoint inhibitor	Therapy	Renal outcome
Anti-PD-1				
Daanen et al. (30)	FSGS, proteinuria	Nivolumab	DC + steroid + MMF	Remission Followed by relapse
Kitchlu et al. (31)	MCD, proteinuria	Pembrolizumab	DC + steroid	Remission (partial)
Lin et al. (26)	Membranous nephropathy (PLA2R neg.), proteinuria	Nivolumab	DC + steroid	Remission (partial)
Jung et al. (33)	AKI, proteinuria and hematuria IgA nephropathy	Nivolumab	DC, steroid and RRT	Recovery (RRT was d/c after 5 months)
Kishi et al. (32)	AKI, proteinuria and hematuria IgA nephropathy	Nivolumab	DC	Remission (complete)
Van den Brom et al. (29)	GPA Dysmorphic erythro-cytes and proteinuria	Pembrolizumab	Cyclosporine and steroid	Remission
Vandiver et al. (37)	AKI	Nivolumab	Steroid	Full recovery
Cortazar et al.*(14)	AKI, no pyuria or hematuria AKI with pyuria AKI with pyuria	Nivolumab Pembrolizumab Pembrolizumab	Steroid Steroid Steroid	Partial recovery Partial recovery Full recovery
Shirali et al.* (17)	AKI with no pyuria or hematuria AKI with proteinuria AKI with pyuria AKI with pyuria	Nivolumab Nivolumab Pembrolizumab Pembrolizumab	Steroid Steroid DC + steroid DC + steroid	Full recovery Full recovery Partial recov-ery + relapse Full recovery
Anti-CTLA-4				
Kitchlu et al. (28,31)	MCD, proteinuria	Ipilimumab	DC + steroid	Remission
Fadel et al.	AKI with proteinuria + DSDNA (lupus nephropathy)	Ipilimumab	DC	DSDNA; not detectable
Izzedine et al. (19)	AKI Granulomatous ATIN	Ipilimumab	Steroid	Full recovery
Voskens et al. (38)	AKI	Ipilimumab	Steroid	Full recovery
Forde et al. (39)	AKI	Ipilimumab	Steroid	Full recovery

(continued)

TABLE 12.1 Reported irAEs and ICI-Associated Renal Toxicity (*continued*)

Reference	Renal manifestation	Checkpoint inhibitor	Therapy	Renal outcome
Anti-CTLA-4				
Cortazar et al.*(14)	AKI with pyuria AKI with pyuria AKI with no pyuria AKI with pyuria AKI with no pyuria or hematuria AKI with pyuria	Ipilimumab Ipilimumab Ipilimumab Ipilimumab Ipilimumab Ipilimumab	Steroid Conservative Steroid Steroid Conservative Steroid	Partial recovery No recovery Dialysis dependent Dialysis dependent Dialysis dependent Partial recovery
Anti-PD-1 + Anti-CTLA-4				
Cusnir et al. (27)	GPA Focal proliferative GN (PR3-ANCA+)	Nivolumab + ipilimumab	Steroids and rituximab	Not Stated
Murakami et al. (25)	AKI secondary to ATIN	Nivolumab + ipilimumab	MMF + steroid	No recovery
Cortazar et al.*(14)	AKI, no proteinuria or pyuria AKI with pyuria AKI with no proteinuria or pyuria AKI with pyuria and hematuria	Nivolumab + ipilimumab Nivolumab + ipilimumab	Steroid Steroid Steroid Steroid + MMF	Full recovery Partial recovery Partial recovery
Shirali et al.*(17)	AKI with no pyuria	Nivolumab + ipilimumab	DC	Partial recovery

*Case series

AKI, acute kidney injury; ANCA, antineutrophil cytoplasmic antibodies; ATIN, acute tubulointerstitial nephritis; DC, immune checkpoint agent was discontinued; FSGS, focal segmental glomerulosclerosis; GN, glomerulonephritis; GPA, granulomatosis with polyangitis; ICI, immune checkpoint inhibitor; irAEs, immune-related adverse events; MCD, minimal change disease; MMF, mycophenolate; MPO, myeloperoxidase; PR3, proteinase 3; RRT, renal replacement therapy.

studies have shown the high prevalence of CKD in patients with solid tumors (40–43). This would be most impactful in patients with renal cell cancer (RCC) where, in 1,114 RCC patients, 22% had CKD stage 3 or higher before nephrectomy, and this percentage increased to 40% for patients older than 70 years (44). CKD patients were excluded from ICI clinical trials and therefore there is limited data about efficacy, toxicity, and overall renal outcomes.

- PD-L1 is expressed in about 20% to 25% of ccRCC tumor cells and was independently associated with metastatic cancer progression (RR, 3.46; $P < .001$) and death from RCC (RR, 4.13; $P < .001$) (45).
- With the expanding use of ICI in treatment of RCC patients we have more data about renal outcomes in this CKD population.
- Clinical trials using nivolumab in metastatic ccRCC was the first of its class to be approved for treatment of metastatic, in 2014, after randomized,

open-label, phase 3 study compared nivolumab with everolimus (Check-Mate 025 study) in patients who had failed prior vascular endothelial growth factor (VEGF) inhibition.
- The median overall survival was 25.0 months with nivolumab and 19.6 months with everolimus (HR, 0.73; 98.5% CI: [0.57–0.93], $p = .0018$) (46). In CheckMate 025, Motzer et al. reported 8% of the RCC patients had an elevation in creatinine and reported as grade 3/4 toxicity (46,47).
- Clinical trials are now underway to investigate anti-VEGF and ICI as a first-line treatment of RCC. With anti-VEGF having potential nephrotoxicity, it would be interesting to see the associated renal outcomes and irAEs (48–50)

ICI USE IN PATIENTS WITH KIDNEY ALLO-TRANSPLANT

- Kidney transplant patients treated with ICI are at high risk of organ rejection, and need to have both an oncologist and transplant nephrologist in close communication for possible organ rejection.
  - Close monitoring of renal function, especially after immunosuppression, is reduced with the diagnosis of cancer.
  - One case in the literature suggests switching tacrolimus to sirolimus, and a higher dose of steroids may have been of benefit in preventing organ rejection while on immunotherapy (51).
  - Organ rejection has been reported with both types of ICI, anti CTLA-4 and anti PD-1. For more information about the use of ICI in patient with organ transplant, see Chapter 15.

MANAGEMENT OF RENAL TOXICITY

The mainstay treatment for renal toxicity associated with ICI has been steroids as is typically done with other organ irAEs (9). However, it has become evident that biomarkers for organ toxicity associated with CPI are much needed to understand novel treatments (52).

There is yet more to be done in the renal realm to characterize the immune biology and potentially develop novel therapies that mitigate the autoimmunity without impacting the positive ICI-induced tumor immunity.

- A baseline urine analysis (UA) and renal function assessment at baseline prior to ICI treatment and before next infusion of ICI would be highly recommended to detect early dysfunction.
- **Stages of Injury Grades (G1–G4 (Table 12.2 and Figure 12.5):** At all stages of renal injury, G1–G4 would recommend *initially holding* CPI and assessing for any other etiologies such as nephrotoxins, infections, pre-renal states, obstruction, heart failure, or pulmonary hypertension.
- *G1 stage renal injury (increased Cr × 1.5 or ≥ 0.3 mg/dL from baseline):* The basic approach with AKI after ICI use is attaining lab and urine analysis, spot protein to creatinine ratio, and urine eosinophils. If proteinuria and/or hematuria is present, then a nephrology consult should be initiated for biopsy consideration, and check serologies for autoimmune disease inducing GN (see Table 12.1). Repeat labs weekly to follow up for renal recovery.

TABLE 12.2 Criteria for Grading the Severity of AKI and Renal Recovery

Grading	Correlated AKIN grading	Criteria	Renal injury outcome	Criteria (14)
G1	Stage 1	Increased Cr × 1.5 or ≥ 0.3 mg/dL	Complete renal recovery	Cr improved to < (baseline Cr + 0.35 mg/dL)
G2	Stage 2	Increased Cr × 2	Partial renal recovery	Cr improved to ≥ (baseline Cr + 0.35 mg/dL) and < Cr ×2 at baseline
G3 G4	Stage 3	Increased Cr × 3 or Cr ≥ 4 mg/dL (with acute rise of ≥ 0.5 mg/dL) Receiving renal replacement therapy	Persistent AKI	Cr ≥ ×2 the baseline Cr or remains on renal replacement therapy

AKI, acute kidney injury; AKIN, acute kidney injury network; Cr, serum creatinine.

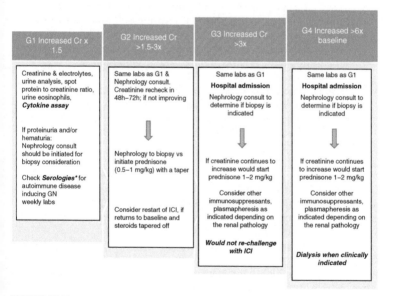

FIGURE 12.5 ICI-induced nephrotoxicity management.

*Serologies to consider: ANA, complement C3, C4, CH50, ANCA, anti-GBM, hepatitis B and C, HIV, immunoglobulins and protein electrophoresis. Rheumatoid Factor (RF)

ANA, antinuclear antibody; ANCA, antineutrophil cytoplasmic antibody; GBM; glomerular basement membrane; GN, glomerulonephritis; HIV, human immunodeficiency virus.

- *G2 stage (increased Cr × 1.5 baseline):* Would recommend same labs as G1 and a nephrology consult. Creatinine recheck in 48 hr to 72 hr; if not improving, in conjunction with nephrology consult, would biopsy versus initiate prednisone (0.5–1 mg/kg) with a taper once creatinine starts to improve over 1 to 2 months based on CKIN (Cancer and Kidney International Network) Workgroup on Immune Checkpoint Inhibitors (47). A kidney biopsy would be indicated to delineate if patient has AIN versus a glomerular process that may require more than steroids.
  - If not improving with steroids and no glomerular disease on biopsy would check cytokine assay and if elevated, we would consider infliximab at 5 mg/kg every two weeks and follow response in conjunction with cytokine assay for further dosing.
  - Repeat basic metabolic panel every 48 hours.

Possible re-challenge would be reasonable once creatinine is at baseline and if all possible contributors to AIN have been discontinued, such as nonsteroidal anti-inflammatory drugs (NSAIDS), proton pump inhibitors (PPIs), and tapered off steroids.

- *G3 (Cr increased > 3× baseline):* Would recommend same as G2 but would need a hospital admission and the same day renal consult to determine if biopsy is indicated; if creatinine continues to increase, would start prednisone/methylprednisolone 1 to 2 mg/kg.
  - Would determine if other immunosuppressants are indicated depending on the renal pathology and plasmapheresis.
  - Would not re-challenge with ICI.
- *G4 (creatinine >6 × baseline):* Patient needs to be admitted with same day nephrology consult and administer prednisone/methylprednisolone 1 to 2 mg/kg. All considerations as above. Dialysis indication when clinically indicated by nephrologist.

CONCLUSION

Given the wide use of ICI across tumor types, physicians should be trained to detect renal complications. The large majority of cases present either with creatinine level impairment due to renal parenchymal damage, the most common being acute interstitial nephritis.

The recommendation for when to obtain renal biopsy is controversial and still a topic open for discussion among experts. Although it is considered to involve highly invasive procedures with risk of bleeding and other complications, it often provides information that can be critical to the optimal management of the renal toxicity, especially when pathology reveals glumeronephropathy in addition to the ATIN, which sometimes require immune suppression regimen different from, or in addition to, steroids. Prompt identification and management are needed to prevent CKD, which would impact the patients' eligibility for future treatments and overall survival.

REFERENCES

1. Eggermont AM, Chiarion-Sileni V, Grob JJ, et al. Adjuvant ipilimumab versus placebo after complete resection of high-risk stage III melanoma (EORTC 18071): a randomised, double-blind, phase 3 trial. *Lancet Oncol.* 2015;16(5):522–530. doi:10.1016/S1470-2045(15)70122-1

2. Weber J, Mandala M, Del Vecchio M, et al. Adjuvant nivolumab versus ipilimumab in resected stage III or IV melanoma. *N Engl J Med.* 2017;377(19):1824–1835. doi:10.1056/NEJMoa1709030

3. Antonia SJ, Villegas A, Daniel D, et al. Durvalumab after chemoradiotherapy in stage III Non-Small-Cell Lung Cancer. *N Engl J Med.* 2017;377(20):1919–1929. doi:10.1056/NEJMoa1709937

4. Brahmer JR, Lacchetti C, Schneider BJ, et al. Management of immune-related adverse events in patients treated with immune checkpoint inhibitor therapy: American Society of Clinical Oncology Clinical Practice Guideline. *J Clin Oncol.* 2018;36(17):1714–1768. doi:10.1200/JCO.2017.77.6385

5. Michot JM, Bigenwald C, Champiat S, et al. Immune-related adverse events with immune checkpoint blockade: a comprehensive review. *Eur J Cancer.* 2016;54:139–148. doi:10.1016/j.ejca.2015.11.016

6. Abdel-Wahab N, Shah M, Suarez-Almazor ME. Adverse events associated with immune checkpoint blockade in patients with cancer: a systematic review of case reports. *PLoS One.* 2016;11(7):e0160221. doi:10.1371/journal.pone.0160221

7. Weber JS, Hodi FS, Wolchok JD, et al. Safety profile of nivolumab monotherapy: a pooled analysis of patients with advanced melanoma. *J Clin Oncol.* 2017;35(7):785–792. doi:10.1200/JCO.2015.66.1389

8. Puzanov I, Diab A, Abdallah K, et al. Managing toxicities associated with immune checkpoint inhibitors: consensus recommendations from the Society for Immunotherapy of Cancer (SITC) Toxicity Management Working Group. *J Immunother Cancer.* 2017;5(1):95. doi:10.1186/s40425-017-0300-z

9. Postow MA. Managing immune checkpoint-blocking antibody side effects. *Am Soc Clin Oncol Educ Book.* 2015;35:76–83.

10. Thompson JA. New NCCN guidelines: recognition and management of immunotherapy-related toxicity. *J Natl Compr Canc Netw.* 2018;16(5S):594–596. doi:10.6004/jnccn.2018.0047

11. Sznol M, Ferrucci PF, Hogg D, et al. Pooled analysis safety profile of nivolumab and ipilimumab combination therapy in patients with advanced melanoma. *J Clin Oncol.* 2017;35(34):3815–3822. doi:10.1200/JCO.2016.72.1167

12. Postow MA, Chesney J, Pavlick AC, et al. Nivolumab and ipilimumab versus ipilimumab in untreated melanoma. *N Engl J Med.* 2015;372(21):2006–2017. doi:10.1056/NEJMoa1414428

13. Weber JS, Gibney G, Sullivan RJ, et al. Sequential administration of nivolumab and ipilimumab with a planned switch in patients with advanced melanoma (CheckMate 064): an open-label, randomised, phase 2 trial. *Lancet Oncol.* 2016;17(7):943–955. doi:10.1016/S1470-2045(16)30126-7

14. Cortazar FB, Marrone KA, Troxell ML, et al. Clinicopathological features of acute kidney injury associated with immune checkpoint inhibitors. *Kidney Int.* 2016;90(3):638–647. doi:10.1016/j.kint.2016.04.008

15. Wanchoo R, Karam S, Uppal NN, et al. Adverse renal effects of immune checkpoint inhibitors: a narrative review. *Am J Nephrol.* 2017;45(2):160–169. doi:10.1159/000455014

16. Clarkson MR, Giblin L, O'Connell FP, et al. Acute interstitial nephritis: clinical features and response to corticosteroid therapy. *Nephrol Dial Transplant.* 2004;19(11):2778–2783. doi:10.1093/ndt/gfh485

17. Shirali AC, Perazella MA, Gettinger S. Association of acute interstitial nephritis with programmed cell death 1 inhibitor therapy in lung cancer patients. *Am J Kidney Dis.* 2016;68(2):287–291. doi:10.1053/j.ajkd.2016.02.057

18. Thajudeen B, Madhrira M, Bracamonte E, et al. Ipilimumab granulomatous interstitial nephritis. *Am J Ther.* 2015;22(3):e84–e87. doi:10.1097/MJT.0b013e3182a32ddc

19. Izzedine H, Gueutin V, Gharbi C, et al. Kidney injuries related to ipilimumab. *Invest New Drugs.* 2014;32(4):769–773. doi:10.1007/s10637-014-0092-7

20. Tivol EA, Borriello F, Schweitzer AN, et al. Loss of CTLA-4 leads to massive lymphoproliferation and fatal multiorgan tissue destruction, revealing a critical negative regulatory role of CTLA-4. *Immunity*. 1995;3(5):541–547. doi:10.1016/1074-7613(95)90125-6

21. Kuehn HS, Ouyang W, Lo B, et al. Immune dysregulation in human subjects with heterozygous germline mutations in CTLA4. *Science*. 2014;345(6204):1623–1627. doi:10.1126/science.1255904

22. Zheng G, Wang Y, Mahajan D, et al. The role of tubulointerstitial inflammation. *Kidney Int Suppl*. 2005(94): S96–S100. doi:10.1111/j.1523-1755.2005.09423.x

23. Jaworska K, Ratajczak J, Huang L, et al. Both PD-1 ligands protect the kidney from ischemia reperfusion injury. *J Immunol*. 2015;194(1):325–333. doi:10.4049/jimmunol.1400497

24. Selamet U, Ziaolhagh A, Lakhani LS, et al. Biopsy proven nephrotoxicity of immune checkpoint inhibitors: MD Anderson Cancer Center experience. New Orleans, LA: American Society of Nephrology Kidney Week, 2017.

25. Murakami N, Borges TJ, Yamashita M, et al. Severe acute interstitial nephritis after combination immune-checkpoint inhibitor therapy for metastatic melanoma. *Clin Kidney J*. 2016;9(3):411–417. doi:10.1093/ckj/sfw024

26. Jonathan T, Lin MS, Steven Salvatore S, et al. Membranous nephropathy related to the checkpoint inhibitor nivolumab. *J Am Soc Nephrol*. 2016;27:102A.

27. Cusnir I, Solez K, Yacyshyn E. Granulomatosis with polyangiitis associated with immune checkpoint blockade: case report and literature review. *J Rheumatol*. 2017;44(Suppl 6):950.

28. Fadel F, El Karoui K, Knebelmann B. Anti-CTLA4 antibody-induced lupus nephritis. *N Engl J Med*. 2009;361(2):211–212. doi:10.1056/NEJMc0904283

29. van den Brom RR, Abdulahad WH, Rutgers A, et al. Rapid granulomatosis with polyangiitis induced by immune checkpoint inhibition. *Rheumatology (Oxford)*. 2016;55(6):1143–1145. doi:10.1093/rheumatology/kew063

30. Daanen RA, Maas RJH, Koornstra RHT, et al. Nivolumab-associated nephrotic syndrome in a patient with renal cell carcinoma: a case report. *J Immunother*. 2017;40(9):345–348. doi:10.1097/CJI.0000000000000189

31. Kitchlu A, Fingrut W, Avila-Casado C, et al. Nephrotic syndrome with cancer immunotherapies: a report of 2 cases. *Am J Kidney Dis*. 2017;70(4):581–585. doi:10.1053/j.ajkd.2017.04.026

32. Kishi S, Minato M, Saijo A, et al. A case of IgA nephropathy after nivolumab therapy for postoperative recurrence of lung squamous cell carcinoma. *Intern Med*. 2018;57(9): 1259–1263. doi:10.2169/internalmedicine.9814-17

33. Jung K, Zeng X, Bilusic M. Nivolumab-associated acute glomerulonephritis: a case report and literature review. *BMC Nephrol*. 2016;17(1):188. doi:10.1186/s12882-016-0408-2

34. Cusnir I, Solez K, Yacyshyn E. Granulomatosis with polyangiitis associated with immune checkpoint blockade: case report and literature review. *J Rheumatol*. 2017;44(6):950–950.

35. Abdel-Wahab N, Shah M, Lopez-Olivo MA, et al. Use of immune checkpoint inhibitors in the treatment of patients with cancer and preexisting autoimmune disease: a systematic review. *Ann Intern Med*. 2018;168(2):121–130. doi:10.7326/M17-2073

36. Danlos FX, Voisin AL, Dyevre V, et al. Safety and efficacy of anti-programmed death 1 antibodies in patients with cancer and pre-existing autoimmune or inflammatory disease. *Eur J Cancer*. 2018;91:21–29. doi:10.1016/j.ejca.2017.12.008

37. Vandiver JW, Singer Z, Harshberger C. Severe hyponatremia and immune nephritis following an initial infusion of nivolumab. *Target Oncol*. 2016;11(4):553–556. doi:10.1007/s11523-016-0426-9

38. Voskens CJ, Goldinger SM, Loquai C, et al. The price of tumor control: an analysis of rare side effects of anti-CTLA-4 therapy in metastatic melanoma from the ipilimumab network. *PLoS ONE*. 2013;8(1):e53745. doi:10.1371/journal.pone.0053745

39. Forde PM, Rock K, Wilson G, et al. Ipilimumab-induced immune-related renal failure—a case report. *Anticancer Res*. 2012;32(10):4607–4608.

40. Launay-Vacher V, Oudard S, Janus N, et al. Prevalence of Renal Insufficiency in cancer patients and implications for anticancer drug management: the renal insufficiency and anticancer medications (IRMA) study. *Cancer*. 2007;110(6):1376–1384. doi:10.1002/cncr.22904

41. Janus N, Oudard S, Beuzeboc P, et al. Prevalence of renal insufficiency in cancer patients: data from the IRMA-2 study. *J Clin Oncol.* 2009;27(15_suppl):9559.

42. Janus N, Launay-Vacher V, Byloos E, et al. Cancer and renal insufficiency results of the BIRMA study. *Br J Cancer.* 2010;103(12):1815–1821. doi:10.1038/sj.bjc.6605979

43. Dogan E, Izmirli M, Ceylan K, et al. Incidence of renal insufficiency in cancer patients. *Adv Ther.* 2005;22(4):357–362. doi:10.1007/BF02850082

44. Canter D, Kutikov A, Sirohi M, et al. Prevalence of baseline chronic kidney disease in patients presenting with solid renal tumors. *Urology.* 2011;77(4):781–785. doi:10.1016/j.urology.2010.11.050

45. Thompson RH, Kuntz SM, Leibovich BC, et al. Tumor B7-H1 is associated with poor prognosis in renal cell carcinoma patients with long-term follow-up. *Cancer Res.* 2006;66(7):3381–3385. doi:10.1158/0008-5472.CAN-05-4303

46. Motzer RJ, Escudier B, McDermott DF, et al. Nivolumab versus Everolimus in Advanced Renal-Cell Carcinoma. *N Engl J Med.* 2015;373(19):1803–1813. doi:10.1056/NEJMoa1510665

47. Murakami N, Motwani S, Riella LV. Renal complications of immune checkpoint blockade. *Curr Probl Cancer.* 2017;41(2):100–110. doi:10.1016/j.currproblcancer.2016.12.004

48. Atkins MB, Plimack ER, Puzanov I, et al. Axitinib in combination with pembrolizumab in patients with advanced renal cell cancer: a non-randomised, open-label, dose-finding, and dose-expansion phase 1b trial. *Lancet Oncol.* 2018;19(3):405–415. doi:10.1016/S1470-2045(18)30081-0

49. Choueiri TK, Larkin J, Oya M, et al. Preliminary results for avelumab plus axitinib as first-line therapy in patients with advanced clear-cell renal-cell carcinoma (JAVELIN Renal 100): an open-label, dose-finding and dose-expansion, phase 1b trial. *Lancet Oncol.* 2018;19(4):451–460. doi:10.1016/S1470-2045(18)30107-4

50. Motzer RJ, Powles T, Atkins MB, et al. IMmotion151: a randomized phase iii study of atezolizumab plus bevacizumab vs sunitinib in untreated metastatic renal cell carcinoma (mRCC). *J Clin Oncol.* 2018;36(6). doi:10.1200/JCO.2018.36.6_suppl.578

51. Barnett R, Barta VS, Jhaveri KD. Preserved renal-allograft function and the PD-1 pathway inhibitor nivolumab. *N Engl J Med.* 2017;376(2):191–192. doi:10.1056/NEJMc1614298

52. Manson G, Norwood J, Marabelle A, et al. Biomarkers associated with checkpoint inhibitors. *Ann Oncol.* 2016;27(7):1199–1206. doi:10.1093/annonc/mdw181

CHAPTER 13

HEMATOLOGIC TOXICITIES OF APPARENT IMMUNE-RELATED ORIGINS

George L. Chen, Caroline Robert, and Alexander M. Lesokhin

INTRODUCTION

The true rate of hematologic toxicities associated with checkpoint inhibitor use is not known, but they are generally rare in comparison to dermatologic, gastrointestinal, and endocrine toxicities. This chapter will review the hematologic toxicities of apparent immune-mediated origin that have been reported in the setting of immune checkpoint blockade and the treatments that were used to manage these toxicities. We also discuss controversies in the assessment of hematologic toxicities.

CLINICAL PRESENTATION AND EPIDEMIOLOGY

There have not yet been large epidemiologic studies of hematologic toxicities after checkpoint inhibitors. Case reports and a case series provide most of the currently available information. The hematologic toxicities which have been reported for checkpoint inhibitors are described below.

- The correlating clinical cases which were reported for each toxicity, the treatment given, and the outcome are presented in Table 13.1.

Aplastic Anemia

This is the absence of hematopoiesis in the bone marrow.

- Signs and symptoms—Infections, fatigue, bleeding, shortness of breath, decrease in white blood cells (WBC), red blood cells (RBC), platelets, and a hypocellular bone marrow.
- Differential diagnosis—Myelodysplastic syndrome, paroxysmal nocturnal hemoglobinuria, tumor involvement of the bone marrow, viral infections, side effects of medication.
- Diagnostic workup—Complete blood count (CBC), peripheral blood smear, and bone marrow biopsy showing decreased cellularity. It is a diagnosis made after excluding other causes for hypocellularity.
- Standard treatment—Immunosuppression with cyclosporine, antithymocyte globulin (ATG), allogeneic hematopoietic cell transplantation.

Published by Springer Publishing Company DOI: 10.1891/9780826172150.0013

TABLE 13.1 Reported Cases of Hematologic Toxicity After Checkpoint Inhibitor Use

Toxicity/reference	Drug	Circumstance	Treatment and outcome
Aplastic anemia (1)	IPI + NIVO × 4 courses followed by NIVO × 5 courses	48-year-old female with metastatic melanoma who developed clinically significant pancytopenia 3 days after last course of NIVO. Found to have a hypoplastic marrow with 10% cellularity.	NIVO was discontinued. Prednisone 1 mg/kg and G-CSF were given daily × 10 days without improvement. The patient suffered a fatal intracerebral hemorrhage on day 11.
Pure red cell aplasia (2)	NIVO × 31 courses	70-year-old female with metastatic melanoma developed normocytic, normochromic anemia, reticulocytopenia, and decreased erythroblasts on bone marrow biopsy 21 months after starting therapy.	NIVO was discontinued. The patient was supported with blood transfusions. Glucocorticoids were initiated and tapered as the anemia recovered without recurrence.
Pure red cell aplasia (3)	IPI 10 mg/kg (reinduction) for progression after initial response to IPI induction and maintenance	55-year-old man with metastatic melanoma developed pure red cell aplasia thought to be antibody mediated after he received two cycles of reinduction IPI.	IPI was discontinued. Prednisone 1 mg/kg/day without response × 4 weeks, then IVIG which rapidly restored reticulocytosis and normalized his hemoglobin.
Autoimmune hemolytic anemia (4)	IPI 3 mg/kg every 3 weeks × 4 courses then NIVO 3 mg/kg every 2 weeks × 5 courses	85-year-old man with metastatic melanoma and known red cell antibodies previously treated without red cell hemolysis who was subsequently treated with NIVO and developed a hemolytic anemia. This case suggests that a breakdown in peripheral tolerance is a cause of hemolysis.	NIVO was discontinued. Supportive care with red blood cell transfusions. High-dose glucocorticoids were given with eventual recovery of the hemoglobin.
Neutropenia (5)	IPI 10 mg/kg every 3 weeks × 4 courses	42-year-old female with metastatic melanoma who developed grade 4 neutropenia 14 days after 4th cycle. The bone marrow was hypocellular with granulocytic hypoplasia. T-cells were not clonal. Parvovirus, EBV, and CMV infections were excluded as causes. Antinuclear, rheumatoid factor, anti-neutrophil cytoplasmic antibodies were all negative. Antineutrophil and platelet antibodies were detected in the patient's serum.	IPI was discontinued. Corticosteroids 1 mg/kg and G-CSF without response Cyclosporine 100 mg and IVIG 1 g/kg × 2 doses over 2 days given with response in WBC the following day. CSA stopped but neutropenia recurrent. IVIG given again with improvement and resolution in 6 days time. WBC dropped again 9 days after 2nd IVIG. Third dose IVIG given 14 days after second dose. Counts fully recovered by 4 weeks.

(continued)

TABLE 13.1 Reported Cases of Hematologic Toxicity After Checkpoint Inhibitor Use (*continued*)

Toxicity/reference	Drug	Circumstance	Treatment and outcome
Neutropenia (6)	NIVO 3 mg/kg every 2 weeks	73-year-old man with a history of non-active Crohn's disease and metastatic lung adenocarcinoma who received five doses of NIVO as 3rd line therapy and then presented with grade 4 neutropenia (<500/mm³) followed 6 days later by fever and colitis confirmed by imaging.	NIVO was discontinued. The patient was admitted and treated with antibiotics, G-CSF, and methylprednisolone 1 mg/kg. Neutrophil counts improved following 1 week of therapy. The patient expired due to arrhythmia 13 days following admission.
Neutropenia (6)	NIVO 3 mg/kg every 2 weeks	74-year-old man with history of follicular lymphoma and metastatic lung adenocarcinoma presented with asymptomatic grade 4 neutropenia following 5 months of NIVO as 4th line therapy.	NIVO was discontinued. The patient was treated with G-CSF and prednisone 1 mg/kg. Neutrophil count recovered after 2 days, however neutropenia recurred with steroid taper. The patient required ongoing steroid therapy for 12 months following the final dose of NIVO. A bone marrow biopsy performed 3 months following presentation with neutropenia ruled out active follicular lymphoma. An increase in activated T cells was observed in the marrow with myeloid maturation defects.
Thrombocytopenia (7)	IPI and NIVO × 1 course	47-year-old female with BRAF mutated recurrent melanoma who developed ITP 15 days after combination therapy	IPI and NIVO were temporarily discontinued. The patient was treated with methylprednisolone and IVIG × 5 days without improvement. Subsequently, she received rituximab and romiplostim. 2 days later, the platelet count began to improve. Four doses of rituximab were given with partial relapse of thrombocytopenia after the second dose. 8 days after the last dose of rituximab the patient was re-challenged with NIVO without relapse of ITP.

(*continued*)

TABLE 13.1 Reported Cases of Hematologic Toxicity After Checkpoint Inhibitor Use (*continued*)

Toxicity/reference	Drug	Circumstance	Treatment and outcome
Thrombocytopenia (7)	NIVO and IPI sequentially	45-year-old female with BRAF wild-type melanoma developed ITP 43 days after neoadjuvant therapy with NIVO in a clinical trial.	NIVO was discontinued. The patient was treated with prednisone × 3 weeks which restored the platelet count to baseline but the thrombocytopenia recurred and a 12-week steroid taper was required. The patient later received ipilimumab monotherapy and developed ITP 8 days later. ITP resolved after treatment with prednisone, IVIG, rituximab, and discontinuation of IPI.
Acquired hemophilia A (8)	IPI 3 mg/kg every 3 weeks × 4 courses	42-year-old man with metastatic melanoma developed hematuria a few days after his fourth injection. Hematuria work up revealed a prolonged PTT which was attributed to a factor VIII inhibitor.	IPI was discontinued. Supportive care was given with blood and clotting factor transfusions, recombinant activated factor VII, and tranexamic acid. Prednisolone was initiated. However, the patient continued to require transfusions suggesting persistence of the factor VIII inhibitor despite prednisone. The patient was transitioned to hospice after two weeks.
Cryoglobulinemia (9)	NIVO 3 mg/kg every 2 weeks	57-year-old man with non-small cell lung cancer s/p left inferior lobectomy who complained of fatigue and acrocyanosis and developed cryoglobulinemia 14 days after his first dose of NIVO.	NIVO was stopped. The patient was treated with prednisone 50 mg/day × 1 week and tapered to 25 mg/day which resulted in disappearance of cryoglobulins after 19 days. NIVO restarted and given a total of 8 cycles without recurrent cryoglobulinemia. NIVO later stopped due to disease progression

(continued)

TABLE 13.1 Reported Cases of Hematologic Toxicity After Checkpoint Inhibitor Use (*continued*)

Toxicity/reference	Drug	Circumstance	Treatment and outcome
Neutrophilia with Sweet's Syndrome (10)	IPI 3 mg/kg every 3 weeks × 4 courses	A 77-year-old woman with metastatic cutaneous melanoma with brain, liver, and lung disease who presented with fever, confusion, and leukocytosis 1 week following her 2nd dose of IPI.	IPI was stopped. The patient was admitted and treated supportively with antibiotics, but developed oliguric renal failure and two weeks following presentation developed erythematous rash on bilateral palms and lateral hands. Biopsy revealed neutrophilic dermatosis consistent with Sweet's syndrome. The patient was treated with methylprednisolone 1 mg/kg. Rash and fever resolved. Confusion and renal function improved. The patient was discharged on a steroid taper.

IPI, ipilimumab; IVIG, intravenous immunoglobulin; NIVO, nivolumab.

Pure Red Cell Aplasia

A condition of severe anemia characterized by a decrease in reticulocytes and near absence of erythroid precursors in the bone marrow. The myeloid, lymphoid, and megakaryocytic lineages are present and appear normal.

- Signs and symptoms—Pallor, decreased exercise tolerance, fatigue, shortness of breath. A slowly declining hematocrit.
  - If early, the patient may be asymptomatic due to physiological compensation for a slowly declining hematocrit (approximately 1/120 of baseline per day)
- Differential diagnosis—Hemolytic anemia, slow hemorrhage.
- Diagnostic workup—Peripheral blood smear showing normochromic normocytic erythrocytes.
  - Normal indirect bilirubin, lactate dehydrogenase (LDH), and haptoglobin, and negative direct antibody (Coombs) test indicating no hemolysis or ineffective erythropoiesis.
  - A low reticulocyte count.
  - Absence of erythroblasts on bone marrow biopsy.
  - Late in the disease course, increased serum iron approaching total iron-binding capacity and a decrease in unsaturated total iron-binding capacity to almost zero as transfer of iron from the plasma to the bone marrow almost ceases.
- Standard treatment—Red cell transfusions if symptomatic.
  - Cessation of any drugs (such as phenytoin, trimethoprim-sulfamethoxazole, zidovudine, chlorpropamide, recombinant human erythropoietins, and mycophenolate mofetil) that may have caused pure red cell aplasia and treatment of any underlying infections.
  - Hematologic consultation to help identify an underlying condition.
  - Glucocorticoids for 1 to 2 months followed by the addition of cyclosporine if no response.
  - If glucocorticoids and cyclosporine are ineffective, or if cyclosporine is contraindicated, then cyclophosphamide is often used. Glucocorticoids are tapered to avoid side effects if cyclophosphamide is used.

Hemolytic Anemia

Decrease in hematocrit due to the destruction of erythrocytes, sometimes immune-mediated.

- Signs and symptoms—Fatigue, shortness of breath.
- Differential diagnosis—Pure red cell aplasia, hemorrhage.
- Diagnostic workup—A decrease in hematocrit with increased reticulocytes not explained by recent bleeding or replenished iron deficiency or other nutritional deficiency.
  - Elevated LDH and total bilirubin, and decreased to undetectable haptoglobin which correlate with hemolysis.
  - Spherocytes on the peripheral blood smear.
  - A positive direct antibody test (Coombs) indicating an immune etiology.

- ◦ Preserved erythropoiesis in the bone marrow.
- Standard treatment—Glucocorticoids and intravenous immunoglobulin (IVIG).
  - ◦ Rituximab or splenectomy for refractory cases.

Leukopenia

Decrease in white blood cell count.

- Signs and symptoms—Fevers, may be asymptomatic, infection. Skin erythema, ulcerations, fissures, tenderness (especially at sites of indwelling catheters and the perirectal and genital areas), gingivitis, ulceration in the mouth, dental pain, an abnormal lung examination, and a decrease in WBCs.
- Differential diagnosis—Drug effect, involvement of the marrow by the underlying malignancy, viral infections.
- Diagnostic workup—CBC, peripheral blood smear, anti-nuclear antibodies (ANA).
- Standard treatment—Directed at underlying cause.

Thrombocytopenia

Decrease in platelet count

- Signs and symptoms—Bleeding, easy bruising. Petechiae, purpura, ecchymosis, mucocutaneous purpura, and decreased platelets.
  - ◦ White blood cells and erythrocytes may also be decreased.
- Differential diagnosis—Disseminated intravascular coagulation, heparin-induced thrombocytopenia, microangiopathic anemia, thrombotic thrombocytopenic purpura, hemolytic uremic syndrome, drug-induced thrombotic microangiopathy.
- Diagnostic workup—CBC, peripheral blood smear, bone marrow biopsy, PT/PTT/international normalized ratio (INR).
- Standard treatment—Glucocorticoids, IVIGs.
- The best predictors for risk of bleeding at specific platelet levels for an individual patient is the platelet level at which the patient bled in the past, and the presence of wet (that is in the mucosal membranes) purpura.
- Thrombotic symptoms in the presence of thrombocytopenia should be immediately referred to a hematologist for workup and evaluation.
  - ◦ A retrospective study of thrombocytopenia (7) in 2,360 patients with melanoma receiving checkpoint inhibitors identified only 11 cases, an incidence of less than 1%. None of these cases had a prior history of thrombocytopenia or idiopathic thrombocytopenia.
  - ◦ In these cases, the average onset of thrombocytopenia was 70 days (range 12–173 days) after the initiation of therapy. The majority of patients did not have clinically significant disease and did not require treatment with the majority of cases resolving spontaneously.
  - ◦ Platelets declined an average of 70% from baseline (range 38%–99%). The average platelet count was 61,000/uL (range <5,000 to 104,000/uL).

- ○ Four out of the 11 required treatment with corticosteroids.
- ○ One relapsed after responding to steroid and was retreated with prednisone with a good response.
- ○ Two did not respond to steroids and were treated with IVIG.
- ○ One patient required rituximab in addition to IVIG.

Acquired Hemophilia A

- Signs and symptoms—Bleeding, sometimes after a surgical procedure, large hematomas, extensive ecchymoses, severe mucosal bleeding including epistaxis, gastrointestinal bleeding, gross hematuria.
  - ○ Spontaneous hemarthroses are unusual in acquired disease although common in hereditary factor VIII deficiency.
- Differential diagnosis—Factor XI or IX deficiencies, inherited factor VIII deficiency, von Willebrand disease, heparin use.
- Diagnostic workup—Prolongation of PTT and a normal PT.
  - ○ Possibilities are deficiencies in factor XI, IX, or VIII, inhibitors of these factors, von Willebrand disease, or heparin use.
  - ○ Heparin use can be ruled out by either redrawing blood from a potentially uncontaminated vein or by checking thrombin time (should be prolonged) and reptilase time (should be normal).
  - ○ Inhibitors can be screened for with a mixing test with testing done immediately and after 1 to 2 hours at 37°C.
  - ○ Correction of aPTT suggests a factor deficiency or von Willebrand disease.
  - ○ Persistent prolongation suggests an inhibitor.
  - ○ The presence of antiphospholipid antibodies is suggested if the aPTT corrects with the addition of phospholipids.
  - ○ If no correction, the Bethesda assay can establish the diagnosis of a factor VIII inhibitor and quantify the antibody titer.
    - ▪ The Bethesda assay consists of mixing serial dilutions of the patient's blood with an equal volume of normal plasma followed by measurement of factor VIII activity with a clotting assay. The reciprocal of the dilution required to achieve 50% factor VIII activity is a measure of how strong the inhibitor is and is the number of Bethesda units.
- Standard treatment—Hematology should be consulted. Provide supportive care by controlling any active bleeding.
  - ○ Treatment options include desmopressin, factor replacement, and agents with factor VIII bypassing activity.
  - ○ The inhibitor can be eliminated by immunosuppression. Either glucocorticoids alone, glucocorticoids plus cyclophosphamide, or glucocorticoids plus rituximab.

Cryoglobulinemia

This is the presence of proteins in the blood which precipitate upon cooling to temperatures lower than 37°C. Many patients with cryoglobulins may be asymptomatic. If patients with cryoglobulinemia have clinical signs of disease (such as small vessel vasculitis), the disorder is called mixed cryoglobulinemia syndrome or essential mixed cryoglobulinemia.

- Signs and symptoms—Palpable purpura, renal disease, arthritis, and arthralgias, peripheral neuropathy, liver disease, Raynaud's phenomenon (acrocyanosis), sicca, hypocomplementemia, spurious leukocytosis, and thrombocytosis if the blood sample is allowed to cool to ≤30°C due to precipitated cryoglobulin particles.
- Differential diagnosis—thrombotic disorders.
- Diagnostic workup—cryocrit, characterization of cryoglobulin, evaluate for hepatitis C and B, and HIV. Evaluate for underlying lymphoproliferative disorders.
  - Blood samples for the cryocrit and cryoglobulin characterization must be specially collected into tubes pre-warmed at 37°C without anticoagulants and kept warm to avoid false-negative (due to loss of cryoglobulin if it precipitates when the tube is inadvertently cooled) or false-positive (due to formation of cryofibrinogen and heparin precipitable complexes) testing.
- Standard treatment—Cryoglobulinemia syndrome or essential mixed cryoglobulinemia can be treated with immunosuppression with rituximab, cyclophosphamide, or pulse glucocorticoids. The underlying disorder should also be treated.

TREATMENT OF THE HEMATOLOGIC TOXICITY

- A common theme in the treatment of the hematologic toxicity was the effective use of glucocorticoids and IVIG when an antibody-mediated mechanism was implicated.
- The presence of clinically significant antibodies may represent a breakdown in peripheral tolerance mechanisms induced by the checkpoint inhibitor, resulting in the presence of pathogenic antibodies (4).
  - IVIG may be effective due to blockage of Fc receptors on reticuloendothelial cells which mediate the clearance of antibody and complement tagged cells.
  - Because the antibodies are distinct from the therapeutic mechanism of checkpoint inhibitors which target the cytotoxic T-lymphocyte antigen 1 (CTLA1) or programmed cell death 1 (PD-1)/programmed cell death ligand 1 (PD-L1) axis in the lymphocyte, it may be possible to manage the toxicity without affecting the therapeutic efficacy.

WHEN TO REFER

Hematologic consultation should be obtained if the cause of hematologic toxicity is not apparent, there is no response to initial treatment, and if additional specialized diagnostic testing is necessary (i.e., bone marrow biopsy).

HEMATOLOGIC TOXICITY ASSESSMENT

The Common Terminology Criteria for Adverse Events (CTCAE) v 5.0 provides a schema for the identification and grading of hematologic toxicity (Table 13.2).

TABLE 13.2 CTCAE v5.0 Grading of Hematologic Toxicities

CTCAE term	Grade 1	Grade 2	Grade 3	Grade 4	Grade 5	Definition
Anemia	Hgb <LLN – 10.0 g/dL; <LLN – 6.2 mmol/L; <LLN – 100 g/L	Hgb <10.0–8.0 g/dL; <6.2–4.9 mmol/L; <100–80 g/L	Hgb <8.0 g/dL; <4.9 mmol/L; <80 g/L; transfusion indicated	Life-threatening consequences; urgent intervention indicated	Death	A disorder characterized by a reduction in the amount of hemoglobin in 100 ml of blood. Signs and symptoms of anemia may include pallor of the skin and mucous membranes, shortness of breath, palpitations of the heart, soft systolic murmurs, lethargy, and fatigability.
Bone marrow hypocellular	Mildly hypocellular or ≤25% reduction from normal cellularity for age	Moderately hypocellular or >25 – <50% reduction from normal cellularity for age	Severely hypocellular or >50 – ≤75% reduction cellularity from normal for age	Aplastic persistent for longer than 2 weeks	Death	A disorder characterized by the inability of the bone marrow to produce hematopoietic elements.
Disseminated intravascular coagulation	–	Laboratory findings with no bleeding	Laboratory findings and bleeding	Life-threatening consequences; urgent intervention indicated	Death	A disorder characterized by systemic pathological activation of blood clotting mechanisms, which results in clot formation throughout the body. There is an increase in the risk of hemorrhage as the body is depleted of platelets and coagulation factors.
Eosinophilia	>ULN and >Baseline	–	Steroids initiated	–	–	A disorder characterized by laboratory test results that indicate an increased number of eosinophils in the blood.

(continued)

TABLE 13.2 CTCAE v5.0 Grading of Hematologic Toxicities (*continued*)

CTCAE term	Grade 1	Grade 2	Grade 3	Grade 4	Grade 5	Definition
Febrile neutropenia	–	–	ANC <1,000/mm³ with a single temperature of >38.3°C (101°F) or a sustained temperature of ≥ 38°C (100.4°F) for more than one hour	Life-threatening consequences; urgent intervention indicated	Death	A disorder characterized by an ANC <1,000/mm³ and a single temperature of >38.3°C (101°F) or a sustained temperature of ≥38°C (100.4°F) for more than 1 hour.
Hemolysis	Laboratory evidence of hemolysis only (e.g., DAT; Coombs'; schistocytes; decreased haptoglobin)	Evidence of hemolysis and ≥2 g decrease in hemoglobin	Transfusion or medical intervention indicated (e.g., steroids)	Life-threatening consequences; urgent intervention indicated	Death	A disorder characterized by laboratory test results that indicate widespread erythrocyte cell membrane destruction.
Hemolytic uremic syndrome	–	–	Laboratory findings with clinical consequences (e.g., renal insufficiency, petechiae)	Life-threatening consequences, (e.g., CNS hemorrhage or thrombosis/ embolism or renal failure)	Death	A disorder characterized by a form of thrombotic microangiopathy with renal failure, hemolytic anemia, and severe thrombocytopenia.
Leukocytosis	–	–	>100,000/mm³	Clinical manifestations of leucostasis; urgent intervention indicated	Death	A disorder characterized by laboratory test results that indicate an increased number of white blood cells in the blood.

(*continued*)

TABLE 13.2 CTCAE v5.0 Grading of Hematologic Toxicities (continued)

CTCAE term	Grade 1	Grade 2	Grade 3	Grade 4	Grade 5	Definition
Thrombotic thrombocytopenic purpura	–	–	Laboratory findings with clinical consequences (e.g., renal insufficiency, petechiae)	Life-threatening consequences, (e.g., CNS hemorrhage or thrombosis/ embolism or renal failure)	Death	A disorder characterized by the presence of microangiopathic hemolytic anemia, thrombocytopenic purpura, fever, renal abnormalities and neurological abnormalities such as seizures, hemiplegia, and visual disturbances. It is an acute or subacute condition.
Activated partial thromboplastin time prolonged	>ULN – 1.5 × ULN	>1.5 – 2.5 × ULN	>2.5 x ULN; bleeding	–	–	A finding based on laboratory test results in which the partial thromboplastin time is found to be greater than the control value. As a possible indicator of coagulopathy, a prolonged PTT may occur in a variety of diseases and disorders, both primary and related to treatment.
CD4 lymphocytes decreased	<LLN – 500/mm³; <LLN – 0.5 x 10e9/L	<500–200/mm³; <0.5–0.2 x 10e9/L	<200–50/mm³; <0.2 x 0.05 – 10e9/L	<50/mm³; <0.05 x 10e9/L	–	A finding based on laboratory test results that indicate a decrease in levels of CD4 lymphocytes in a blood specimen.
Fibrinogen decreased	<1.0 – 0.75 x LLN; if abnormal, <25% decrease from baseline	<0.75 – 0.5 x LLN; if abnormal, 25%–<50% decrease from baseline	<0.5 – 0.25 x LLN; if abnormal, 50%–<75% decrease from baseline	<0.25 x LLN; if abnormal, 75% decrease from baseline; absolute value <50 mg/dL	–	A finding based on laboratory test results that indicate a decrease in levels of fibrinogen in a blood specimen.

(continued)

TABLE 13.2 CTCAE v5.0 Grading of Hematologic Toxicities (continued)

CTCAE term	Grade 1	Grade 2	Grade 3	Grade 4	Grade 5	Definition
Haptoglobin decreased	<LLN	–	–	–	–	A finding based on laboratory test results that indicate a decrease in levels of haptoglobin in a blood specimen.
Hemoglobin increased	Increase in >0–2 g/dL	Increase in >2–4 g/dL	Increase in >4 g/dL	–	–	A finding based on laboratory test results that indicate increased levels of hemoglobin above normal.
INR increased	>1.2 – 1.5; >1 – 1.5 x baseline if on anticoagulation; monitoring only indicated	>1.5 – 2.5; >1.5 – 2.5 x baseline if on anticoagulation; dose adjustment indicated	>2.5; >2.5 x baseline if on anticoagulation; bleeding	–	–	A finding based on laboratory test results that indicate an increase in the ratio of the patient's prothrombin time to a control sample in the blood.
Investigations – Other, specify	Asymptomatic or mild symptoms; clinical or diagnostic observations only; intervention not indicated	Moderate; minimal, local or noninvasive intervention indicated; limiting age-appropriate instrumental ADL	Severe or medically significant but not immediately life-threatening; hospitalization or prolongation of existing hospitalization indicated; limiting self care ADL	Life-threatening consequences; urgent intervention indicated	Death	–

(continued)

TABLE 13.2 CTCAE v5.0 Grading of Hematologic Toxicities (*continued*)

CTCAE term	Grade 1	Grade 2	Grade 3	Grade 4	Grade 5	Definition
Lymphocyte count decreased	<LLN – 800/mm³; <LLN – 0.8 x 10e9/L	<800–500/mm³; <0.8 – 0.5 x 10e9 /L	<500–200/mm³; <0.5 – 0.2 x 10e9 /L	<200/mm³; <0.2 x 10e9 /L	–	A finding based on laboratory test results that indicate a decrease in number of lymphocytes in a blood specimen.
Lymphocyte count increased	–	>4,000/mm³–20,000/ mm³	>20,000/mm³	–	–	A finding based on laboratory test results that indicate an abnormal increase in the number of lymphocytes in the blood, effusions or bone marrow.
Neutrophil count decreased	<LLN – 1,500/mm³; <LLN – 1.5 x 10e9/L	<1,500–1000/mm³; <1.5–1.0 x 10e9/L	<1,000–500/mm³; <1.0–0.5 x 10e9/L	<500/mm³; <0.5 x 10e9/L	–	A finding based on laboratory test results that indicate a decrease in number of neutrophils in a blood specimen.
Platelet count decreased	<LLN – 75,000/mm³; <LLN – 75.0 x 10e9/L	<75,000–50,000/mm³; <75.0–50.0 x 10e9/L	<50,000–25,000/ mm³; <50.0–25.0 x 10e9/L	<25,000/mm³; <25.0 x 10e9/L	–	A finding based on laboratory test results that indicate a decrease in number of platelets in a blood specimen.
White blood cell decreased	<LLN – 3,000/mm³; <LLN – 3.0 x 10e9/L	<3,000–2,000/mm³; <3.0 – 2.0 x 10e9 /L	<2,000–1,000/ mm³; <2.0 – 1.0 x 10e9/L	<1,000/mm³; <1.0 x 10e9/L	–	A finding based on laboratory test results that indicate a decrease in number of white blood cells in a blood specimen.

ADL, activities of daily living; ANC, absolute neutrophil count; CNS, central nervous system; CTCAE, common terminology criteria for adverse events; DAT, direct antiglobulin test; Hgb, hemoglobin; LLN, lower limit of normal; PTT, partial thromboplastin time; ULN, upper limit of normal.

- Grading of thrombocytopenia may not fully reflect the clinical severity of the decrease in platelets because it is based upon absolute numbers of platelets.
  - Relative changes in the platelet count may occur with checkpoint inhibitors and this would not be captured with current CTCAE grading.
- Although platelet counts tend to be stable in a narrow range in individuals over time, there is wide variability in the population median levels.
  - The absolute change in platelet count in a patient with baseline higher levels of platelets who experiences a 50% decrease may not be low enough to trigger CTCAE grading but may portend a clinically significant adverse effect from the checkpoint inhibitor.
- Immune-related hematologic toxicities need to be differentiated from changes in laboratory parameters that normally occur while initiating checkpoint inhibitor therapy.
  - Lymphocytosis, eosinophilia, neutrophilia, and monocytosis (as opposed to cytopenias) have been observed and may not be clinically significant although they may be prognostic for disease response to checkpoint inhibitors (11).
- Causal attribution may also be complicated by the underlying malignancy which may also cause cytopenias if the bone marrow is involved. The underlying malignancy may also cause laboratory abnormalities which will confound the diagnostic workup of toxicity.
  - For example, LDH can be elevated at baseline in melanoma and if not noted, may by misleading in an evaluation of hemolytic anemia.

CONCLUSION

Toxicities from immune checkpoint inhibitors involving hematologic system are relatively infrequent, eminently manageable when discovered prior to a serious event. Therefore, as in other organ-specific toxicities, early detection, proper grading using CTCAE 4.0 criteria and appropriate intervention are the key to success.

- In all patients receiving immune checkpoint inhibitors (ICIs), routine monitoring for clinical signs of bleeding, anemia, and infection is recommended.
- All patients should have a baseline CBC with differential (CBC+diff.), including red blood cell count, white blood cell count, and platelets with report on both absolute and relative frequencies of blood cell subgroups including neutrophils, lymphocytes, monocytes, eosinophils, and any immature cells.
- Complete blood cell count with differential should be repeated before each cycle, and at any time during treatment if clinical symptoms warrant it.
- Once an immune-mediated hematologic toxicity is diagnosed, appropriate treatment should be started promptly.

○ For patients with severe complications (i.e., bleeding), uncertain etiology of their abnormalities, poor response to initial therapy or in need of additional testing (bone marrow biopsy), hematology consultation is appropriate and necessary.

REFERENCES

1. Helgadottir H, Kis L, Ljungman P, et al. Lethal aplastic anemia caused by dual immune checkpoint blockade in metastatic melanoma. *Ann Oncol.* 2017;28:1672–1673. doi:10.1093/annonc/mdx177

2. Yuki A, Takenouchi T, Takatsuka S, et al. A case of pure red cell aplasia during nivolumab therapy for cardiac metastatic melanoma. *Melanoma Res.* 2017;27:635–637. doi:10.1097/CMR.0000000000000392

3. Gordon IO, Wade T, Chin K, et al. Immune-mediated red cell aplasia after anti-CTLA-4 immunotherapy for metastatic melanoma. *Cancer Immunol Immunother.* 2009;58:1351–1353. doi:10.1007/s00262-008-0627-x

4. Kong BY, Micklethwaite KP, Swaminathan S, et al. Autoimmune hemolytic anemia induced by anti-PD-1 therapy in metastatic melanoma. *Melanoma Res.* 2016;26:202–204. doi:10.1097/CMR.0000000000000232

5. Akhtari M, Waller EK, Jaye DL, et al. Neutropenia in a patient treated with ipilimumab (anti-CTLA-4 antibody). *J Immunother.* 2009;32:322–324. doi:10.1097/CJI.0b013e31819aa40b

6. Turgeman I, Wollner M, Hassoun G, et al. Severe complicated neutropenia in two patients with metastatic non-small-cell lung cancer treated with nivolumab. *Anticancer Drugs.* 2017;28:811–814. doi:10.1097/CAD.0000000000000520

7. Shiuan E, Beckermann KE, Ozgun A, et al. Thrombocytopenia in patients with melanoma receiving immune checkpoint inhibitor therapy. *J Immunother Cancer.* 2017;5:8. doi:10.1186/s40425-017-0210-0

8. Delyon J, Mateus C, Lambert T. Hemophilia A induced by ipilimumab. *N Engl J Med.* 2011;365:1747–1748. doi:10.1056/NEJMc1110923

9. Pellegrino B, Musolino A, Tiseo M. Anti-PD-1-related cryoglobulinemia during treatment with nivolumab in NSCLC patient. *Ann Oncol.* 2017;28:1405–1406. doi:10.1093/annonc/mdx126

10. Pintova S, Sidhu H, Friedlander PA, et al. Sweet's syndrome in a patient with metastatic melanoma after ipilimumab therapy. *Melanoma Res.* 2013;23:498–501. doi:10.1097/CMR.0000000000000017

11. Hopkins AM, Rowland A, Kichenadasse G, et al. Predicting response and toxicity to immune checkpoint inhibitors using routinely available blood and clinical markers. *Br J Cancer.* 2017;117:913–920. doi:10.1038/bjc.2017.274

CHAPTER 14

OCULAR TOXICITIES CAUSED BY IMMUNE DYSREGULATION

Liliya Golas and Dimitra Skondra

INTRODUCTION

Ocular toxicities related to immune checkpoint inhibitor (ICI) use arise from immune dysregulation leading to immune reactions against normal ocular and orbital tissues. Incidence of ocular immune-related adverse events (irAEs) is reported to be less than 1% (1–2). However, with variable severity of inflammation, these ocular toxicity events may be vision-threatening if not addressed promptly (3). Awareness, early detection, and prompt intervention are crucial to ensure that the most common mild to moderate inflammatory ophthalmic toxicities do not lead to more severe inflammation and vision-threatening consequences. Clinicians should be aware that the differential diagnosis of ophthalmological symptoms may include neurological immune toxicity like cranial nerve palsy and/or encephalitis, and progression of disease including brain and leptomenengial metastases.

Ocular toxicities may be subdivided into orbital and ocular inflammation. irAEs may affect any anatomic segment of the eye, leading to a panoply of associated symptoms.

- From anterior to posterior ocular structures affected, ocular toxicity may cause dry eye, peripheral ulcerative keratitis (PUK), episcleritis, scleritis, uveitis (both anterior and posterior), Vogt–Koyanagi–Harada-(VKH)-like syndrome with serous retinal detachments, optic nerve edema, giant cell arteritis, and orbital inflammation.
- One of the most common ocular irAEs is uveitis (anterior more than posterior or panuveitis).
  - Few studies report greater incidence of uveitis and episcleritis in patients who also developed colitis (4,5).

Time of onset of ocular toxicities varies greatly, from 1 to 2 weeks following the first infusion to months after the last infusion. However, the median occurrence is about 2 months after initiation of ICI treatment (1,6).

PARTS OF EYE AFFECTED

Orbit

- Orbital soft tissues, lacrimal gland, and extraocular muscles may be affected in ocular irAEs.
  - Therefore, orbital inflammation may manifest as a variety of symptoms, ranging from eyelid edema and erythema, ptosis, proptosis, limited or painful extraocular movements, decrease in vision, conjunctival chemosis or injection, and eye pain.

Published by Springer Publishing Company DOI: 10.1891/9780826172150.0014

- With limited confines of the bony orbit, significant inflammation may cause the eye to be pushed forward, leading to limited motility and double vision, proptosis, incomplete lid closure, corneal or conjunctival exposure, and in extreme cases corneal decompensation or perforation.
- Significant pressure on the optic nerve may lead to irreversible optic neuropathy.

Cornea/Conjunctiva/Episclera

- The outermost barriers of the eye may be affected by immune dysregulation.
- Corneal involvement may manifest in dry eye, PUK, leading to photophobia, eye redness, eye pain, tearing, and blurry vision.
- In severe cases, if left untreated it may lead to corneal scarring, infections, and even perforation.
- Conjunctival and episcleral inflammation may lead to pain, foreign body sensation, and erythema.

Uvea

Uvea is a pigmented layer of the eye, which includes the iris, ciliary body, and choroid, inflammation of any of which leads to the diagnosis of uveitis. Uveitis is further divided into anterior, intermediate, posterior, and panuveitis, based on which part of the uvea is predominantly affected.

- With anterior uveitis, inflammation is mainly confined to the anterior segment of the eye between the iris and the cornea and is diagnosed with a careful slit lamp examination.
  - Anterior uveitis quickly leads to eye erythema, pain, photophobia, and decrease in vision.
  - With uncontrolled prolonged inflammation, the iris may become adherent to the capsule of the lens causing irregular pupil and may lead to elevated intraocular pressures by disrupting normal aqueous flow within the eye.
- Posterior uveitis results from inflammation of the vitreous cavity, retina, or choroid.
  - Symptoms may include floaters and light flashes, variable degrees of decrease in vision.
  - Contrasted with anterior uveitis and iridocyclitis, early posterior uveitis may be painless, which may delay diagnosis and treatment.
  - Full evaluation for posterior or panuveitis includes a careful dilated eye exam, potentially ocular ultrasonography, fluorescein angiography, and optical coherence tomography (OCT) among other tests.

Retina

- Retina is the innermost, neurosensory layer of the eye, inflammation of which frequently leads to a decrease in vision, metamorphopsia, scotomas, and a decrease in color vision.

- Inflammation of the retina may lead to edema, scarring or epiretinal membrane formation, optic nerve swelling, serous retinal detachments as seen in VKH-like syndrome, and exudative detachments.
- Choroidal inflammation affects the overlying retina, as choroidal vasculature is the blood supply of the outer retina.
- Untreated retinal inflammation frequently leads to permanent retinal and optic nerve damage and significant vision loss.

SPECIFIC DRUGS

Ipilimumab

To date, more than 25 cases of ocular toxicity related to ipilimumab use have been published in literature, including orbital inflammation, retinopathy with serous retinal detachments, VKH-like syndrome, optic nerve edema, anterior and posterior uveitis, choroidal neovascular membrane, PUK, and Tolosa–Hunt syndrome (3,5,7–27).

- Most cases report complete resolution of ocular irAE with topical or systemic steroids.

Pembrolizumab

There are seven case reports of pembrolizumab-related ocular toxicities reported in literature that mainly include anterior uveitis, posterior uveitis, and retinal vasculitis, with multiple cases developing macular edema due to inflammation (28–34).

- Treatments ranged from topical to systemic and intraocular steroids.

Nivolumab

There are 10 case reports of nivolumab-related ocular toxicity, ranging from dry eye syndrome to anterior and posterior uveitis and VKH syndrome (35–44). One patient's dry eye led to corneal perforation.

- Treatment modalities ranged from topical lubrication to intraocular and topical steroids and mydriatics.
- Majority of ocular irAE cases report full resolution with topical, intraocular, and/or systemic steroids.
  - However, there are reports of residual visual field or vision loss despite initiation of appropriate treatment.

No ocular irAEs due to newer ICIs, such as atezolizumab, durvalumab, and avelumab have been reported to date.

DIAGNOSTIC EVALUATION

Prompt referral to an ophthalmologist should be initiated with any visual complaints or signs of ocular involvement like eye redness or proptosis, even in absence of visual complaints by the patient. However, some of the tests may be performed at the oncology clinic visit.

- Visual acuity and color vision (each eye separately) while patient is wearing reading glasses if appropriate may be checked with a near vision chart and color vision chart, which are readily available on smartphones.
- Pupils should be checked to determine if they are equal, round, and reactive and whether an afferent pupillary defect is present.
- Conjunctival injection should be noted and may indicate dry eye, episcleritis, keratitis, and/or uveitis.
- Extraocular movements should be checked as well, as they may be limited in cases with orbital inflammation.
- Once the patient is seen by an ophthalmologist, intraocular pressure, presence, and grade of ocular inflammation checked with slit lamp exam and dilated fundus exam to evaluate the optic nerve and retina will be performed in addition to other functional and imaging tests like Humphrey visual field, fundus photos, fluorescein angiogram, OCT, and ultrasonography.

MANAGEMENT

- Any visual symptoms, including eye pain, dryness, decrease or distortion in vision, redness, and diplopia, should lead to an immediate referral for full evaluation by an ophthalmologist.
  - Accurate diagnosis and severity grading are paramount in management decisions and treatment choices.
- Prescription of topical ocular or systemic steroids prior to a full ophthalmic exam should be avoided unless systemic steroids are indicated for non-ophthalmic toxicity, as they may mask true grade of inflammation or exacerbate potentially unrelated infectious processes, such as herpetic keratitis/uveitis or orbital cellulitis.
- Patients with orbital inflammation will likely require systemic steroids.
- Topical lubrication may be necessary in these cases as well where incomplete lid closure or proptosis of the eye leads to ocular surface exposure.
- Dry eye syndrome requires topical lubrication, in some cases along with cyclosporine drops.
- Majority of patients with mild or moderate anterior uveitis can be managed with topical steroids and mydriatics to prevent scarring down of the iris to the lens capsule.
  - For intermediate, posterior, and panuveitis on the other hand, topical steroids may not be adequate to control inflammation.
  - These patients frequently require intraocular or periocular steroids and/or systemic steroids after infectious etiology have been excluded.
- Ocular steroid treatments, both topical and intra-/periocular, may lead to elevated intraocular pressure as well as cataract formation and should be carefully managed by an ophthalmologist.
  - Special care should be taken in patients with preexisting eye conditions, such as glaucoma.
  - Once inflammation is controlled, slow taper of steroid medications will be initiated by the ophthalmologist with close follow-up monitoring for rebound inflammation or recurrence.

- Decision on whether to permanently discontinue ICI therapy should be made in collaboration with the oncology team and the ophthalmologist and should depend on grade/severity of ocular toxicity, patient's systemic response to ICI treatments, ocular response to local or systemic steroids, and the degree of ocular damage from irAE.
  - Some patients can be considered to be restarted on the ICI therapy once complete or near-complete resolution of ocular irAEs is achieved depending on the grade of the ocular toxicity and response to ICI treatment and under close ophtalmological follow-up.
  - For patients with rebound or persistent ocular inflammation despite local or systemic steroids and discontinuation of ICI treatment, steroid-sparing immunomodulatory treatments infliximab or mycophenolate may be required (45).

The Common Terminology Criteria for Adverse Events (CTCAE) (46) developed by the National Cancer Institute (NCI) provides grading criteria for irAEs. According to CTCAE, uveitis and episcleritis inflammatory reactions can be divided into 4 grades. The Society for Immunotherapy of Cancer (SITC) Toxicity Management Working Group has recently published management recommendations, summarized in Table 14.1 (47).

TABLE 14.1 Management Recommendations by SITC Toxicity Management Working Group

Grade	CTCAE description		Management
	Uveitis	Episcleritis	
1	• Asymptomatic • Clinical or diagnostic observations only		• Continue immunotherapy • Referral to Ophthalmology within 1 week • Start lubricating drops
2	• Anterior uveitis • Requiring medical treatment	• Symptomatic • Limiting instrumental ADL • VA 20/40 or better	• Hold immunotherapy • Referral to Ophthalmology within 2 days • Do not initiate steroid treatment prior to formal eye exam • Treatment coordination with ophthalmologist (cycloplegic drops, topical/systemic steroids)
3	• Posterior uveitis • Panuveitis • May be initially asymptomatic	• Symptomatic • Limiting self-care ADL • VA worse than 20/40	• In most cases permanent discontinuation of immunotherapy may be required. • Urgent ophthalmology referral prior to initiating treatment • Treatment coordination with ophthalmologist (systemic/intravitreal steroids/periocular steroids/topical steroids as recommended) • Select cases with ocular toxicity control on local/topical/systemic steroid therapy may be considered to restart immunotherapy.

(continued)

TABLE 14.1 Management Recommendations by SITC Toxicity Management Working Group (*continued*)

Grade	CTCAE description		Management
	Uveitis	Episcleritis	
4	• Blindness • VA 20/200 or worse in affected eye		• Permanent discontinuation of immunotherapy • Urgent ophthalmology referral prior to initiating any treatment • Treatment coordination with ophthalmologist (systemic steroids/intravitreal/periocular or topical steroids as recommended)

ADL, activities of daily living; CTCAE, common terminology criteria for adverse events; SITC, The Society for Immunotherapy of Cancer; VA, visual acuity.

COLLABORATION

Patient education and awareness about possible ocular irAEs should take place prior to starting the ICI therapy.

• Patients should be advised to immediately contact their medical team if they experience ocular pain or redness, light sensitivity, decrease in vision, floaters, flashing lights, changes in color vision, distortion in vision, visual field changes, pain with eye movements or proptosis, diplopia, and eyelid edema.
• Patients with colitis or diarrhea as irAEs should be strongly considered for a referral to the ophthalmologist due to the reports of concomitant uveitis/episcleritis in these patients (4,5).

Close treatment coordination with patient's ophthalmologist will help with early detection and management of ocular irAEs and may prevent serious sequelae of untreated ocular or orbital inflammation and possibly vision loss.

DISCUSSION

Ocular toxicity is a rare AE of ICI therapy and represents a significant challenge for clinicians and patients alike. If unrecognized, ocular irAEs may lead to blindness. Thus, it is imperative that clinicians inform patients to report any ocular symptoms so they may be evaluated promptly and receive appropriate therapy. It is equally important that clinicians recognize symptoms do not always correlate with the severity of the condition, and superficial eye evaluation performed in most oncologist's offices is not adequate to determine extent of the conditions. Consultation with an ophthalmologist should be considered early. Continued observation by ophthalmology to determine response to first-line topical or systemic steroid therapy is critical as, rarely, initiation of other immune suppressive agents may be required.

REFERENCES

1. Antoun J, Titah C, Cochereau I. Ocular and orbital side-effects of checkpoint inhibitors: a review article. *Curr Opin Oncol.* 2016;28(4):288–294. doi:10.1097/cco.0000000000000296

2. Villadolid J, Amin A. Immune checkpoint inhibitors in clinical practice: update on management of immune-related toxicities. *Trasl Lung Cancer Res.* 2015;4(5):560–575. doi:10.3978/j.issn.2218-6751.2015.06.06

3. Miserocchi M, Cimminiello C, Mazzolla M, et al. New onset uveitis during CTLA-4 blockade therapy with ipilimumab in metastatic melanoma patient. *Can J Ophthalmol.* 2015;50:e2–e4. doi:10.1016/j.jcjo.2014.10.010

4. Scarpati GDL, Fusciello C, Perri F, et al. Ipilimumab in the treatment of metastatic melanoma: management of adverse events. *Onco Targets Ther.* 2014;7:203–209. doi:10.2147/ott.s57335

5. Robinson MR, Chan CC, Yang JC, et al. Cytotoxicty lymphocyte-associated antigen 4 blockade in patients with metastatic melanoma: a new cause of uveitis. *J Immunother.* 2004;27(6):478–479. doi:10.1097/00002371-200411000-00008

6. Tarhini A. Immune-mediated adverse events associated with ipilimumab CTLA-4 blockade therapy: the underlying mechanisms and clinical management. *Scientifica.* 2013;2013:1–19. doi:10.1155/2013/857519

7. Borodic G, Hinkle DM, Cia Y. Drug-induced grave's disease from CTLA-4 receptor suppression. *Ophthal Plast Reconstr Surg.* 2011;27(4):e87–e88. doi:10.1097/iop.0b013e3181ef72a1

8. Crews J, Agawal A, Jack L, et al. Ipilimumab-associated retinopathy. *Ophthalmic Surg Lasers Imaging Retina.* 2015;46(6):658–660. doi:10.3928/23258160-20150610-10

9. Crosson JN, Laird PW, Debiec M, et al. Koyanagi-Harada-like syndrome after CTLA-4 inhibition with ipilimumab for metastatic melanoma. *J Immunother.* 2015;38(2):80–84. doi:10.1097/cji.0000000000000066

10. Fierz FC, Meier F, Chaloupka K, et al. Intraocular inflammation associated with new therapies for cutaneous melanoma—case series and review. *Klin Monatsbl Augenheilkd.* 2016;233(4):540–544. doi:10.1055/s-0042-102668

11. Hahn L, Pepple KL. Bilateral neuroretinitis and anterior uveitis following ipilimumab treatment for metastatic melanoma. *J Ophthalmic Inflamm Infect.* 2016;6(1):14. doi:10.1186/s12348-016-0082-3

12. Henderson AD, Thomas DA. A case of orbital inflammatory syndrome secondary to ipilimumab. *Ophthal Plast Reconstr Surg.* 2015;31(3):e68–e70. doi:10.1097/iop.0000000000000081

13. Lecouflet M, Verschoore M, Giard C, et al. Orbital myositis associated with ipilimumab. *Ann Dermatol Venereol.* 2013;140(6–7):448–451. doi:10.1016/j.annder.2013.02.029

14. Liao B, Shroff S, Kamiya-Matsuoka C, et al. Atypical neurological complications of ipilimumab therapy in patients with metastatic melanoma. *Neuro Oncol.* 2014;16(4):589–593. doi:10.1093/neuonc/nou001

15. Mantopoulos D, Kendra KL, Letson AD, et al. Bilateral choroidopathy and serous retinal detachments during ipilumumab treatment for cutaneous melanoma. *JAMA Ophthalmol.* 2015;133(8):965–967. doi:10.1001/jamaophthalmol.2015.1128

16. McElnea EE. Thyroid-like ophthalmopathy in a euthyroid patient receiving ipilimumab. *Orbit.* 2014;33(6):424–427. doi:10.3109/01676830.2014.949792

17. Min L, Vaidya A, Becker C. Thyroid ophthalmopathy related to melanoma biological therapy. *Eur J Endocrinol.* 2011;164(2):303–307. doi:10.1530/eje-10-0833

18. Modjtahedi BS, Maibach H, Park S. Multifocal bilateral choroidal neovascularization in a patient on ipilimumab for metastatic melanoma. *Cutan Ocul Toxicol.* 2013;32(4):341–343. doi:10.3109/15569527.2013.781618

19. Nallapaneni NN, Mourya R, Bhatt VR, et al. Ipilimumab-induced hypophysitis and uveitis in a patient with metastatic melanoma and history of ipilimumab-induced skin rash. *J Natl Compr Canc Netw.* 2014;12(8):1077–1081. doi:10.6004/jnccn.2014.0105

20. Papavasileoiou E, Prasad S, Freitag SK, et al. Ipilimumab-induced ocular and orbital inflammation—a case series and review of literature. *Ocul Immunol Inflamm.* 2015;24(2):140–146. doi:10.3109/09273948.2014.1001858.

21. Sohrab MA, Desai RY, Chambers CB, et al. Re: "Drug-induced Graves disease from CTLA-4 receptor suppression." *Ophthal Plast Reconstr Surg*. 2013;29(3):239–240. doi:10.1097/iop.0b013e3182895795

22. Voskens C, Cavallaro A, Erdmann M, et al. Anti-cytotoxic T-cell lymphocyte antigen-4-induced regression of spinal cord metastases in association with renal failure, atypical pneumonia, vision loss, and hearing loss. *J Clin Oncol*. 2012;30(33):e356–e357. doi:10.1200/jco.2011.41.4359

23. Voskens CJ, Goldinger SM, Loquai C, et al. The price of tumor control: an analysis of rare side effects of anti-CTLA-4 therapy in metastatic melanoma from the ipilimumab network. *PLoS ONE*. 2013;8(1):e53745. doi:10.1371/journal.pone.0053745

24. Wilson MA, Guld K, Galetta S, et al. Acute visual loss after ipilimumab treatment for metastatic melanoma. *J Immunother Cancer*. 2016;4:66. doi:10.1186/s40425-016-0170-9

25. Wong RK, Lee JK, Huang JJ. Bilateral drug (ipilimumab) induced vitritis, choroiditis, and serous retinal detachments suggestive of Vogt-Koyanagi-Harada syndrome. *Retin Cases Brief Rep*. 2012;6(4):423–426. doi:10.1097/icb.0b013e31824f7130

26. Yeh OL, Francis CE. Ipilimumab-associated bilateral optic neuropathy. *J Neuroophthalmol*. 2015;35(2):144–147. doi:10.1097/WNO.0000000000000217

27. Numata S, Iwata Y, Okumura R, et al. Bilateral anterior uveitis and unilateral facial palsy due to ipilimumab for metastatic melanoma in an individual with human leukocyte antigen DR4: a case report. *J Dermatol*. 2018;45(1):113–114. doi:10.1111/1346-8138.13779

28. Aaberg MT, Aaberg TM. Pembrolizumab administration associated with posterior uveitis. *Retin Cases Brief Rep*. 2017;11(4):348–351. doi:10.1097/ICB.0000000000000368

29. Abu Samra K, Valdes-Navarro M, Lee S, et al. A case of bilateral uveitis and papillitis in a patient treated with pembrolizumab. *Eur J Ophthalmol*. 2016;26(3):e46–e48. doi:10.5301/ejo.5000724

30. Basilious A, Lloyd JC. Posterior subcapsular cataracts and hypotony secondary to severe pembrolizumab induced uveitis: case report. *Can J Ophthalmol*. 2016;51(1):e4–e6. doi:10.1016/j.jcjo.2015.09.008

31. Diem S, Keller F, Ruesch R, et al. Pembrolizumab-triggered uveitis: an additional surrogate marker for responders in melanoma immunotherapy? *J Immunother*. 2016;39(9):379–382. doi:10.1097/cji.0000000000000143

32. Hanna KS. A rare case of pembrolizumab-induced uveitis in a patient with metastatic melanoma. *Pharmacotherapy*. 2016;36(11):e183–e188. doi:10.1002/phar.1839

33. Manusow JS, Khoja L, Pesin N, et al. Retinal vasculitis and ocular vitreous metastasis following complete response to PD-1 inhibition in a patient with metastatic cutaneous melanoma. *J Immunother Cancer*. 2014;2(1):41. doi:10.1186/s40425-014-0041-1

34. Bricout M, Petre A, Amini-Adle M, et al. Vogt-Koyanagi-Harada-like syndrome complicating pembrolizumab treatment for metastatic melanoma. *J Immunother*. 2017;40(2):77–82. doi:10.1097/CJI.0000000000000154.

35. Aria T. Case of acute anterior uveitis and Vogt-Koyanagi-Harada syndrome-like eruptions induced by nivolumab in a melanoma patient. *J Dermatol*. 2017;44(8):975–976. doi:10.1111/1346-8138.13612

36. De Velasco G, Bernas B, Choueiri TK. Autoimmune arthropathy and uveitis as complications of programed death 1 inhibitor treatment. *Arthritis Rheumatol*. 2016;68(2):556–557. doi:10.1002/art.39406

37. Karlin J, Gentzler R, Golen J. Bilateral anterior uveitis associated with nivolumab therapy. *Ocul Immunol Inflamm*. 2016;26(2):283–285. doi:10.1080/09273948.2016.1215473

38. Nguyen AT, Elia M, Materin MA, et al. Cyclosporine for dry eye associated with nivolumab: a case progressing to corneal perforation. *Cornea*. 2016;35(3):399–401. doi:10.1097/ico.0000000000000724

39. Theillac C, Straub M, Breton AL, et al. Bilateral uveitis and macular edema induced by nivolumab: a case report. *BMC Ophthalmol*. 2017;17(1):227. doi:10.1097/ico.0000000000000724

40. Baughman DM, Lee CS, Snydsman BE, et al. Bilateral uveitis and keratitis following nivolumab treatment for metastatic melanoma. *Med Case Rep (Wilmington)*. 2017;3(2):8. doi:10.21767/2471-8041.100044. Epub 2017 Apr 14.

41. Richardson DR, Ellis B, Mehmi I, et al. Bilateral uveitis associated with nivolumab therapy for metastatic melanoma: a case report. *Int J Ophthalmol.* 2017;10(7):1183–1186. doi:10.18240/ijo.2017.07.28

42. Matsuo T, Yamasaki O. Vogt-Koyanagi-Harada disease-like posterior uveitis in the course of nivolumab (anti-PD-1 antibody), interposed by vemurafenib (BRAF inhibitor), for metastatic cutaneous malignant melanoma. *Clin Case Rep.* 2017;5(5):694–700. doi:10.1002/ccr3.911

43. Kanno H, Ishida K, Yamada W, et al. Uveitis induced by programmed cell death protein 1 inhibitor therapy with nivolumab in metastatic melanoma patient. *J Infect Chemother.* 2017;23(11):774–777. doi:10.1016/j.jiac.2017.04.007

44. Brouwer NJ, Haanen JBAG, Jager MJ. Development of ocular rosacea following combined ipilimumab and nivolumab treatment for metastatic malignant skin melanoma. *Ocul Oncol Pathol.* 2017;3(3):188–192. doi:10.1159/000455150

45. Prete M, Dammacco R, Fatone MC, et al. Autoimmune uveitis: clinical, pathogenetic, and therapeutic features. *Clin Exp Med.* 2016;16(2):125–136. doi: 10.1007/s10238-015-0345-6. Epub 2015 Mar 28.

46. U.S. Department of Health and Human Services. Common Terminology Criteria for Adverse Events (CTCAE) Version 4.03.2010. https://www.eortc.be/services/doc/ctc/CTCAE_4.03_2010-06-14_QuickReference_5x7.pdf

47. Puzanov I, Diab A, Abdallah K, et al. Managing toxicities associated with immune checkpoint inhibitors: consensus recommendations from the Society for Immunotherapy of Cancer (SITC) Toxicity Management Working Group. *J Immunother Cancer.* 2017;5:95. doi:10.1186/s40425-017-0300-z

SAFETY AND REGULATION OF IMMUNE CHECKPOINT INHIBITORS IN SPECIAL PATIENT POPULATIONS

Douglas B. Johnson, Ryan Sullivan, and Paolo A. Ascierto

INTRODUCTION

Immunotherapies, particularly immune checkpoint inhibitors (ICI), have revolutionized the treatment landscape for numerous solid cancers. Despite the broad activity and generally favorable toxicity profile, there remains substantial concern to treat a number of perceived high-risk patient groups. As such, clinicians still frequently struggle with the decision to administer these agents in particular populations, especially those excluded from clinical trials.

- Patients perceived to be at high risk of immune activation include patients with prior autoimmune disorders, solid organ, or hematopoietic stem cell transplant, and perhaps chronic viral infection or immunosuppression.
- In addition, patients with clinically relevant comorbidities or conditions that may variably impact the ability to receive systemic therapy may also prompt uncertainty, including organ dysfunction, pregnancy, poor performance status, extremes of age (pediatric and very elderly populations), and brain metastases.

In this chapter, we will review the available evidence of ICI safety in these populations.

AUTOIMMUNE DISORDERS

Excluded from essentially all clinical trials, patients with autoimmune disorders present intriguing test cases of the role of specific immune checkpoints in autoimmunity. A simplistic view would posit that, since immune suppression treats these disorders, immune activation would invariably lead to disease flares, and perhaps immune-related adverse events (irAEs). The clinical experience, however, has been more nuanced.

- A large series of 30 melanoma patients treated with anti-cytotoxic T-lymphocyte antigen 4 (CTLA-4) (ipilimumab) with preexisting autoimmune disease was evaluated (1).
  - This cohort included a fairly diverse set of diseases, including rheumatoid arthritis, inflammatory bowel disease, psoriasis, and lupus, most of which were receiving immunosuppressants at baseline.

Published by Springer Publishing Company DOI: 10.1891/9780826172150.0015

- ○ A minority of patients experienced flares of their autoimmune disease (27%) and/or irAEs (33%), with a 20% response rate.
- ○ One patient with a long delay in seeking care died of a colitis flare.
- A similar group of 52 melanoma patients with autoimmune disease treated with anti-programmed cell death 1 (PD-1) was also evaluated (2).
  - ○ Similar rates of autoimmune exacerbations (30%; with 4% drug discontinuation) and irAEs (29%; 8% discontinued treatment) were observed in this cohort.
  - ○ No patient died of either autoimmune flares or irAEs, and events responded to standard treatment algorithms.
  - ○ Notably, rheumatologic diseases tended to flare more than gastrointestinal or neurologic diseases (no flares).
  - ○ The response rate mirrored that observed in unselected melanoma patients (33%) (3).
- In a large systematic review that summarized the evidence on adverse events (AEs) associated with the use of ICIs in patients with preexisting autoimmune diseases, the authors identified a total of 123 patients from published case reports, series, and retrospective studies through September 2017. They reported a higher rate of autoimmune diseases exacerbation (36%–62%) and new onset irAEs (26%–42%). Most patients responded to immunosuppression, but 17.1% required immunotherapy discontinuation. Few patients died because of AEs (autoimmune flare or irAEs) and/or progressive cancer (4).

In Europe, prospective data of the REISAMIC registry compared 45 patients with preexisting autoimmune diseases to 352 patients without autoimmune diseases who received anti-PD-1 agents over the same period. Among patients with autoimmune diseases, 24.4% had autoimmune diseases flare and 22.2% had new onset irAEs. Most patients responded to immunosuppression, but approximately 10% required immunotherapy discontinuation. No significant differences were observed between patients with and without preexisting autoimmune diseases in the objective response and overall survival (OS) rates (5). Taken together, these studies suggest that autoimmune disorders are not an absolute contraindication to the use of ICIs. Much of the risk in those patients is owing to an increased rate of autoimmune disease exacerbation, not necessarily to an increased risk of irAEs. However, the still ongoing checkmate CA209-172 study will prospectively evaluate a cohort of patients affected by auto-immune disease and treated with nivolumab for advanced melanoma. This study will provide additional information about this group of patients.

- Despite the lack of prospective, high-quality data, we posit that most patients can safely receive these therapies with close monitoring.
- We would be more hesitant to offer combined immune checkpoint blockade (e.g., combination ipilimumab and nivolumab) in these patients, and would have a careful discussion of the potentially high risks and benefits in patients with prior life-threatening autoimmunity (e.g., acute demyelinating polyneuropathy, myasthenia gravis).

Another frequently asked question for this patient cohort is how to manage concurrent immunosuppressants in this population.

- In the larger cohort of PD-1 inhibitor treatment in the context of autoimmune disease, it is notable that patients on active immunosuppression appeared to have lower response rates to anti-PD-1 compared with those of immunosuppression (15% vs. 44%), although numbers are small and not statistically significantly different.
- There is essentially no data to guide practice here but a general sense (and clear theoretical concern) that immunosuppression may blunt treatment response.
- Our approach is to co-manage patients with rheumatology (or other appropriate specialties) and minimize immunosuppression to replace dose steroids (10 mg or less) and other immunosuppressives that likely have minimal T-cell effects (e.g., budesonide, hydroxychloroquine). However, the use of higher doses of corticosteroids and other aggressive immunosuppressives such as tumor necrosis factor inhibitors and other anti-cytokine agents, has been also reported (4). Additional data are needed to characterize which approach is most effective and the decision should be based on the risks and benefits for individual cases.

TRANSPLANT

While autoimmune disorders are life-threatening at times, rejection of a transplanted organ is by definition life-threatening, thus this condition potentially represents the highest risk situation for ICI use.

- One small clinical trial evaluated the safety of ipilimumab in patients with relapsed hematologic malignancies following allogeneic stem cell transplant (n = 29) (6).
  - Grade 3/4 irAEs (including one death) were observed in 21% and 14% had graft-versus-host disease (GVHD)—no deaths.
- Another fairly large retrospective series evaluated the effects of anti-PD-1 in lymphoma patients following allogeneic transplant (n = 31) (7).
  - This study observed a high response rate (77%), but frequent GVHD (55%), with 26% of patients dying from GVHD.
- The evidence for immune checkpoint inhibition following solid organ transplantation is limited to case reports and small series. A systematic review of the literature identified a high graft rejection rate that occurred shortly after initiation of immunotherapy in 50% of kidney transplant, 44% of liver transplant, and 25% of cardiac transplant recipients (8).
  - Intriguingly, in both solid organ and hematopoietic stem cell transplants, a suggestion of higher rates of complication with PD-1 inhibition has been observed, compared with anti-CTLA-4 (which is typically a more toxic therapy).
  - More data are needed, however, to more conclusively report rejection rates with any available regimens.

Thus, in our view, ICIs can be considered in these patients although an extremely high risk of organ rejection (or GVHD) must be considered and discussed with the patient. It remains unclear whether prophylactic low-dose immunosuppression or other factors (e.g., time from transplant, lack of prior rejection/GVHD) influence this risk.

ORGAN DYSFUNCTION

While initial studies uniformly excluded patients with impaired liver or kidney function, several more recent studies allowed patients with mild organ dysfunction.

- One phase II study evaluated 119 patients treated with atezolizumab with moderate renal dysfunction (glomerular filtration rate 30 to 60 mL/min) (9).
  - Response rates (23%) and incidence of grade 3/4 treatment-related AEs (16%) were generally consistent with other atezolizumab studies.
- A phase I/II study of nivolumab evaluated 214 patients with hepato-cellular carcinoma (HCC) in the dose-escalation portion, and reported a 20% response rate (10).
  - Patients with child-pugh scores of ≤7 were permitted, although essentially all patients enrolled had scores of 6 or below.
  - Grade 3/4 treatment-related AEs occurred in only 4% of patients and no liver-specific safety signal was identified.
- A retrospective study also assessed 19 patients with more severe renal (creatinine >2, including three patients on hemodialysis), hepatic (bili-rubin >3), and cardiac (ejection fraction <45%) dysfunction (11).
  - This study reported only three grade 3/4 irAEs, but several patients were hospitalized for fluid-volume overload.
  - It was not clear whether the natural history of these disorders, increased fluid from infusions, or drug-induced systemic inflammation triggered these events.
  - Regardless, we do not consider even more advanced organ dysfunction as a contraindication to ICIs, but would recommend close monitoring of fluid-volume status.

CHRONIC VIRAL INFECTIONS

Patients infected with HIV, hepatitis B (HBV), or hepatitis C (HCV) were always excluded from ICI clinical trials, Recently, in several trials these restrictions have been modified and do not necessarily exclude these patient populations.

- Importantly, a number of preclinical models suggest that the PD-1/ programmed cell death ligand 1 (PD-L1) axis is critical for chronic viral infection maintenance, and these therapies have been considered potential treatments for chronic viral infections (12).
  - Nonetheless, the interactions between these chronic infections and safety/efficacy were not clear, leading to their exclusion from clinical trials.

- Subsequently, the largest study to evaluate this population is the afore-mentioned study of nivolumab in HCC (10).
  - Equivalent safety and efficacy was observed in patients with HBV (n = 51) and HCV (n = 50) compared with non-infected patients.
- Several case reports and small series have also suggested that these agents are safe in patients with HIV (13–16). The interim data from the ongoing phase I clinical trial (NCT02595866) evaluating the use of pembrolizumab in patients with HIV suggested no significant risk (17). One could postulate that patients with severely depressed CD4 T-cell counts could potentially:
  - Have difficulty responding to treatment due to lack of a competent immune system
  - Have increased risk of immune reconstitution inflammatory syndrome (IRIS), particularly if paired with initiation of antiretroviral therapy
  - Regardless, we do not consider HIV or even AIDS as a contraindication to immune checkpoint inhibition, but clearly more data are needed to characterize the safety and efficacy of these agents.

PREGNANCY

Metastatic cancer during pregnancy may lead to very challenging treatment and medical decisions.

- The PD-1/PD-L1 axis appears to play a critical role in inducing and maintaining fetal tolerance.
  - The placenta, in fact, is often used as positive control for PD-L1 expression.
- Extremely limited clinical data around the use of immunotherapies during pregnancy exists.
  - Animal data suggest that inhibition increases the risk of spontaneous abortions, but not the risk of birth defects in surviving animals.
- The Food and Drug Administration has labeled anti-PD-1 agents as category D whereas ipilimumab is category C.

POOR PERFORMANCE STATUS

While every clinical trial requires regular assessment of patient performance status, there has not been any correlation made between poor performance status and more severe or frequent irAEs due to immunotherapy. In fact, in the setting of higher tumor burden and/or increasing tumor aggressiveness, toxicity may be less common. The justification of this statement comes from two pieces of evidence divined from clinical trial evidence in patients with melanoma.

- First, patients with resected, stage III/IV melanoma have higher grade 3/4/5 ipilimumab-associated toxicity than patients with unresectable stage III/IV melanoma (18–20).

- ○ Specifically, across two adjuvant trials of patients with melanoma treated with ipilimumab 10 mg/kg, 409 of 924 (44%) patients developed grade 3 or higher toxicity compared to 124 of 364 (34%) patients with unresectable stage III/IV therapy treated with 10 mg/kg ipilimumab.
- ○ When a simple Fischer exact test is performed, the two-tailed p-value is 0.0009, clearly statistically and significantly different.
  - ▪ Since this phenomenon has not previously been studied, nor to the authors' knowledge, even been evaluated with an analysis such as the abovementioned Fischer exact test calculation, there obviously is no proven explanation for this difference.
- ○ One may hypothesize that patients treated in the adjuvant setting may have a more responsive immune system, while patients with advanced disease have a more compromised immune activation; indeed, in the setting following curative intent surgery (e.g., resected, high-risk melanoma) patients either have no disease (those who never recur) or have minimal residual disease (those who will recur) below the limits of radiographic detection at the time of adjuvant therapy.
- ○ In this setting, there likely are no major tumor microenvironments established that can produce factors (such as cytokines, chemokines, etc.) that may be immunosuppressive, as happens in the unresectable and/or metastatic setting.
  - ▪ In fact, it is hypothesized here that the reason why unresectable/metastatic disease patients have less toxicity is that their tumor is producing substances that protect them from autoimmune toxicity.
- In the Checkmate CA209-172 study, nivolumab after ipilimumab failure in advanced melanoma, a specific cohort of patients with performance status 2 was enrolled (21).
  - ○ In this cohort, the overall response rate (ORR), as expected, was lower than that observed in the intent-to-treat population (15% versus 32% respectively) with no additional signal of toxicity.
  - ○ A second line of evidence to support that this hypothesis can be found in the same study in the cohorts with normal, elevated (> upper limit of normal [ULN]), and very elevated (>2 × ULN) lactate dehydrogenase (LDH) (21).
  - ○ Even if the ORR was better in the normal LDH cohort (36%, 26%, and 10% respectively), no toxicity differences were found among the groups.
  - ○ Since elevated LDH typically is associated with more aggressive disease and is a strong negative predictor of survival in melanoma patients, an interesting set of conclusions can be made.
- Further evidence in such direction come from the Checkmate 067 trial that randomized patients to one of three treatments: nivolumab alone or in combination with ipilimumab versus ipilimumab alone (22).
  - ○ In all patients randomized, grade three or greater toxicity is seen in 28%, 21%, and 59% respectively, in the above cohorts.
- In a pooled analysis of this data and that of other frontline trials involving ipilimumab/nivolumab or nivolumab, Checkmate 069

(randomizing patients to either ipilimumab or a combination of ipilimumab plus nivolumab) (23) and Checkmate 066 (randomizing patients to nivolumab or dacarbazine) (24), with respect to LDH levels:

- Patients with an LDH greater than the ULN, compared with those with a normal LDH and independent of treatment, had a poorer performance status, lower response rate, and poorer progression-free survival.
- In patients treated with combination therapy, grade 3/4 toxicity was greater in patients with a normal LDH (60%) than in patients with an elevated LDH (49%) and those with an LDH greater than two times the ULN (37%).
- There did not appear to be a major difference in toxicity between patients treated with ipilimumab or nivolumab according to LDH level.

ADVANCED AGE

Compared to chemotherapy, ICI therapy is well tolerated (25). Furthermore, other than autoimmune conditions, immune-related toxicity is not likely to occur in patients with chronic organ dysfunction, although those conditions themselves may be associated with increased hospitalization due to the underlying condition (11).

- Additionally, it seems fair to say that ICIs are not more likely to cause significant problems in patients with poor performance status, but the ramifications of toxicity may be more profound in a patient with a significant comorbid condition.
  - For example, a patient with critical aortic stenosis likely will have much more trouble in the setting of high-grade, high-volume diarrhea than a patient with normal cardiac function. This also appears to be the case for older patients.
- A retrospective analysis of the Surveillance Epidemiology and End Results (SEER) and Texas Cancer Registry (TCR) linked with Medicare data between March 2011 and December 2013 evaluated all elderly melanoma patients (65 years or older) treated with ipilimumab (26).
  - The incidence of irAEs in elderly patients was comparable to all melanoma patients treated with ipilimumab, but hypothyroidism was reported more frequently than in clinical trials. Elderly patients with severe irAEs seemed to have the highest risk of death while elderly patients with nonsevere irAEs had improved OS compared to patients without irAEs.
- In the largest series studying the influence of age on ICI efficacy and toxicity, 254 patients with unresectable/metastatic melanoma who received anti-PD-1/PD-L1 therapy were analyzed retrospectively (27).
  - There was no difference in progression free or OS, across four age groups (<50, 50–64, 65–74, ≥75), a finding not predicted by preclinical models of immune senescence (28,29).

- We have also observed responses even at extreme old age (30).
  - Furthermore, there was no significant difference in the development or severity of irAEs across these age groups.
- In addition, in a retrospective analysis from the Italian ipilimumab expanded access program, 188 elderly patients (>70 years old) were enrolled with an immune-related disease control rate (irDCR) of 38%, and the 1- and 2-year progression-free survival (PFS) rates of 21% and 12%, respectively (31).
  - Ipilimumab treatment at classical dosage of 3 mg/kg was generally well tolerated with no new signal of toxicity.
  - Based on these results, the risk/benefit ratio clearly favors treating elderly melanoma patients with ICIs (particularly single-agent anti-PD-1 or PD-L1 therapy), however, noncancer related comorbidities should be taken into account. It is unclear if this will hold true for every indication of these agents and careful attention to this issue must continue to be made.

BRAIN METASTASES

Another special population of patients that may have unique response and toxicity considerations compared are those with metastatic disease in the brain.

- Remarkably, in trials of patients with brain metastases treated with ipilimumab, anti-PD1 inhibitors (including pembroliumab and nivolumab) and combination ipilimumab plus nivolumab have demonstrated significant responses at a slightly lower rate than in patients without central nervous system (CNS) disease.
- Importantly, there do not appear to be major autoimmune toxicities that occur in this population at a higher rate than in other patient populations without brain metastases (32–37).
- One issue that remains to be determined is if the rate of radionecrosis is higher in patients treated with concurrent or sequential stereotactic radiosurgery and ICI therapy (38).

CONCLUSION

The lack of data on the safety and efficacy of ICIs in these patient populations represent a major clinical challenge. At present, there are no consensus recommendations on how oncologists should intervene in these patients. Although there are no absolute contraindications, the treatment decision requires a multidisciplinary approach that carefully balances between potential benefits and risks until more robust data become available to better guide our practice.

REFERENCES

1. Johnson DB, Sullivan RJ, Ott PA, et al. Ipilimumab therapy in patients with advanced melanoma and preexisting autoimmune disorders. *JAMA Oncol.* 2016;2:234–240. doi:10.1001/jamaoncol.2015.4368

2. Menzies AM, Johnson DB, Ramanujam S, et al. Anti-PD-1 therapy in patients with advanced melanoma and preexisting autoimmune disorders or major toxicity with ipilimumab. *Ann Oncol*. 2016;28(2):368–376. doi:10.1093/annonc/mdw443

3. Weber JS, Hodi FS, Wolchok JD, et al. Safety profile of nivolumab monotherapy: a pooled analysis of patients with advanced melanoma. *J Clin Oncol*. 2017;35:785–792. doi:10.1200/jco.2015.66.1389

4. Abdel-Wahab N, Shah M, Lopez-Olivo MA, et al. Use of immune checkpoint inhibitors in the treatment of patients with cancer and preexisting autoimmune disease: a systematic review. *Ann Intern Med*. 2018;168:121–130. doi:10.7326/m17-2073

5. Danlos FX, Voisin AL, Dyevre V, et al. Safety and efficacy of anti-programmed death 1 antibodies in patients with cancer and pre-existing autoimmune or inflammatory disease. *Eur J Cancer*. 2018;91:21–29. doi:10.1016/j.ejca.2017.12.008

6. Davids MS, Kim HT, Bachireddy P, et al. Ipilimumab for patients with relapse after allogeneic transplantation. *N Engl J Med*. 2016;375:143–153. doi:10.1056/nejmoa1601202

7. Haverkos BM, Abbott D, Hamadani M, et al. PD-1 blockade for relapsed lymphoma post-allogeneic hematopoietic cell transplant: high response rate but frequent GVHD. *Blood*. 2017;130:221–228. doi:10.1182/blood-2017-01-761346

8. Abdel-Wahab N, Abudayyeh A, Shah M, et al. Allo-immunity and graft rejection after checkpoint inhibitor therapy (CPI) in solid organ transplant (SOT) recipients. *J Clin Oncol*. 2018;36:3082. doi:10.1200/jco.2018.36.15_suppl.3082

9. Balar AV, Galsky MD, Rosenberg JE, et al. Atezolizumab as first-line treatment in cisplatin-ineligible patients with locally advanced and metastatic urothelial carcinoma: a single-arm, multicentre, phase 2 trial. *Lancet*. 2017;389:67–76. doi:10.1016/s0140-6736(16)32455-2

10. El-Khoueiry AB, Sangro B, Yau T, et al. Nivolumab in patients with advanced hepatocellular carcinoma (CheckMate 040): an open-label, non-comparative, phase 1/2 dose escalation and expansion trial. *Lancet*. 2017;389:2492–2502. doi:10.1016/s0140-6736(17)31046-2

11. Kanz BA, Pollack MH, Johnpulle R, et al. Safety and efficacy of anti-PD-1 in patients with baseline cardiac, renal, or hepatic dysfunction. *J Immunother Cancer*. 2016;4:60.

12. Grabmeier-Pfistershammer K, Stecher C, Zettl M, et al. Antibodies targeting BTLA or TIM-3 enhance HIV-1 specific T cell responses in combination with PD-1 blockade. *Clin Immunol*. 2017;183:167–173. doi:10.1016/j.clim.2017.09.002

13. McCullar B, Alloway T, Martin M. Durable complete response to nivolumab in a patient with HIV and metastatic non-small cell lung cancer. *J Thorac Dis*. 2017;9:E540–E542. doi:10.21037/jtd.2017.05.32

14. Davar D, Wilson M, Pruckner C, et al. PD-1 blockade in advanced melanoma in patients with hepatitis C and/or HIV. *Case Rep Oncol Med*. 2015;2015:1–5. doi:10.1155/2015/737389

15. Marra A, Scognamiglio G, Peluso I, et al. Immune checkpoint inhibitors in melanoma and HIV infection. *Open AIDS J*. 2017;11:91–100. doi:10.2174/1874613601711010091

16. Ostios-Garcia L, Faig J, Leonardi GC, et al. Safety and efficacy of PD-1 inhibitors among HIV-positive patients with non-small cell lung cancer. *J Thorac Oncol*. 2018;13:1037–1042. doi:10.1016/j.jtho.2018.03.031

17. 32nd Annual Meeting and Pre-Conference Programs of the Society for Immunotherapy of Cancer (SITC 2017): late-breaking abstracts. *J Immunother Cancer*. 2017;5:89. doi:10.1186/s40425-017-0297-3

18. Eggermont AM, Chiarion-Sileni V, Grob JJ, et al. Prolonged survival in stage III melanoma with ipilimumab adjuvant therapy. *N Engl J Med*. 2016;375:1845–1855. doi:10.1056/nejmoa1611299

19. Weber J, Mandala M, Del Vecchio M, et al. Adjuvant nivolumab versus ipilimumab in resected stage III or IV melanoma. *N Engl J Med*. 2017;377:1824–1835. doi:10.1056/nejmoa1709030

20. Ascierto PA, Del Vecchio M, Robert C, et al. Ipilimumab 10 mg/kg versus ipilimumab 3 mg/kg in patients with unresectable or metastatic melanoma: a randomised, double-blind, multicentre, phase 3 trial. *Lancet Oncol*. 2017;18:611–622. doi:10.1016/s1470-2045(17)30231-0

21. Schadendorf D, Ascierto PA, Haanen JBAG, et al. Efficacy and safety of nivolumab (NIVO) in patients with advanced melanoma (MEL) and poor prognostic factors who progressed on or after ipilimumab (IPI): Results from a phase II study (CheckMate 172). *J Clin Oncol.* 2017;35:9524. doi:10.1200/jco.2017.35.15_suppl.9524

22. Wolchok JD, Chiarion-Sileni V, Gonzalez R, et al. Overall survival with combined nivolumab and ipilimumab in advanced melanoma. *N Engl J Med.* 2017;377:1345–1356. doi:10.1056/nejmoa1709684

23. Postow MA, Chesney J, Pavlick AC, et al. Nivolumab and Ipilimumab versus Ipilimumab in Untreated Melanoma. *N Engl J Med.* 2015;372(21):2006–2017. doi:10.1056/nejmoa1414428

24. Robert C, Long GV, Brady B, et al. Nivolumab in previously untreated melanoma without BRAF mutation. *N Engl J Med.* 2015;372(4):320–330.

25. Ribas A, Puzanov I, Dummer R, et al. Pembrolizumab versus investigator-choice chemotherapy for ipilimumab-refractory melanoma (KEYNOTE-002): a randomised, controlled, phase 2 trial. *Lancet Oncol.* 2015;16(8):908–918. doi:10.1016/s1470-2045(15)00083-2.

26. Mian I, Yang M, Zhao H, et al. Immune-related adverse events and survival in elderly patients with melanoma treated with ipilimumab. *J Clin Oncol.* 2016;34:3047. doi:10.1200/jco.2016.34.15_suppl.3047

27. Betof AS, Nipp RD, Giobbie-Hurder A, et al. Impact of age on outcomes with immunotherapy for patients with melanoma. *Oncologist.* 2017;22:963–971. doi:10.1634/theoncologist.2016-0450

28. Padron A, Hurez V, Gupta HB, et al. Age effects of distinct immune checkpoint blockade treatments in a mouse melanoma model. *Exp Gerontol.* 2018;105:146–154. doi:10.1016/j.exger.2017.12.025

29. Kaur A, Webster MR, Marchbank K, et al. sFRP2 in the aged microenvironment drives melanoma metastasis and therapy resistance. *Nature.* 2016;532:250–254. doi:10.1038/nature17392

30. Johnpulle RA, Conry RM, Sosman JA, et al. Responses to immune checkpoint inhibitors in nonagenarians. *Oncoimmunology.* 2016;5(11):e1234572. doi:10.1080/2162402x.2016.1234572

31. Chiarion Sileni V, Pigozzo J, Ascierto PA, et al. Efficacy and safety of ipilimumab in elderly patients with pretreated advanced melanoma treated at Italian centres through the expanded access programme. *J Exp Clin Cancer Res.* 2014;33:30. doi:10.1186/1756-9966-33-30

32. Margolin K, Ernstoff MS, Hamid O, et al. Ipilimumab in patients with melanoma and brain metastases: an open-label, phase 2 trial. *Lancet Oncol.* 2012;13:459–465. doi:10.1016/s1470-2045(12)70090-6

33. Goldberg SB, Gettinger SN, Mahajan A, et al. Pembrolizumab for patients with melanoma or non-small-cell lung cancer and untreated brain metastases: early analysis of a non-randomised, open-label, phase 2 trial. *Lancet Oncol.* 2016;17:976–983. doi:10.1016/s1470-2045(16)30053-5

34. Queirolo P, Spagnolo F, Ascierto PA, et al. Efficacy and safety of ipilimumab in patients with advanced melanoma and brain metastases. *J Neurooncol.* 2014;118:109–116. doi:10.1007/s11060-014-1400-y

35. Di Giacomo AM, Ascierto PA, Queirolo P, et al. Three-year follow-up of advanced melanoma patients who received ipilimumab plus fotemustine in the Italian Network for Tumor Biotherapy (NIBIT)-M1 phase II study. *Ann Oncol.* 2015;26:798–803. doi:10.1093/annonc/mdu577

36. Tawbi HA, Forsyth PA, Algazi A, et al. Combined nivolumab and ipilimumab in melanoma metastatic to the brain. *N Engl J Med.* 2018;379:722–730. doi:10.1056/nejmoa1805453

37. Long GV, Atkinson V, Lo S, et al. Combination nivolumab and ipilimumab or nivolumab alone in melanoma brain metastases: a multicentre randomised phase 2 study. *Lancet Oncol.* 2018;19:672–681. doi:10.1016/s1470-2045(18)30139-6

38. Johnson DB, Friedman DL, Berry EG, et al. Survivorship in immune therapy: assessing chronic immune toxicities, health outcomes, and functional status among long-term ipilimumab survivors at a single referral center. *Cancer Immunol Res.* 2015;3(5):464–469. doi:10.1158/2326-6066.cir-14-0217.

CHAPTER 16

CANCER-RELATED FATIGUE IN PATIENTS OF IMMUNE CHECKPOINT INHIBITOR THERAPY

Eric D. Hansen, Michelle Walter, and Amy A. Case

INTRODUCTION

Many patients on immune checkpoint inhibitor (ICI) therapy will experience cancer-related fatigue, a troubling symptom which can significantly impact quality of life. The National Comprehensive Cancer Network (NCCN) definition of fatigue includes the following key components: (a) it is "distressing and persistent"; (b) it can be physical, emotional, or cognitive; (c) it is out of proportion to recent activity; and (d) it interferes with daily functioning (1). Associated features may include diminished concentration, diminished motivation, insomnia or hypersomnia, nonrestorative sleep, and short-term memory deficits (2). Of note, many of these symptoms are also present in depression, and it can be difficult to differentiate whether patients have cancer-related fatigue, depression, or both (3).

Fatigue is one of the most distressing symptoms affecting cancer patients' quality of life. For some patients, fatigue may be more problematic than pain, nausea, or vomiting, and it is more challenging to treat (1,4). For patients with metastatic cancer, fatigue can rob them of time and participation in the events and activities that make their life meaningful, all the more distressing when they know that their time may be limited by their incurable disease (1).

CANCER-RELATED FATIGUE/ICI-RELATED FATIGUE MECHANISMS, PATHOPHYSIOLOGY, AND RISK FACTORS

The etiology of cancer-related fatigue is still being investigated. The strongest predictor of post-treatment fatigue for patients treated with traditional chemotherapy is pretreatment fatigue (5–7).

- Physical inactivity and elevated body mass index are also risk factors for cancer-related fatigue (5,8,9).
- Patients who have poor coping skills and engage in negative self-statements are more likely to experience fatigue during and after treatment (5,10).
- Inflammation has been linked with cancer-related fatigue, both during and posttreatment.

Published by Springer Publishing Company DOI: 10.1891/9780826172150.0016

- ○ It is thought that peripheral inflammatory cytokines alter the central nervous system to produce symptoms of fatigue (5,11).
  - ▪ Several inflammatory markers (IL-6, IL1 receptor antagonist, tumor necrosis factor (TNF-α), and C-reactive proteins) have been shown to be associated with cancer-related fatigue, although the results have been inconsistent (11,12).
- ○ Studies that have evaluated longitudinal changes in inflammatory markers have shown more consistent associations with cancer-related fatigue (5).
  - ▪ Elevated levels of several inflammatory markers (IL-1 RA, sTNF-RII, neopterin, soluble IL-6 receptor) have also been associated with patients who experience persistent posttreatment fatigue, up to 5 years after completion of treatment (13).
- Alterations in the immune system have also been associated with cancer-related fatigue.
  - ○ Patients with elevated CD4+ and CD56+ T-cells, and decreased activated T-cells and myeloid dendritic cells, are more likely to have persistent fatigue post-treatment (5,11,14).
  - ○ An elevated white blood cell count has also been reported to be associated with cancer-related fatigue, although the results are not consistent (5,15).
- Additional proposed mechanisms of cancer-related fatigue under study include hypothalamic–pituitary–adrenal axis dysregulation, circadian rhythm desynchronization, skeletal muscle wasting, and genetic dysregulation (1).
- The mechanism of ICI-induced fatigue is also unclear. Immune-related adverse events are thought to be primarily T-cell-mediated, but the role B-cells, granulocytes, and cytokines may play is still under investigation (16).

ICI-RELATED FATIGUE INCIDENCE

Fatigue is a widespread symptom in patients with cancer and associated with more advanced disease (1,17).

- For patients treated with ICI therapy, a systematic review of phase II and III trials revealed an incidence of all-grade treatment-associated fatigue varying from 14% to 42%; high-grade (grade ≥ 3) treatment-associated fatigue varied between 1% and 11% (18).
- However, placebo-controlled studies of ICI therapy show that while rates of fatigue are higher in the therapy arms, there is still a significant background rate of fatigue due to the disease itself in the placebo arms (Table 16.1) (18–20).

ICI-RELATED FATIGUE EVALUATION AND MANAGEMENT

There are four key components of the evaluation and treatment of cancer related fatigue which also applies to ICI-induced fatigue: **screening**, **primary evaluation**, **intervention**, and **re-evaluation** (1).

TABLE 16.1 Incidence of Fatigue in ICI Therapy Versus Placebo

Study	Therapy arm	Overall fatigue (%)	Grade 3 fatigue (%)	Grade 4 fatigue (%)
Kwon 2014 (19)	Ipilimumab	38	9	2
	Placebo	31	8	1
Eggermont 2015 (20)	Ipilimumab	38	2	<1
	Placebo	29	1	<1

Screening of Fatigue

Fatigue is underrecognized in cancer patients. Cancer patients may not think it is important enough to mention to their physicians unless they are directly asked. They may also be afraid that their treatment will be altered if they report fatigue (1).

- Patients should be screened systematically at initiation of therapy, and periodically re-screened throughout the duration of their treatment.
- The NCCN and American Society of Clinical Oncology (ASCO) guidelines identify 14 commonly used tools to assess cancer-related fatigue (1,21). The shortest is the NCCN problem list, which comprises a single dichotomous yes/no question.
  - If fatigue is present, it should be rated from 0 to 10, with 0 being no fatigue and 10 being worst fatigue.
  - If a numeric scale is used, most commonly patients are grouped into no fatigue (0), mild fatigue (1–3), moderate fatigue (4–6), and severe fatigue (7–10).
  - For patients who have difficulty rating their fatigue using a numeric scale, it may be easier to have them rate their fatigue as mild, moderate, or severe.
  - The single item scale is a useful initial screen; however, it can be difficult to capture the subtle aspects of fatigue with a single numeric scale question. Especially for patients with moderate to severe fatigue, it can be helpful to use a more thorough assessment tool (22).
- Unidimensional tools, which primarily focus on the physical effects of fatigue, include the FACT-F (Functional Assessment of Cancer Therapy-Fatigue), the EORTC QLQ C30 (European Organization for Research and Treatment of Cancer Quality-of-Life Questionnaire Core 30), and the POMS-F (Profile of Mood States-Fatigue).
- Multidimensional tools, which also measure the cognitive or emotional symptoms of fatigue, include the BFI (Brief Fatigue Inventory), the Visual Analogue Fatigue Scale, the Fatigue Questionnaire, the Chalder Fatigue Scale, the FSI (Fatigue Symptom Inventory), the MFI-20 (20-item Multidimensional Fatigue Inventory), the MFSI-30 (Multidimensional Fatigue Symptom Inventory 30-item short form), the Revised Piper Fatigue Scale, and the Schwartz Cancer Fatigue Scale (1,21).

○ While all of the multidimensional tools evaluate the physical aspects of fatigue thoroughly, there is much more variability in how thoroughly they assess the cognitive and emotional components of fatigue (23).

Evaluation of Fatigue

The first step in evaluating fatigue is to take a careful history and physical, to determine whether a specific etiology can be determined, especially a potentially reversible cause.

- A description of the fatigue should include onset, duration, change over time, associated factors, interference with function, as well as associated physical, cognitive, and psychological symptoms (1).
  ○ It is also important to recognize that fatigue often significantly impacts a patient's functional status at home and to assess their safety and level of caregiver support at home (1,24).
- The next step is to determine whether fatigue is related to recurrence or progression of the patient's underlying malignancy. Many patients will assume this is the cause of their worsening fatigue.
  ○ It helps relieve a patient's anxiety if it has been determined that their fatigue is not due to progression or recurrence of their malignancy and then they may be educated about the other possible causes of their fatigue.
- In further determining the etiology of fatigue, it is important to rule out other potential causes (Table 16.2).
  ○ Fatigue often presents as a symptom cluster together with pain, sleep disturbance, depression, and anxiety. Patients with fatigue should be assessed for these symptoms, which if treated often lead to improvement in fatigue as well (1,25).
  ○ It is also important to rule out other conditions which may contribute to fatigue; these include hypoxemia, anemia, obstructive sleep apnea, systemic infection, organ dysfunction (heart, lung, liver, kidney), electrolyte disturbance (hypokalemia, hyponatremia, hypomagnesemia, hypercalcemia), deconditioning, and nutritional deficiency.
  ○ Patients' medications should also be reviewed as it is common, especially in a cancer patient population, to have pain medications, anxiety medications, anti-emetics, and other sedating medications which may contribute to fatigue.
- If after evaluating for the above, no clear etiology of fatigue has been identified, the ICI may be contributing.
  ○ There are multiple ICI toxicities which can lead to fatigue, although fatigue can present as an isolated side effect (Table 16.2).
  ○ These toxicities are endocrine (hypothyroidism, hypoadrenalism, and hypopituitarism), gastrointestinal (diarrhea, colitis hepatitis), renal (nephritis/nephrotic syndrome), or pulmonary (pneumonitis).

TABLE 16.2 Etiologies of Fatigue

Symptoms frequently experienced concurrently with fatigue	Pain Depression Anxiety Insomnia
Conditions which can contribute to fatigue	Hypoxemia Obstructive sleep apnea Anemia Systemic infection Organ dysfunction 　　Heart failure 　　Liver insufficiency 　　Renal insufficiency 　　Reduced pulmonary function Electrolyte disturbance 　　Hypokalemia 　　Hyponatremia 　　Hypomagnesemia 　　Hypercalcemia Nutritional deficiency Deconditioning Sedating medications
ICI toxicities which may contribute to fatigue	Endocrine 　　Hypothyroidism 　　Hypoadrenalism 　　Hypopituitarism Gastrointestinal 　　Diarrhea 　　Colitis Hepatitis Nephritis/nephrotic syndrome Pneumonitis

Treatment of Fatigue

Fatigue is a challenging symptom to recognize and treat. There is often not one medication or nonpharmacologic strategy which will resolve fatigue on its own. Patients need a supporting strategy which is multimodal. Despite the fact that there are treatment guidelines for fatigue, they are often underutilized (26).

Nonpharmacologic Strategies

- First, patients should be counseled on energy conservation. Prioritizing activities and setting realistic expectations are critical to help patients maximize their activities when their energy levels are best and also have realistic expectations about what they are able to do, as when they are not met it may be distressing.
  - Energy-level diaries can be helpful to give patients a sense of when their energy level will be best throughout the day (1).
  - One trial of an energy conservation counseling intervention showed improvement in patients' fatigue (27).

- Both exercise and psychological support interventions have been shown to be effective in the treatment of cancer-related fatigue.
  - A recent meta-analysis which was comprised of 113 studies including 11,525 patients revealed that exercise and psychological interventions both significantly improved fatigue levels for patients, while pharmacologic interventions did not (28).
- A Cochrane review published in 2012 that included 56 studies (4,068 participants) supported exercise, specifically aerobic exercise, as an effective treatment for cancer-related fatigue.
  - The benefit was most pronounced in patients with solid tumors (29).
  - Successful interventions generally were of moderate intensity (approximately 55%–75% of maximum heart rate), aerobic exercise, ranging from 10 to 60 minutes in duration, 3 to 6 days per week (30).
- A meta-analysis has confirmed that exercise has consistently been shown to be an effective treatment for cancer-related fatigue.
  - Although the population studied was cancer survivors, exercise was effective both during and posttreatment (31).
- Patients can be referred to exercise specialists, such as a physical therapist or physical medicine and rehabilitation specialist, to help tailor an exercise regimen. Referral is especially encouraged in patients who have cardiovascular or pulmonary comorbidities, have undergone recent surgery, or have specific functional deficits due to their cancer.
  - Caution must be taken with patients who have bone metastases, thrombocytopenia, anemia, active infection, or are at increased risk for falls (1).
- Other physical interventions which are under active investigation include yoga, acupuncture, and massage therapy.
  - Several randomized controlled trials support the utility of yoga in reducing fatigue in patients undergoing chemotherapy or radiation (32,33).
  - Several small, randomized controlled studies suggest possible benefit for acupuncture and massage therapy to treat cancer-related fatigue, though this needs to be confirmed by larger studies (34–36).
- Psychosocial interventions for cancer-related fatigue can primarily be grouped into three main categories: cognitive behavioral therapy/ behavioral therapy, psychoeducational therapies, and supportive expressive therapy (1,23).
  - Cognitive behavioral therapy/behavioral therapy, which includes stress management, problem solving, and relaxation training, has quality evidence to support its use for cancer-related fatigue (37–39).
  - Psychoeducational therapies, which include coping strategies, education about cancer symptoms and management, and emotional adjustment training, also have evidence to support their use to improve cancer-related fatigue (40,41).
  - Supportive expressive therapies, which include support groups and journal writing to facilitate expression of emotions, need further study to support their use (1).

- Nutrition evaluation and consultation for patients at risk of deficiency is also important.
  - Inadequate nutritional intake can lead to nutritional deficiencies, as well as dehydration and electrolyte imbalances, all of which contribute to fatigue (1).

Pharmacologic Interventions

Although there has been intense interest in finding a medication which effectively treats cancer-related fatigue, no easy cure has yet been identified. Furthermore, in evaluating the literature, it is important to note that there is a significant placebo response in patients involved with studies of treatments for cancer-related fatigue; one study suggested that the placebo response rate is as high as 56% (42).

Psychostimulants

Methylphenidate and modafinil have been studied as treatment for cancer-related fatigue with mixed results.

- Two systematic reviews suggest benefit for methylphenidate, particularly in patients treated long term with methylphenidate, although the treatment effects are small and several of the individual studies did not find any benefit (43,44).
- Side effects of methylphenidate include anorexia, vertigo, anxiety, and nausea and may limit use in a cancer patient population where anorexia, anxiety, and nausea are frequent symptoms.
- Although there are some positive studies showing benefit for modafinil, overall the evidence is mixed and quite limited in quality.
- The NCCN guidelines recommend cautious use of methylphenidate but do not recommend modafinil due to lack of evidence (1).

Dietary Supplements

Several dietary supplements have also been studied for the treatment of fatigue.

- A randomized controlled trial involving 364 patients evaluated Wisconsin ginseng (panax quinquefolius, 2,000 mg daily) showed patient improvement in fatigue at 8 weeks (as measured by the MFSI-30), particularly in those undergoing active treatment (45).
  - A study of a different kind of ginseng, panax ginseng, failed to find benefit (46).
  - Further study is needed to confirm the benefit of ginseng for treating cancer-related fatigue and to determine whether the type of ginseng strain is important in its efficacy for treating fatigue.
- Coenzyme Q and l-carnitine have also been studied, but failed to show benefit (47,48).

CONCLUSION

Cancer-related fatigue is one of the most challenging symptoms for clinicians to manage. Although the etiologies are under active investigation, inflammatory cytokines and changes in the immune system have both been linked to cancer-related fatigue and likely explain the mechanism behind ICI-related fatigue. Patients should be screened regularly throughout their treatment and after completion of the treatment.

For those identified as having fatigue, it is important to perform a thorough evaluation for possible reversible causes. If ICI therapy is thought to be the cause of a patient's fatigue, it is important to institute a multimodal approach, including nonpharmacologic strategies focusing on consistent light exercise as tolerated, cognitive behavioral therapy, psychoeducational strategies, and energy conservation. Although pharmacologic options are limited, there is some evidence to support trials of ginseng or methylphenidate for refractory cancer-related fatigue, after consideration of the risk–benefit profile for each patient.

REFERENCES

1. National Comprehensive Cancer Network. Cancer-Related Fatigue (Version 1.2018). https://www.nccn.org/professionals/physician_gls/pdf/fatigue.pdf

2. Reisfield GM, Wilson GR. Fast Facts and Concepts #173. Cancer-Related Fatigue. 2007. https://www.mypcnow.org

3. Traeger L, Braun IM, Greer JA, et al. Parsing depression from fatigue in patients with cancer using the fatigue symptom inventory. *J Pain Symptom Manage.* 2011;42(1):52–59. doi:10.1016/j.jpainsymman.2010.10.262

4. Hinds PS, Quargnenti A, Bush AJ, et al. An evaluation of the impact of a self-care coping intervention on psychological and clinical outcomes in adolescents with newly diagnosed cancer. *Eur J Oncol Nurs.* 2000;4(1):6–17; discussion 18–19. doi:10.1054/ejon.1999.0051

5. Bower JE. Cancer-related fatigue—mechanisms, risk factors, and treatments. *Nat Rev Clin Oncol.* 2014;11(10):597–609. doi:10.1038/nrclinonc.2014.127

6. Geinitz H, Zimmermann FB, Thamm R, et al. Fatigue in patients with adjuvant radiation therapy for breast cancer: long-term follow-up. *J Cancer Res Clin Oncol.* 2004;130(6):327–333. doi:10.1007/s00432-003-0540-9

7. Goedendorp MM, Gielissen MF, Verhagen CA, et al. Development of fatigue in cancer survivors: a prospective follow-up study from diagnosis into the year after treatment. *J Pain Symptom Manage.* 2013;45(2):213–222. doi:10.1016/j.jpainsymman.2012.02.009

8. Winters-Stone KM, Bennett JA, Nail L, et al. Strength, physical activity, and age predict fatigue in older breast cancer survivors. *Oncol Nurs Forum.* 2008;35(5):815–821. doi:10.1188/08.ONF.815-821

9. Andrykowski MA, Donovan KA, Laronga C, et al. Prevalence, predictors, and characteristics of off-treatment fatigue in breast cancer survivors. *Cancer.* 2010;116(24):5740–5748. doi:10.1002/cncr.25294

10. Jacobsen PB, Andrykowski MA, Thors CL. Relationship of catastrophizing to fatigue among women receiving treatment for breast cancer. *J Consult Clin Psychol.* 2004;72(2):355–361. doi:10.1037/0022-006X.72.2.355

11. Seruga B, Zhang H, Bernstein LJ, et al. Cytokines and their relationship to the symptoms and outcome of cancer. *Nat Rev Cancer.* 2008;8(11):887–899. doi:10.1038/nrc2507

12. Collado-Hidalgo A, Bower JE, Ganz PA, et al. Inflammatory biomarkers for persistent fatigue in breast cancer survivors. *Clin Cancer Res.* 2006;12(9):2759–2766. doi:10.1158/1078-0432.CCR-05-2398

13. Bower JE, Ganz PA, Aziz N, et al. Fatigue and proinflammatory cytokine activity in breast cancer survivors. *Psychosom Med.* 2002;64(4):604–611.

14. Bower JE, Ganz PA, Aziz N, et al. T-cell homeostasis in breast cancer survivors with persistent fatigue. *J Natl Cancer Inst.* 2003;95(15):1165–1168.

15. Alexander S, Minton O, Andrews P, et al. A comparison of the characteristics of disease-free breast cancer survivors with or without cancer-related fatigue syndrome. *Eur J Cancer.* 2009;45(3):384–392. doi:10.1016/j.ejca.2008.09.010

16. Naidoo J, Page DB, Li BT, et al. Toxicities of the anti-PD-1 and anti-PD-L1 immune checkpoint antibodies. *Ann Oncol.* 2015;26(12):2375–2391. doi:10.1158/2326-6066.CIR-15-0123

17. Abrahams HJ, Gielissen MF, Schmits IC, et al. Risk factors, prevalence, and course of severe fatigue after breast cancer treatment: a meta-analysis involving 12 327 breast cancer survivors. *Ann Oncol.* 2016;27(6):965–974. doi:10.1093/annonc/mdw099

18. Abdel-Rahman O, Helbling D, Schmidt J, et al. Treatment-associated fatigue in cancer patients treated with immune checkpoint inhibitors; a systematic review and meta-analysis. *Clin Oncol (R Coll Radiol).* 2016;28(10):e127–e138. doi:10.1016/j.clon.2016.06.008

19. Kwon ED, Drake CG, Scher HI, et al. Ipilimumab versus placebo after radiotherapy in patients with metastatic castration-resistant prostate cancer that had progressed after docetaxel chemotherapy (CA184-043): a multicentre, randomised, double-blind, phase 3 trial. *Lancet Oncol.* 2014;15(7):700–712. doi:10.1016/S1470-2045(14)70189-5

20. Eggermont AM, Chiarion-Sileni V, Grob JJ, et al. Adjuvant ipilimumab versus placebo after complete resection of high-risk stage III melanoma (EORTC 18071): a randomised, double-blind, phase 3 trial. *Lancet Oncol.* 2015;16(5):522–530. doi:10.1016/S1470-2045(15)70122-1

21. Bower JE, Bak K, Berger A, et al. Screening, assessment, and management of fatigue in adult survivors of cancer: an American Society of Clinical Oncology clinical practice guideline adaptation. *J Clin Oncol.* 2014;32(17):1840–1850. doi:10.1200/JCO.2013.53.4495

22. Stone PC, Minton O. Cancer-related fatigue. *Eur J Cancer.* 2008;44(8):1097–1104. doi:10.1016/j.ejca.2008.02.037

23. Kangas M, Bovbjerg DH, Montgomery GH. Cancer-related fatigue: a systematic and meta-analytic review of non-pharmacological therapies for cancer patients. *Psychol Bull.* 2008;134(5):700–741. doi:10.1037/a0012825

24. Luciani A, Jacobsen PB, Extermann M, et al. Fatigue and functional dependence in older cancer patients. *Am J Clin Oncol.* 2008;31(5):424–430. doi:10.1097/COC.0b013e31816d915f

25. de Raaf PJ, de Klerk C, Timman R, et al. Systematic monitoring and treatment of physical symptoms to alleviate fatigue in patients with advanced cancer: a randomized controlled trial. *J Clin Oncol.* 2013;31(6):716–723. doi:10.1200/JCO.2012.44.4216

26. Pearson EJ, Morris ME, McKinstry CE. Cancer-related fatigue: a survey of health practitioner knowledge and practice. *Support Care Cancer.* 2015;23(12):3521–3529. doi:10.1007/s00520-015-2723-8

27. Barsevick AM, Dudley W, Beck S, et al. A randomized clinical trial of energy conservation for patients with cancer-related fatigue. *Cancer.* 2004;100(6):1302–1310. doi:10.1002/cncr.20111

28. Mustian KM, Alfano CM, Heckler C, et al. Comparison of pharmaceutical, psychological, and exercise treatments for cancer-related fatigue: a meta-analysis. *JAMA Oncol.* 2017;3(7):961–968. doi:10.1001/jamaoncol.2016.6914

29. Cramp F, Byron-Daniel J. Exercise for the management of cancer-related fatigue in adults. *Cochrane Database Syst Rev.* 2012;11:CD006145. doi:10.1002/14651858.cd006145.pub3

30. Mustian KM, Sprod LK, Janelsins M, et al. Exercise recommendations for cancer-related fatigue, cognitive impairment, sleep problems, depression, pain, anxiety, and physical dysfunction: a review. *Oncol Hematol Rev.* 2012;8(2):81–88. doi:10.17925/ohr.2012.08.2.81

31. Speck RM, Courneya KS, Masse LC, et al. An update of controlled physical activity trials in cancer survivors: a systematic review and meta-analysis. *J Cancer Surviv.* 2010;4(2):87–100. doi:10.1007/s11764-009-0110-5

32. Taso CJ, Lin HS, Lin WL, et al. The effect of yoga exercise on improving depression, anxiety, and fatigue in women with breast cancer: a randomized controlled trial. *J Nurs Res.* 2014;22(3):155–164. doi:10.1097/jnr.0000000000000044

33. Chandwani KD, Perkins G, Nagendra HR, et al. Randomized, controlled trial of yoga in women with breast cancer undergoing radiotherapy. *J Clin Oncol.* 2014;32(10):1058–1065. doi:10.1200/JCO.2012.48.2752

34. Balk J, Day R, Rosenzweig M, et al. Pilot, randomized, modified, double-blind, placebo-controlled trial of acupuncture for cancer-related fatigue. *J Soc Integr Oncol.* 2009;7(1):4–11.

35. Molassiotis A, Sylt P, Diggins H. The management of cancer-related fatigue after chemotherapy with acupuncture and acupressure: a randomised controlled trial. *Complement Ther Med.* 2007;15(4):228–237. doi:10.1016/j.ctim.2006.09.009

36. Ahles TA, Tope DM, Pinkson B, et al. Massage therapy for patients undergoing autologous bone marrow transplantation. *J Pain Symptom Manage*. 1999;18(3):157–163. doi:10.1016/s0885-3924(99)00061-5

37. Jacobsen PB, Meade CD, Stein KD, et al. Efficacy and costs of two forms of stress management training for cancer patients undergoing chemotherapy. *J Clin Oncol*. 2002;20(12):2851–2862. doi:10.1200/JCO.2002.08.301

38. Montgomery GH, David D, Kangas M, et al. Randomized controlled trial of a cognitive-behavioral therapy plus hypnosis intervention to control fatigue in patients undergoing radiotherapy for breast cancer. *J Clin Oncol*. 2014;32(6):557–563. doi:10.1200/JCO.2013.49.3437

39. Luebbert K, Dahme B, Hasenbring M. The effectiveness of relaxation training in reducing treatment-related symptoms and improving emotional adjustment in acute non-surgical cancer treatment: a meta-analytical review. *Psychooncology*. 2001;10(6):490–502. doi:10.1002/pon.537

40. Boesen EH, Ross L, Frederiksen K, et al. Psychoeducational intervention for patients with cutaneous malignant melanoma: a replication study. *J Clin Oncol*. 2005;23(6):1270–1277. doi:10.1200/jco.2005.05.193

41. Gaston-Johansson F, Fall-Dickson JM, Nanda J, et al. The effectiveness of the comprehensive coping strategy program on clinical outcomes in breast cancer autologous bone marrow transplantation. *Cancer Nurs*. 2000;23(4):277–285. doi:10.1097/00002820-200008000-00004

42. de la Cruz M, Hui D, Parsons HA, Bruera E. Placebo and nocebo effects in randomized double-blind clinical trials of agents for the therapy for fatigue in patients with advanced cancer. *Cancer*. 2010;116(3):766–774. doi:10.1002/cncr.24751

43. Gong S, Sheng P, Jin H, et al. Effect of methylphenidate in patients with cancer-related fatigue: a systematic review and meta-analysis. *PLoS ONE*. 2014;9(1):e84391. doi:10.1371/journal.pone.0084391

44. Minton O, Richardson A, Sharpe M, et al. Psychostimulants for the management of cancer-related fatigue: a systematic review and meta-analysis. *J Pain Symptom Manage*. 2011;41(4):761–767. doi:10.1016/j.jpainsymman.2010.06.020

45. Barton DL, Liu H, Dakhil SR, et al. Wisconsin Ginseng (*Panax quinquefolius*) to improve cancer-related fatigue: a randomized, double-blind trial, N07C2. *J Natl Cancer Inst*. 2013;105(16):1230–1238. doi:10.1093/jnci/djt181

46. Yennurajalingam S, Tannir NM, Williams JL, et al. A double-blind, randomized, placebo-controlled trial of panax ginseng for cancer-related fatigue in patients with advanced cancer. *J Natl Compr Canc Netw*. 2017;15(9):1111–1120. doi:10.6004/jnccn.2017.0149

47. Lesser GJ, Case D, Stark N, et al. A randomized, double-blind, placebo-controlled study of oral coenzyme Q10 to relieve self-reported treatment-related fatigue in newly diagnosed patients with breast cancer. *J Support Oncol*. 2013;11(1):31–42.

48. Cruciani RA, Dvorkin E, Homel P, et al. l-carnitine supplementation in patients with advanced cancer and carnitine deficiency: a double-blind, placebo-controlled study. *J Pain Symptom Manage*. 2009;37(4):622–631. doi:10.1016/j.jpainsymman.2008.03.021

CHAPTER 17

COST EFFECTIVENESS AND FINANCIAL TOXICITY IN NEW CANCER THERAPIES

Christine Kohn, Natalia Shcherbakova, and Alberto J. Montero

INTRODUCTION

While research advances in the last decade have produced new cancer therapies with significant and durable benefits, rising costs associated with novel oncologic medications are so substantial that the term "financial toxicity" is both well established in the medical literature, and a generally accepted adverse event related to cancer care (1). In our current healthcare environment, policy makers, providers, and patients alike need sound evidence as a framework within which to determine the value of different therapeutic alternatives in oncology.

Health economics, the application of economic principles and methods to health and healthcare, has become a growing field with the objective of contributing to our understanding of healthcare utilization, quality, and costs. The ECHO (Economic, Clinical, and Humanistic Outcomes) model has been used to understand the true impact of new and standard healthcare interventions (2), and a health economic evaluation assists decision-makers in determining the value of medical interventions and appropriately allocating limited healthcare resources. The central task of economic evaluations is to identify, measure, value, and compare the costs and consequences of the alternatives being considered (3). The value of a healthcare intervention is thought of as the ratio between its cost (in monetary units) and effectiveness (in relevant outcome measures—the outcomes measured and comparisons made differ depending on the type of analysis) (4).

Distinct economic evaluation designs illustrate the various approaches in assessing the value of a range of healthcare interventions. Table 17.1 presents a summary of four main health economic analyses. A cost-minimization analysis (CMA), used when interventions have equivalent outcomes, identifies the least costly alternative but is uncommon in the medical literature and is rarely an appropriate method of analysis when sampled data on costs and effects are available (5). A cost–benefit analysis (CBA) compares the value of all resources consumed from a new healthcare intervention or program to the benefits or outcomes gained. Both costs and consequences are valued in monetary units, allowing decision-makers to evaluate competing alternatives on the basis of whether the cost is worth the benefit (6). A cost-effectiveness analysis (CEA) compares costs to the effectiveness of an intervention by measuring outcomes in nonmonetary natural units such as cases cured, life-years saved, or an appropriate disease-specific outcome (7).

Published by Springer Publishing Company DOI: 10.1891/9780826172150.0017

TABLE 17.1 Types of Pharmacoeconomic Studies

Study type	Measurement of outcomes	Measurement of costs
Cost-minimizations analysis	Assumed to be equivalent and are not measured	Monetary units
Cost-effectiveness analysis	Natural units (life years gained, remission achieved, etc.)	Monetary units
Cost-utility analysis	Quality-adjusted life years	Monetary units
Cost–benefit analysis	Monetary units	Monetary units

A cost-utility analysis (CUA), considered a subtype of CEA, incorporates patient preferences or quality of life by evaluating outcomes in terms of preference-weighted measures of health, typically reporting a utility measure or quality-adjusted life year (QALY). Utility is the value or worth placed on a particular health state as measured by the preferences of individuals or society and is expressed as a numerical value from 0 to 1, 0 representing death and 1 representing perfect health (3). QALYs are calculated by multiplying the utility of a health state by the time spent in that health state. As such, a year of life lived in perfect or full health is equal to a QALY of 1.0 (1 year of life × 1 utility = 1 QALY), while a QALY of less than one is attained by a year of life lived in a state other than perfect health (utility < 1). By incorporating morbidity and mortality into a single unit, CUA allows for the comparison of diverse cancer therapies that affect quantity and quality of life in various ways.

CEAs and CUAs typically report an incremental cost-effectiveness ratio (ICER), which is used to assess the comparative monetary value between the interventions studied. An ICER is calculated as the ratio of the differences in costs to the differences in effectiveness measures of the two therapies being compared. ICERs are most useful when a new medication is more expensive but also more effective. When interpreting an ICER, the results of a CUA are compared to a predetermined threshold ICER or willingness-to-pay (WTP) threshold, below which an intervention is considered as "cost-effective" and can be adopted or funded; if the ICER is greater than the WTP threshold, an intervention is not considered cost-effective and is unlikely to be recommended for adoption. In the medical literature, a threshold of $50,000–$150,00 per QALY in the United States has been a commonly used benchmark (8). The threshold used in the United Kingdom is £20,000–30.000 per QALY (9), and in Australia $30.000 per QALY (10). The World Health Organization's recommended threshold for ICER is three times the per capita gross domestic product (GDP) in order for a therapy to be deemed "cost-effective" (11).

PERSPECTIVE, COSTS, AND SENSITIVITY ANALYSIS

The study perspective from which an economic evaluation is performed determines the components (e.g., direct medical costs, direct nonmedical costs, and indirect/productivity costs) and valuation of included costs (12). There are many perspectives including the payer (third-party payer or a government payer such as Medicare), provider, institution or hospital, healthcare system, patient, and societal perspective (12). For example, an analysis that takes a payer perspective will calculate the costs to the payer—that is, the actual charges allowed by the payer for medical products and services rendered. This perspective typically includes direct medical costs, which are the actual resources attributed to the delivery of medical care for detecting, preventing, or treating a disease. These include hospitalizations, medications, clinic visits, and ancillary services (6). A societal perspective—the net total of the different cost components to society—is considered the broadest perspective in terms of included costs and consequences, and includes patients' lost productivity and the expenses involved in providing and receiving medical care. It is important to understand the perspective of an economic analysis because even within the same disease state, costs and outcomes can vary widely depending on the perspective chosen.

In an economic evaluation, costs and consequences are estimated by a number of assumptions within a range of possible values. It is thus important to identify, calculate, and evaluate uncertainty by performing a sensitivity analysis in order to determine the degree to which the results of the analysis may vary with changes to these variables.

FINANCIAL TOXICITY

Financial toxicity describes the patient-level impact related to the very high cost of cancer treatment. In the United States, cancer ranks among the five most expensive diseases (13). Rising cancer-related costs are in part owed to advances in treatments. Better therapeutic options come at a price: patients receive expensive chemotherapy and immunotherapy agents, as well as supportive agents, all of which are, at least in part, passed on to patients (14). In addition, in the U.S. insurance costs continue to rise annually, with premiums for family coverage having increased 19% since 2012 and 55% since 2007 (15). Prescription drug costs have also steadily increased: new medications are introduced at higher prices, while most existing therapies have themselves experienced substantial price increases. A study of 32 oral cancer medications found that since 2000, the mean monthly costs rose from less than $2,000 to greater than $11,000 in 2014 (16). In addition to such objective financial burden findings, subjective financial distress affects patients' well-being and quality of care. Indeed, higher out-of-pocket costs are associated with higher rates of medication nonadherence and discontinuation (1,17–19). A retrospective cohort study found that cancer patients were 2.65 times more likely to go bankrupt than people without cancer (20). Nearly a third of cancer survivors in a 2016 study reported experiencing increased financial burden, a problem associated with lower health-related quality of life, increased risk of depressed mood, and a higher frequency of worrying about cancer recurrence (21).

Financial discussions between physicians and patients should be a critical element of treatment selection in cancer care, and should be incorporated into decision making in the same way other toxicities and treatment effects are discussed (22). In a survey of medical oncologists, most (80%) felt that it was important to be explicit about the impact of treatment choices on patients' finances, although only 42% discussed chemotherapy costs always or most of the time (23). Almost one-third of oncologists reported a high degree of discomfort in discussing treatment costs with patients (23). Another study found that while patients varied in their desire to discuss costs with doctors, those who did believe these conversations beneficial in helping to reduce their costs (24).

While there is currently no single solution for eradicating the impact of cancer-related financial toxicity in its entirety, several strategies have been suggested to ease patients' financial burden. These include, among others: decreasing out-of-pocket costs, using patient-reported outcomes that include screening for financial distress and establishing cost-conscious clinical practice guidelines (17).

SUMMARY OF ECONOMIC STUDIES OF IMMUNE CHECKPOINT INHIBITORS

For the past five years cancer drugs continued to comprise over 30% of all annual new drug approvals by the U.S. Food and Drug Administration (FDA) (25–29). This increase in FDA approved oncologic medications has led to a rapidly rising share of cancer therapeutics in overall U.S. drug spending. Currently, anti-neoplastic medications are the second leading drug class (preceded by diabetes therapeutics) in terms of spending in the United States, and in 2016 comprised 10% of the $323 billion spent on pharmaceuticals (30). Monoclonal antibody agents comprised nearly a third of cancer drug spending in recent years (31). To date, FDA approved six agents in the new class of immune checkpoint inhibitors (ICIs)— nivolumab, permbrolizumab, ipilimumab, atezolizumab, avelumab, and durvalumab (32). The costs associated with the use of each of these agents exceed $100,000 (33). For example, the anti-cytotoxic T-lymphocyte antigen 4 (CTLA-4) monoclonal antibody ipilimumab (Yervoy®), FDA approved in 2011, entered the market at a price of $120,000 per course of treatment (34). In 2014, anti-programmed cell death ligand 1 (PD-L1) monoclonal antibodies, *nivolumab* and *pembrolizumab*, which are largely interchangeable in relation to safety and efficacy (35), were approved for the treatment of melanoma at a price of $158,000 and $126,000 per annual treatment, respectively.

Thus far, only a few economic studies have been published examining the cost-effectiveness of ICIs in the United States (36,37). One study examined cost-effectiveness of several ICIs and their combinations in advanced melanoma (36). That study found that, for treatment-naïve patients, pembrolizumab followed by ipilimumab was a more effective and less costly treatment compared to chemotherapy followed by ipilimumab and nivolumab or ipilimumab alone followed by nivolumab. Moreover, this study found that, compared to dacarbazine alone, the incremental cost-effectiveness ratio associated with using nivolumab followed by ipilimumab was $90,871 per QALY. By contrast, first-line nivolumab and ipilimumab followed by carboplatin and paclitaxel as second-line therapy was associated with a cost of $198,867 per QALY as compared to dacarbazine. Another study stratified the cost-effectiveness analyses of checkpoint inhibitors in lung cancer by whether a biomarker testing (PD-L1) is used as a predictive marker to identify patients most likely to benefit (37). The ICER for all patients with nonsquamous tumors treated with nivolumab or atezolizumab as second line as compared to dacarbazine was $187,685 and $215,802, respectively. When the authors recalculated the treatments' ICERs among only patients with PD-L1 positive tumors, the values decreased by up to 65%, thus improving significantly the value of the therapies. In the same study, pembrolizumab was found to have an ICER of $98,421. This is likely due to the fact that pembrolizumab in non-small cell lung cancer was only tested in patients with PD-L1 expressing tumors, and hence patients unlikely to benefit from treatment were excluded on the basis of this biomarker.

Several commentaries and letters from practicing clinicians have emerged in the literature focused on the unsustainable costs of new cancer agents, including ICI agents (38–42). A number of them have pointed out that the key driver of costs of new immune checkpoint agents are dosing schedules—whether the drugs are administered using flat doses or by weight (41,42). A randomized controlled trial of pembrolizumab showed comparable outcomes for patients administered doses between 2 mg/kg and 10 mg/kg (43). However, the monthly costs of these two treatment regimens can differ several-folds between $9,000 for a 2 mg/kg every 3 weeks regimen and $46,000 for 10 mg/kg every 3 weeks (41). A follow-up budget impact analyses from a societal standpoint showed annual savings of nearly $1 billion associated with the use of personalized dosing schedule (2 mg/kg) of pembrolizumab as compared to using a fixed non-weight based dose of 200 mg (44).

CANCER DRUG VALUE ASSESSMENT, UNITED STATES

The American Society of Clinical Oncology (ASCO) with the input from key stakeholders including clinicians, patients, payers, and pharmaceutical manufacturers has developed a cancer value framework that incorporates three key elements: clinical benefit or efficacy, toxicity or safety, and cost (45). This framework is physician-guided and contains two versions, one to be used for potentially curative treatments (adjuvant or neo-adjuvant therapy), the other for advanced cancer. The net health benefit (NHB) for a therapy is then calculated by summing the scores for clinical benefit, toxicity, and any bonus points for drugs with a survival curve tail. The maximum NHB score is 100 for curative intent therapies and 130 for palliative intent therapies. The outcome metric of clinical benefit in the curative setting can have a categorical 1–5 score, which is based on the hazard ratio (HR) for overall survival (OS) when the evaluated therapy is compared to the standard of care. Alternatively, when OS is not available, the HR for disease-free survival (DFS) is used. The score is then multiplied by 16 (for OS) or 15 (for DFS). This means that a therapy with a maximum clinical benefit score of 5 earns 80 points (16×5) out of 100 possible. In other words, the larger element of value for a therapy is attributed to its improvement of survival. In a context of advanced disease, the calculation of benefit is somewhat similar. The categorical score is also 1–5 and is based on the HR, or relative difference in risk, between evaluated therapy and standard of care. The score for toxicity for both curative and advanced cancer scenarios can take a value from −20 to +20 and is measured as the relative toxicity of the therapy against a comparator based on the frequency of all adverse events. The points awarded for the evaluated regimen are then divided by the points for the standard of care and multiplied by 20. Both drug acquisition cost per month of therapy and patient monthly cost are used in the context of the advanced disease. In the context of curative treatment, same costs but for the total duration of therapy are used.

CANCER DRUG VALUE ASSESSMENT, EUROPE

The European Society for Medical Oncology (ESMO) has developed a similar tool to the ASCO's value assessment tool titled the Magnitude of Clinical Benefit Scale (ESMO-MCBS) (46). The scale integrates data on HRs, prognosis, and absolute treatment magnitude. These values (for HR the lower limit of the confidence interval is used conservatively) are then compared with the prespecified thresholds to determine if the evaluated therapy is beneficial. The studies to which ESMO-MCBS scale can be applied include randomized trials, comparative observational cohort studies, and meta-analyses. The scale, similar to ASCO's approach, has two forms: to be used in the curative (form 1) and advanced (form 2) settings, respectively. The scores for curative treatments receive values A, B, and C, with A and B grades considered significant improvements. The scores for advanced disease treatments receive grades 1 to 5, with 4 to 5 considered significant improvements. The ESMO recommends that therapies receiving high scores should promptly undergo cost-effectiveness and value assessment.

Table 17.2 provides a summary of ASCO and ESMO value frameworks.

When evaluated, the agreement between the two frameworks was fair, driven by differing grading algorithms (47). On the other hand, the relationship between the magnitude of the clinical benefit as measured by both frameworks and monthly drug costs was significant and inverse (47). The incremental drug cost for treatments that met the ESMO benefit threshold was $2,981 as compared to $8,621 for treatments that failed to meet the threshold (47). The correlation between the ASCO net benefit score and the monthly drug costs was −0.207 ($p = .039$) again pointing to significantly higher costs for less effective treatments (47).

CANCER DRUG VALUE, DEVELOPING COUNTRIES

The immunotherapies for the treatment of cancer have revolutionized cancer treatment landscape in the developed countries albeit at

TABLE 17.2 Comparison of Value Frameworks of ASCO and ESMO

Characteristic	ASCO framework	ESMO framework
Clinical benefit	Score 1–5 based on the improvement of overall (or progression free) survival or response rate	Grades A, B, C or scores 1–5 based on improvement in overall/progression-free survival /quality of life improvement
Toxicity	Score –20 to +20 based on the difference of the evaluated treatment and standard of care	Evaluated concomitantly with clinical benefit with grade/score increased/decreased based on toxicity profile
Cost	Drug acquisition cost and patient co-pay per month/per treatment	Evaluated concomitantly with clinical benefit/toxicity with grade/score increased/decreased based on increase/decrease in treatment costs

ASCO, American Society of Clinical Oncology; ESMO, European Society of Medical Oncology.

substantial costs to both patients and healthcare systems (41,48). On the other hand, patients in developing countries not only lack access to the recently approved products such as immunotherapies, but also to standard chemotherapies, even though most are currently available as generic drugs (49,50).

CONCLUSION

Given the climbing proportion of cancer drugs in the annual FDA new drug approvals, the costs for new oncologic agents, including checkpoint inhibitors, likely will continue to rise. This is largely due to market-driven mechanisms rather than value-driven pricing mechanisms, when interchangeable agents' prices, or worse prices for therapies with lower overall benefit, tend to be significantly higher (35,47). The development of value frameworks by key stakeholders in both the United States and Europe is the first step in making treatment decisions based on the value of a given therapy. The early findings from applying these frameworks to currently used therapies, as well as identifying striking negative relationships between treatment benefits and costs, may in the long term force clinicians, policy makers, and payers to abandon agents with substantial costs and low benefits. In addition, as shown in several economic studies to date, relying upon biomarkers in the selection of patients for therapy may significantly improve cost-effectiveness ratios and, hence, value associated with checkpoint inhibitor treatments. Moreover, applying weight-based rather than flat dosing regimens to eligible patients may further decrease waste and improve value. Considering the opportunity costs associated with a healthcare intervention, if resources are directed to treatments that lack evidence of value, these resources are no longer available to be spent on proven beneficial and cost-effective alternatives. In a nutshell, this is why advocacy and action from clinicians, payers, and policymakers is crucial in promoting value-based cancer care.

REFERENCES

1. Zafar SY, Abernethy AP. Financial toxicity, Part I: a new name for a growing problem. *Oncology (Williston Park)*. 2013;27:80–149.

2. Gunter MJ. The role of the ECHO model in outcomes research and clinical practice improvement. *Am J Manag Care*. 1999;5:S217–S224;

3. Drummond M, Sculpher M, Torrance G, et al. *Methods for the Economic Evaluation of Health Care Programmes*. 3rd Ed. Oxford, UK: Oxford University Press; 2005.

4. Toscani M, Pizzi L. Measuring and improving the intervention. In: Patterson R, Ed. *Changing Patient Behavior: Improving Outcomes In Health and Disease Management*. San Francisco, CA: Jossey Bass; 2001.

5. Briggs AH, O'Brien BJ. The death of cost-minimization analysis? *Health Econ*. 2001;10:179–184. doi:10.1002/hec.584.

6. Eisenberg JM. Clinical economics. a guide to the economic analysis of clinical practices. *JAMA*. 1989;262:2879–2886.

7. National Institute for Health and Clinical Excellence. The Guidelines Manual—Process and Methods [PMG6]. https://www.nice.org.uk/Process/Pmg6/Chapter/Assessing-Cost-Effectiveness

8. Institute for Clinical and Economic Review. Modifications to the ICER Value Assessment Framework for Treatments for Ultra-Rare Diseases. 2017. https://icer-review.org/wp-content/uploads/2017/11/ICER-Adaptations-of-Value-Framework-for-Rare-Diseases.pdf.

9. Mccabe C, Claxton K, Culyer AJ. The NICE cost-effectiveness threshold: what it is and what that means. *Pharmacoeconomics*. 2008;26:733–744. doi:10.2165/00019053-200826090-00004

10. Managing uncertainty in the assessment of medicines for listing on the pharmaceutical pharmaceutical benefits scheme. 2008. http://www.pbs.gov.au/info/general/working-groups/amwg/amwg-interim-report-attachment-b

11. Bertram MY, Lauer JA, De Joncheere K, et al. Cost-effectiveness thresholds: pros and cons. *Bull World Health Organ*. 2016;94:925–930. doi:10.2471/blt.15.164418

12. Husereau D, Drummond M, Petrou S, et al. Consolidated health economic evaluation reporting standards (CHEERS) statement. *BMJ*. 2013;346:F1049. doi:10.1136/bmj.F1049

13. Soni A. Trends in the five most costly conditions among the U.S. Civilian Institutionalized Population, 2002 and 2012. Statistical brief 470. Rockville, MD: agency for Healthcare Research and Quality; 2015. https://meps.ahrq.gov/data_files/publications/st470/stat470.shtml

14. PDQ Cancer information summaries [Internet]. Bethesda (MD): National Cancer Institute (US). [Date Unknown]. Financial Toxicity and Cancer Treatment (PDQ®)–Health Professional Version; [Updated May 3, 2017]. https://www.ncbi.nlm.nih.gov/Pubmed-health/PMH0032652/

15. The Henry J. Kaiser Family Foundation. 2017 Employer Health Benefits Survey. https://www.Kff.Org/Report-Section/Ehbs-2017-Summary-Of-Findings/

16. Dusetzina SB. Drug pricing trends for orally administered anticancer medications reimbursed by commercial health plans, 2000–2014. *JAMA Oncol*. 2016;2:960–961. doi:10.1001/Jamaoncol.2016.0648

17. Zafar SY, Abernethy AP. Financial Toxicity, Part II: how can we help with the burden of treatment-related costs? *Oncology (Williston Park)*. 2013;27:253–254, 6.

18. Bestvina CM, Zullig LL, Yousuf Zafar S. The implications of out-of-pocket cost of cancer treatment in the USA: a critical appraisal of the literature. *Future Oncol*. 2014;10:2189–2199. doi:10.2217/Fon.14.130

19. Kaisaeng N, Harpe SE, Carroll NV. Out-of-pocket costs and oral cancer medication discontinuation in the elderly. *J Manag Care Spec Pharm*. 2014;20:669–675. doi:10.18553/Jmcp.2014.20.7.669s

20. Ramsey S, Blough D, Kirchhoff A, et al. Washington State Cancer Patients found to be at greater risk for bankruptcy than people without a cancer diagnosis. *Health Aff (Millwood)*. 2013;32:1143–1152. doi:10.1377/Hlthaff.2012.1263

21. Kale HP, Carroll NV. Self-reported financial burden of cancer care and its effect on physical and mental health-related quality of life among US cancer survivors. *Cancer*. 2016;122:283–289. doi:10.1002/Cncr.29808

22. Ubel PA, Abernethy AP, Zafar SY. Full disclosure—out-of-pocket costs as side effects. *N Engl J Med*. 2013;369:1484–1486. doi:10.1056/Nejmp1306826

23. Schrag D, Hanger M. Medical oncologists' views on communicating with patients about chemotherapy costs: a pilot survey. *J Clin Oncol*. 2007;25:233–237. doi:10.1200/JCO.2006.09.2437

24. Zafar SY, Chino F, Ubel PA, et al. The utility of cost discussions between patients with cancer and oncologists. *Am J Manag Care*. 2015;21:607–615.

25. Mullard A. 2016 FDA drug approvals. *Nat Rev Drug Discov*. 2017;16:73–76. doi:10.1038/Nrd.2017.14

26. Mullard A. 2015 FDA Drug approvals. *Nat Rev Drug Discov*. 2016;15:73–76. doi:10.1038/Nrd.2016.15

27. Mullard A. 2014 FDA Drug approvals. *Nat Rev Drug Discov*. 2015;14:77–81. doi:10.1038/Nrd4545

28. Mullard A. 2013 FDA Drug approvals. *Nat Rev Drug Discov*. 2014;13:85–89. doi:10.1038/Nrd4239

29. Mullard A. 2012 FDA Drug approvals. *Nat Rev Drug Discov*. 2013;12:87–90. doi:10.1038/Nrd3946

30. Medicines Use and Spending in the U.S. a review of 2016 and outlook to 2021: IMS Health; 2017. https://www.Iqvia.Com/Institute/Reports/Medicines-Use-And-Spending-In-The-Us-A-Review-Of-2016

31. IMS Health Study: U.S. drug spending growth reaches 8.5 percent in 2015 IMS Health 2016. http://www.Imshealth.Com/En/About-Us/News/Ims-Health-Study-Us-Drug-Spending-Growth-Reaches-8.5-Percent-In-2015

32. Jardim DL, De Melo Gagliato D, Giles FJ, et al. Analysis of drug development paradigms for immune checkpoint inhibitors. *Clin Cancer Res*. 2017;24(8):1785–1794. doi:10.1158/1078-0432.CCR-17-1970

33. Davis MP, Panikkar R. Checkpoint inhibitors, palliative care, or hospice. *Curr Oncol Rep*. 2018;20:2. doi:10.1007/S11912-018-0659-0

34. Sledge G. Musings of a cancer doctor: the cost of drugs. *Oncology Times*. 2011;33:32,4.

35. Prasad V, Kaestner V. Nivolumab and pembrolizumab: monoclonal antibodies against programmed cell death-1 (PD-1) that are interchangeable. *Semin Oncol*. 2017;44:132–135. doi:10.1053/J.Seminoncol.2017.06.007

36. Kohn CG, Zeichner SB, Chen Q, et al. Cost-effectiveness of immune checkpoint inhibition in BRAF wild-type advanced melanoma. *J Clin Oncol*. 2017;35:1194–1202. doi:10.1200/JCO.2016.69.6336

37. Aguiar PN Jr, Perry LA, Penny-Dimri J, et al. The effect of PD-L1 testing on the cost-effectiveness and economic impact of immune checkpoint inhibitors for the second-line treatment of NSCLC. *Ann Oncol*. 2017;29(4):1078–1078.doi:10.1093/Annonc/Mdx478

38. Kelly RJ, Smith TJ. Checkpoint inhibitors in lung cancer are not immune from cost-effectiveness analysis. *J Thorac Oncol*. 2016;11:1814–1816. doi:10.1016/J.Jtho.2016.07.028.

39. Goldstein DA, Stemmer SM, Gordon N. The cost and value of cancer drugs – are new innovations outpacing our ability to pay? *ISR J Health Policy Res*. 2016;5:40. doi:10.1186/S13584-016-0097-0

40. Goldstein DA. Opposition to value-based cancer care-interests of patients or conflicts of interest? *Mayo Clin Proc*. 2016;91:1842–1843. doi:10.1016/J.Mayocp.2016.10.001

41. Andrews A. Treating with checkpoint inhibitors-figure $1 Million Per patient. *Am Health Drug Benefits*. 2015;8:9.

42. Bach PB, Saltz LB. Raising the dose and raising the cost: the case of pembrolizumab in lung cancer. *J Natl Cancer Inst*. 2017;109:djx125. doi:10.1093/Jnci/Djx125

43. Robert C, Schachter J, Long GV, et al. Pembrolizumab versus ipilimumab in advanced melanoma. *N Engl J Med*. 2015;372:2521–2532. doi:10.1056/Nejmoa1503093

44. Goldstein DA, Gordon N, Davidescu M, et al. A phamacoeconomic analysis of personalized dosing Vs fixed dosing of pembrolizumab in firstline PD-L1-positive non-small cell lung cancer. *J Natl Cancer Inst*. 2017;109:djx063. doi:10.1093/Jnci/Djx063

45. Schnipper LE, Davidson NE, Wollins DS, et al. Updating the American Society of Clinical Oncology value framework: revisions and reflections in response to comments received. *J Clin Oncol*. 2016;34:2925–2934. doi:10.1200/JCO.2016.68.2518

46. Cherny NI, Sullivan R, Dafni U, et al. A standardised, generic, validated approach to stratify the magnitude of clinical benefit that can be anticipated from anti-cancer therapies: the European Society for Medical Oncology magnitude of clinical benefit scale (ESMO-MCBS). *Ann Oncol.* 2015;26:1547–1573. doi:10.1093/Annonc/Mdv249

47. Del Paggio JC, Sullivan R, Schrag D, et al. Delivery of meaningful cancer care: a retrospective cohort study assessing cost and benefit with the ASCO and ESMO frameworks. *Lancet Oncol.* 2017;18:887–894. doi:10.1016/S1470-2045(17)30415-1

48. Zafar SY, Peppercorn JM, Schrag D, et al. The financial toxicity of cancer treatment: a pilot study assessing out-of-pocket expenses and the insured cancer patient's experience. *Oncologist.* 2013;18:381–390. doi:10.1634/Theoncologist.2012-0279

49. Gyawali B. Me, too. *J Glob Oncol.* 2016;2:99–104. doi:10.1200/JGO.2015.000588

50. Mehta PS, Wiernikowski JT, Petrilli JA, et al. Essential medicines for pediatric oncology in developing countries. *Pediatr Blood Cancer.* 2013;60:889–891. doi:10.1002/Pbc.24476

INDEX